Educating the 21st Century Nurse

Challenges and Opportunities

Edited by Vernice D. Ferguson

NLN Press • New York
Pub. No. 14-7467

The views expressed in this publication represent the views of the authors and do not necessarily reflect the official views of the National League for Nursing.

Library of Congress Cataloging-in-Publication Data

Educating the 21st century nurse: challenges and opportunities/
  edited by Vernice D. Ferguson.
     p. cm.
  Includes bibliographical references and index.
  Pub. no. 14-7467.
  ISBN 0-88737-746-7
  1. Nursing—Study and teaching. I. Ferguson, Vernice.
RT71.E37 1997
610.73'071—dc21   97-20342
                                      CIP

This book was set in Goudy Old Style by Bi-Comp, Inc. The editor and designer was Nancy Jeffries. The printer was BookCrafters. The cover was designed by Gerard Associates.

Printed in the United States of America

Educating the 21st Century Nurse

Challenges and Opportunities

This book is dedicated to the nurses, their teachers, mentors and role models who will lead the profession into the 21st century with a relevant and responsive practice and a commanding presence in the health care arena.

Contents

Acknowledgments

The 21st century is upon us and with it are challenges and opportunities in abundance as the education of nurses for a demanding future takes shape. The contributors to this book were asked to consider one area of focus about which they felt strongly, which deserved attention and would be worth sharing with other nurses as the education of nurses for tomorrow's practice is considered. For some, their chapters are an outgrowth of their research and study, for others, their experiences in interacting with today's students, while for still others their chapters are expressions of their principal work experience, knowledge and observations of today's health care realities and the gaps to be filled so ably by nurses.

I offer my special thanks to these contributors who have shared their thoughts so generously with us.

Thanks are in order as well for Nancy Jeffries, Senior Editor of NLN Press, whose editorial services, advice and consultation assured the publication of this book. I am grateful to Sylvia Johnson, Administrative Assistant in the School of Nursing at the University of Pennsylvania for her invaluable assistance as well.

I am grateful to Dr. Claire Fagin and her husband Sam for funding the Fagin Family Chair in Cultural Diversity at the School of Nursing, University of Pennsylvania. I have been privileged to hold this chair for four and a half years and through it have served as editor for this book and the earlier, Case Studies in Cultural Diversity: A Workbook.

I am appreciative as well to Ms. Susan Sherman, President of the Independence Foundation, for funding an initiative geared toward preparing nurses for community focused health care as accommodation of cultural diversity proceeds.

May the sharing of these ideas be instructive as we prepare nurses for a relevant future.

Vernice D. Ferguson
Editor

Contributors

Charlotte F. Beason, EdD, RN is a Program Director in the Nursing Strategic Healthcare Group, Department of Veterans Affairs (DVA), Washington, DC. She has had extensive experience in the management of national academic and employee education programs for nurses and associated health professionals. Dr. Beason has been actively engaged in national health care reform efforts on the White House Task Force on Health Care Reform and within the DVA. Her activities have included co-chairing the national committee which recommended the restructuring of DVA's national employee education system.

Jane M. Brennan, DNSc, RN is an Assistant Professor of Nursing in the College of Nursing at Widener University where she works primarily with undergraduate baccalaureate nursing students of diverse cultural and ethnic backgrounds. She is an ANA certified gerontological nurse with clinical interest in adult health care. Dr. Brennan serves as a volunteer with the Main Line Interfaith Hospitality Network for the homeless. She is a contributor to the recent book from the NLN Press, *Case Studies in Cultural Diversity: A Workbook*.

Paulette R. Cournoyer, DNSc, RN, CS is a Program Director in the Department of Veterans Affairs (DVA) Headquarters Nursing Strategic Healthcare Group decentralized to the Brockton/West Roxbury, Massachusetts VA Medical Center. She is a graduate of St. Anselm College in New Hampshire and received her Master's and Doctor of Nursing Science degrees from Boston University. She is a certified clinical nurse specialist in adult psychiatric and mental health nursing. Her publications and presentations have primarily focused on clinical nursing research. She is a research reviewer for several nursing journals and organizations. Dr. Cournoyer represents the DVA on the National Institute of Nursing Research's National Advisory Council for Nursing Research.

Danielle N. DeVoss, MA is a Research Assistant for the Family Care Research Program at Michigan State University. Ms. DeVoss edits and produces newsletters distributed to physicians and patients involved in the Family Care Research Program (FCRP) studies and policy statements distributed to local, state, and federal agencies, organizations, and legislators.

Elizabeth L. Dickason, EdD, RN is an Assistant Professor of Nursing in the College of Nursing at Widener University. Her current research is focused on the health beliefs of employed women. While in the process of conducting a study of the breast cancer screening behaviors of women, Dr. Dickason is presenting programs to a diverse racial and ethnic group of women geared to facilitating their participation in breast self exam, clinical breast exam and mammography screening. She is a contributor to the recent book from the NLN Press, *Case Studies in Cultural Diversity: A Workbook.*

Ann Doherty, MSN, RN, PhD candidate is completing requirements for a doctorate of jurisprudence at the Greenwich University in Hawaii and the doctor of public health and human services degree at Columbia Pacific University. She has held positions as project Director for WHO Healthy Cities, Philadelphia. Ms. Doherty has served as a nurse consultant to the Ministry of Health of Zambia, the British National Health Services of the United Kingdom, the University of Space Industry and Medicine, Beijing, China, and with the Pan American Health Organization.

Juanita W. Fleming, PhD, RN, FAAN is a Special Assistant to the President for Academic Affairs at the University of Kentucky and Professor of Nursing. She has had a long and distinguished career in maternal-child nursing and education. She has functioned as a clinical educator, researcher, evaluator, consultant and administrator. Her scholarly productivity is evidenced by her publications, grant activity, invited presentations, her work as a reviewer, member of study sections, and her professional memberships. Her contributions are recognized by the many honors and awards she has received.

Barbara A. Given, PhD, RN, FAAN is a Professor and the Associate Director for the Cancer Prevention and Control Division of the Michigan State University Cancer Center, and Director of Research for the Michigan State University for Managed Care. Dr. Given has served as an advisor to the National Center for Nursing Research (NIH) and has chaired the Expert Panel on Aging of the American Academy of Nursing. She is a productive scholar with many publications to her credit along with numerous national and international presentations.

Charles W. Given, PhD is a Professor and the Associate Chair for Research for the Michigan State University College of Human Medicine, Department of Family Practice. Dr. Given was designated as Michigan State University's Outstanding Faculty in 1996. Dr. Given serves as a grant reviewer for the Agency for Health Care Policy and Research (AHCPR) and National Institute of Aging (NIA). In addition, he serves as an advisor to the State Office of Services to the Aging.

Shirlee Drayton-Hargrove, PhD, RN, CRRN is an Assistant Professor of Nursing in the Department of Nursing, College of Allied Health Professions at Temple University. She provides instruction on the graduate and undergraduate level. Dr. Drayton-Hargrove teaches the core graduate course, "Health Issues of Underserved and Diverse Populations" at the University. Her areas of expertise include multicultural issues, leadership, interaction analysis and rehabilitative aspects of care. She is a contributor to the recent book from the NLN Press, *Case Studies in Cultural Diversity: A Workbook.*

Constance Holleran, MSN, RN, FAAN is Senior Fellow–International in the School of Nursing, University of Pennsylvania. She served with distinction as the Deputy Executive Director for the American Nurses Association in Washington, DC and as Executive Director of the International Council of Nurses in Geneva, Switzerland, a post she held for 15 years. Among her numerous honors and awards is an honorary Doctor of Social Science degree from Villanova University.

Beatrice Adderley-Kelly, PhD, RN is an Associate Professor in the College of Nursing at Howard University, Washington, DC. All of her professional life has been devoted to working with populations of diverse cultural backgrounds. The curriculum at the Howard University College of Nursing, which focuses on cultural diversity, enables Dr. Adderley-Kelly to teach cultural diversity throughout the curriculum and to educate students to provide health care to culturally diverse clients. A project at the University afforded her the opportunity to travel to two African countries where she worked with nursing educators and practicing nurses on curriculum design. Dr. Adderley-Kelly's research focuses on vulnerable populations, particularly low income elderly African-American women.

Norma M. Lang, PhD, RN, FAAN, FRCN is the Margaret Bond Simon Dean and Professor at the University of Pennsylvania School of Nursing. She is former President of the American Nurses' Foundation and remains active in professional affairs. Dr. Lang is a consultant to the International Council of Nurses in Geneva, Switzerland for the development of an International Classification of Nursing Practice. Her research interests include quality assurance, patient outcomes, peer review and the Nursing Minimum Data Set. She is a fellow of the American Academy of Nursing, the Institute of Medicine, the College of Physicians of Philadelphia and is an honorary fellow of the Royal College of Nursing of the United Kingdom.

Barbara Mallory, MSN, RN is a nurse consultant for the City of Philadelphia and a faculty member at Temple University School of Nursing. She has extensive experience in community/public health nursing and currently serves as the Administrative Liaison for the Philadelphia Department of Public Health to the MercyCARE Mobile Health Program.

Kathleen A. McCormick, PhD, RN, FAAN, FACMI, FRCNA is Senior Science Advisor, Center for Information Technology, Agency for Health Care Policy and Research, DHHS. In that capacity she has developed a new program in computerized decision support systems. Dr. McCormick served as Director, Office of the Forum for Quality and Effectiveness in Health Care responsible for developing the methodologies and process of clinical practice guidelines. She is co-author of *Essentials of Computers for Nurses, 2nd ed.*

Gloria J. McNeal, MSN, RN, CS, PhD candidate is the Program Director of the Mercy Health Corporation Comprehensive Mobile Health System in Bala Cynwyd, Pennsylvania. In this position she is responsible for the design, implementation and evaluation of a fleet of high tech mobile health vans that deliver primary health services to underserved populations living in Philadelphia and surrounding counties. Prior to this position she held a dual appointment in the Department of Nursing at Thomas Jefferson University serving as assistant professor and acting track coordinator for critical care/trauma and clinical assistant professor.

Andrea Mengel, PhD, RN is head of the Department of Nursing at Community College of Philadelphia. She has a bachelor's degree in nursing from the Pennsylvania State University, a master's degree in psychiatric nursing and a PhD in higher education from the University of Pennsylvania. She chairs the National League for Nursing's Council of Associate Degree Programs, Accreditation Committee and has been appointed to the National League for Nursing Accrediting Committee.

Donna Gentile O'Donnell, MSN, RN is currently a pre-doctoral student at the University of Pennsylvania School of Nursing. Ms. O'Donnell is the Deputy Commissioner of Public Health for Policy and Planning for the City of Philadelphia. Her contributions to nursing have been recognized by both Villanova University which named her the recipient of the Nursing Alumni Medallion, and the Pennsylvania Public Health Association, which honored her with the Rodale Award in 1994. As principal author of the Philadelphia ICARE Immunization Project, the Clinton Administration funded her initiative at $1 million, which provided immunizations for over 5,000 children.

Freida Outlaw, DNSc, RN is an Assistant Professor and Program Director for Adult Psychiatric Mental Health and Special Populations at the University of Pennsylvania School of Nursing. Her post doctoral training focused on the psychosocial adjustment to illness of African Americans with special emphasis on the role of religion and prayer as coping strategies. As a family therapist, Dr. Outlaw works with low income families. Her current research focuses on mother-son HIV risk reduction interventions. She is a contributor to the recent book from the NLN Press, *Case Studies in Cultural Diversity: A Workbook.*

Dolores S. Patrinos, MA, RN is an Assistant Professor in the Nursing Department, College of Allied Health Professions at Temple University. She was the principal investigator of a five-year project, *Nursing Career Opportunities Program* (NCOP) for students from under represented minorities and economically disadvantaged backgrounds. Ms. Patrinos, while working in Open, Inc., in Philadelphia, taught community youths who were providing community health services to senior citizens in north Philadelphia. She is a contributor to the recent book from the NLN Press, *Case Studies in Cultural Diversity: A Workbook.*

A. Phylip Pritchard, BA, RGN, RMN is Chief Administrator of the Federation of European Cancer Societies in Brussels, Belgium. He has published widely and is well known nationally and internationally for his editorship of *The Royal Marsden Hospital Manual of Clinical Nursing Procedures* and volume one of *Oncology for Nurses and Health Care Professionals.* He was the founding editor of the *European Journal of Cancer Care.* He is an appointed member of the board of directors of the International Society of Nurses in Cancer Care and is a member of the International Union Against Cancer's Nursing Project Committee. He served as temporary advisor for the WHO study group on Nursing Beyond the Year 2000.

Kathy Redmond, MSc, RGN is College Lecturer, Department of Nursing Studies at University College in Dublin, Ireland. She is a distinguished cancer nurse who has served as the Irish representative, board member and president of the European Oncology Nursing Society and is an appointed member to the board of directors of the International Society of Nurses in Cancer Care. She was a member of the working party which developed the core curriculum for a post basic course in cancer nursing for the European Commission.

Susan Sherman, MA, RN is President of the Independence Foundation, a private philanthropy based in Philadelphia with a mission that includes supporting nurse managed health care delivery systems where services are not ordinarily available. She has taught nursing, headed an associate degree nursing program, consulted privately and through the National League for Nursing (NLN), and was chairperson of the National League for Nursing's, Council of Associate Degree Programs and member of the NLN Board of Governors.

Donna Tartasky, PhD, RN is Associate Dean for Special Projects and Partnerships in the School of Nursing at Southern Illinois University at Edwardsville, Edwardsville, IL. She was an Assistant Professor in the College of Nursing at Villanova University where she taught community nursing at the undergraduate and graduate level. She served as a manuscript reviewer for *Public Health Nursing*. Dr. Tartasky is the recipient of two grants for a *Community Based Assessment of Adult Minority Asthmatics*. She is a contributor to the recent book from the NLN Press, *Case Studies in Cultural Diversity: A Workbook*.

Patricia W. Underwood, PhD, RN is an Associate Professor in the Kirkhof School of Nursing at Grand Valley State University in Allendale, Michigan. With 30 years of experience in BSN and MSN education, she has initiated several innovative programs including a summers only MSN program for nurse educators and a community-based, intensive model for educating women's health nurse practitioners. Her work with MSN students relative to community coalition building was spurred by an initiative of the W.K. Kellogg Foundation and the American Nurses Association aimed at preparing nurse leaders to promote collaboration within communities to address health problems.

Nancy M. Valentine, PhD, MPH, RN, FAAN is Chief Consultant, Nursing Strategic Healthcare Group, Office of Patient Care Services of the Department of Veterans Affairs and directs policy development governing nursing services for the Department's 171 medical centers which includes 63,000 nursing staff. She holds adjunct faculty positions at Catholic University School of Nursing, Georgetown University School of Nursing, the Massachusetts General Hospital Institute of Health Professions and the Harvard Medical School. She is President of the American Psychiatric Nurses Association. Dr. Valentine is a presenter at national and international meetings and has authored numerous publications.

About the Editor

Vernice D. Ferguson, MA, RN, FAAN, FRCN had a long and distinguished career in federal service. Until her retirement in December 1992, she served as the Assistant Chief Medical Director for Nursing Programs of the Department of Veterans Affairs, the leadership role for more than 60,000 nursing personnel. Prior to this assignment, Ms. Ferguson was the Chief of the Nursing Department at the Clinical Center, the National Institutes of Health and served as Chief Nurse at the VA Medical Center, Madison, Wisconsin and West Side Chicago, Illinois.

Ms. Ferguson is a fellow of the American Academy of Nursing and Past President. She is an honorary fellow of the Royal College of Nursing of the United Kingdom, the second American nurse so honored. She is Past President of Sigma Theta Tau International and is Immediate Past President of the International Society of Nurses in Cancer Care.

Her honors and awards are numerous including the Lavinia Dock Prize for highest scholastic standing and honors in clinical practice from Bellevue-New York University, the Mary Mahoney Award of the American Nurses Association, the Jean McVicar Outstanding Nurse Executive Award of the National League for Nursing, the Distinguished Service Award of the Department of Health and Human Services, and the Exceptional Service Award of the Department of Veterans Affairs. She is the recipient of two fellowships and seven honorary doctorates.

Most recently she was Senior Fellow in the School of Nursing at the University of Pennsylvania where she held the Fagin Family Chair in Cultural Diversity.

Foreword

As we enter the 21st century, it is important that we as nurses are prepared to face the new challenges the millennium will bring. Three of the changes which we can predict with assurance are that the demographics of the United States are shifting with increased representation of minorities and women; that major transitions in health care will continue; and that the number of individuals with chronic illness will expand. It is further predicted that the science of nursing will advance along with the changes and challenges. The rapid approach of the year 2000 causes us to focus more readily on change than might normally be our inclination. We are very fortunate that Vernice Ferguson and the authors she has assembled in this volume give us an excellent springboard for our own contemplation of the future. By preparing us insightfully for emerging trends, they position us to seize opportunities and take control.

There is a great deal to be learned from these cogent essays. They expand our understanding of the forces, especially the cultural forces, which impact health care delivery. These authors sharpen our thinking about multiculturalism in our profession, in the populations we serve, and in the communities where we live. As nursing continues its movement back into the community and increases its use of distance learning to reach students, these authors provide valuable insights and broaden our multicultural competence and understanding.

All of us in nursing—teachers, researchers, practitioners, administrators, policymakers, students—will have new perspectives on the forces affecting nursing after reading this volume. It is the nursing students—the practitioners and nursing leaders of the 21st century—who will be especially enriched by *Educating the 21st Century Nurse—Challenges and Opportunities*. This important collection of articles will empower them to take advantage of opportunities for nursing with a keen appreciation of the issues and trends affecting health care delivery in the future.

Norma M. Lang
Dean, School of Nursing
University of Pennsylvania

Introduction

N*ewness and change surround* us. At another period of profound social change, which we experienced in the United States during the turbulent 1960s, a commentator of the times wrote, "changes are coming faster and faster—in a sense change has become a way of life. The only people who will live successfully in tomorrow's world are those who can accept and enjoy temporary systems" (Farson, 1969). His thoughts are reflected across the world as nations in increasing numbers recognize that change, often bold and relentless, is evident.

A century earlier during a period of strife, turbulence and change in our national life, the President of the United States uttered words so fitting to our present. He said, "The dogmas of the quiet past are inadequate to the stormy present. The occasion is piled high with difficulty, and we must rise to the occasion. As our case is new, so we must think and act anew . . ." (Lincoln, 1862).

Once again as newness and change become the constant in our lives another President has spoken. In his State of the Union Address to the Congress of the United States and the American people in 1997, President Clinton placed education at the heart of his economic agenda. The choice has resonated well with the American public, ahead of reducing the deficit, protecting Social Security and Medicare and reducing crime. Peter Hart, the pollster, has stated that concerns about education are at the top of the national agenda in a way the pollsters have not seen in over a generation.

A Wall Street/NBC News poll revealed that 50 percent of all adults said education is *essential* to getting ahead in life, while a third of the respondents said it is very important. Only 1 percent said education is either not very important or not at all important in being successful. The poll also underscored the fact that while the concern with education is a cross cutting issue for all groups polled by occupation or education, there was an upscale tilt. Professional, upper income adults and those with a college education were much more likely than others to consider education essential in getting ahead. Women, who are not as prevalent in these groups, place a higher emphasis on education than men. In an era of increased racial concern, it was noted that there was very little difference between whites and blacks (Hunt, 1997).

RESPONSES TO NEWNESS AND CHANGE

In this nation we look to the federal government, academic institutions and the philanthropic community primarily to provide direction and support at times of profound change. One need only reflect on our national response to Russia when it launched Sputnik. We quickly recognized that world leadership in the space age was inextricably linked to major new program initiatives and funding, primarily for enhanced science education at all levels. Our major investment in science education assured our ability to compete globally as a world class power.

The health care delivery system and its financing provide a dramatic example of the newness and wide ranging change which affects all segments of the population. Once again we look to government, academe and philanthropic foundations to be in the forefront of our response to the profound change. The striking and continuing changes are affecting all of the professions engaged in preparing health care professional students for a relevant future. One of the greatest challenges facing nursing is to move rapidly to assure that its practitioners possess the knowledge and skills required in this new environment, while assuring that research efforts proceed which fit the new realities—measuring outcomes, assessing and meeting the needs of diverse populations and collaboration. With the significant shift in the United States health care system from a fragmented fee-for-service system toward an integrated financial and delivery system, new skills are required as health care costs and care are managed. While we are engaged in these pursuits we must not lose sight of nursing's social obligation to the public as the education of nurses for a new century is shaped. We need to remind ourselves continually and assist others as well in realizing that the marketplace is not the only valid reference point for assessing, delivering and evaluating health care services.

Practicing with the community requires a new orientation as the knowledge, skills and behaviors required of nurses shifts markedly. Nurses in the community will be providing nursing services in many instances over a protracted period of time and often to people who differ in many ways from themselves.

We have come to realize that our total reliance on the western world view of health care practices dominated by aggressive treatment and the wide use of technology is not adequate as we respond to a rapidly changing and culturally diverse society. In this nation of immigrants, which in the past was dominated by cultural groups from Europe, we are informed that the present minority population will become the majority population of the 21st century. It is predicted that by the year 2000, 50 percent of the population of the United States, or more than 135 million people will be people of color. Some 32 million people will speak languages other than English at home. The Census Bureau (1997) predicts that in the year 2050, one American in 20 will be over 85, one in five will be retired and the face of the nation will be far more Asian and Hispanic.

Understanding family systems, accommodating the needs of an ever growing population of elders, working with the increasing number of individuals with chronic conditions as they learn to manage their lives, and whenever possible, averting the occurrence of illness, while coordinating the vast array of services required, are increasingly important functions for the new nurse. Challenges abound as the more predictable and supportive environment of the hospital, once the center of the health care delivery system, gives way to a more expansive and uncontrolled environment, the larger community.

In this new environment there is increased focus on the consumers of health care services as individuals and as members of a family and community, and their ultimate empowerment as they take charge of their lives. The prevention of disease becomes more prominent as a critical strategy to improve the quality of life as well as reduce the cost of care as healthier communities emerge. It is instructive to note the shift in funding priorities of the four largest foundations active in the health care arena. The Henry J. Kaiser Family Foundation, Pew Charitable Trusts, the Robert Wood Johnson Foundation and the W. K. Kellogg Foundation are providing substantial funds for the development and testing of innovative solutions to problems which are increasingly visible as the focus in health care shifts from acute to primary care. Families and neighborhoods, access to basic health care for all, the chronically ill, the disabled, the elderly, substance abusers, disadvantaged children, low income and minority Americans, are among the targeted populations that are receiving increased attention (Sabatino, 1991).

Throughout the latter half of the 20th century we have witnessed the increase in the number of health care professions, the growth of specialty areas and the dominance of the acute care hospital which for many years was viewed as the center of the nation's health care system. The orientation of the health care system toward disease, its diagnosis and treatment commanded center stage with most health care expenditures resulting from this practice pattern. Both medical and nursing education were based on principles supporting scientifically based disciplines. Evident in the practice models was an absence of multiculturalism. Since the majority of those being served came from Europe, a eurocentric ethos prevailed. Now as multiculturalism takes hold and an increasing number of Americans claim African, Asian, Hispanic and Native American ancestry, the melting pot phenomenon no longer holds as consumers of health care expect their uniqueness to be regarded and understood as care is provided. The continuing proliferation of newness creates an urgency for the academic community as the future success of nursing is assured.

As we shift from the centrality of the hospital which remains notable for illness care, we soon recognize that the education of nurses must change to accommodate the increased expectations of nurses as practitioners, educators, researchers, managers and administrators as well as policy shapers. No longer must the professional nurse feel frustrated as the profession's independent function is compromised. The opportunity is now afforded to enhance collaborative and satisfying relationships between and among other health care providers and to form partnerships with those being served assuring their maximum independence and empowerment. As new partnerships are forged with the recipients of nursing services, the helping (behavioral) model so well known to nurses who practice in rehabilitation, mental health and substance abuse programs is replacing the medical model, the dominant model used in hospitals, as more appropriate.

With these changes have come a large place for alternative and complementary therapies as well as holistic health care practices. Increasingly, consideration is being given to the mind and body interface. Our educational preparation, however, has been based on the explanatory model of illness causation. It is a model which states that all conditions of health and illness have a measurable cause and effect. Our orientation to scientific evidence has resulted in the eradication of some diseases and the amelioration of many others. The results of the phenomenal success in the treatment of illness, however, have created a marked increase in an aging population and an increasing number of individuals with chronic conditions. Disease prevention and health promotion were not adequately dealt with, nor was the focus on individuals and families in relation to their communities in our earlier advances.

A variety of practice settings await tomorrow's nurse including the rapidly growing home care arena, nurse managed centers and integrated managed care systems. Programmatic emphasis on subacute and chronic care, primary prevention, family centered care, sophisticated information and communications technology, coupled with a culturally responsive care provider, offer unparalleled opportunities for nursing. With the diversity in nursing roles, we are challenged to think creatively as we make unprecedented contributions to improving the public's health at a time of great chaos and opportunity. Linking educational efforts and research priorities to reform goals can position nursing as an essential player in the change process.

EDUCATING NURSES FOR FUTURE SUCCESS

> In all things success depends on previous prepa-
> ration and without such preparation there is
> sure to be failure.
>
> *Confucius*

No one can predict with certainty how nursing will look in the 21st century. Some major trends, however, are becoming apparent. Illuminating them lends direction to the nursing profession as planning for the future takes place.

The contributors to this book have written in a compelling way about many of the considerations in educating the 21st century nurse, all geared toward achieving greater success as the public is served. From the guideposts in an information age to the competencies required of the new warriors, we have been provided with views that remind us of the need for reinventing the education of future nurses. Each author captures some facet of what will be required as nursing education recreates itself to match the new fundamentals. As we stretch our thinking and action well beyond what we ever imagined, we will have repositioned nursing in keeping with the dynamic times and befitting the many talents that nurses bring to the workplace.

Immigration patterns and the magnitude of adjustments required, unmatched in the history of the United States, demand major attention as education responds to the new realities. Hence, it is not surprising that many of the authors addressed the need for cultural competence as nurses continue to meet the public's need. The underrepresentation of racial and ethnic minorities in nursing is appreciated as the requirement that all nurses attain the competencies to provide acceptable care to culturally diverse populations in a variety of settings is accommodated.

The rapid changes in health care are likewise transforming relationships among patients, health care institutions, nurses and other health care providers, as well as payers of these services. It is encouraging to note that as these changes take place, new coalitions and alliances are emerging between two principal groups of providers, physicians and nurses. When these partnerships form, the agenda moves forward more quickly and with a more adequate response from those who have so much to offer within the same forum.

We are learning a great deal about what will be required for success in the 21st century. The educational process continues to inform as the necessary preparation takes place. As it proceeds, success for nursing is assured.

Vernice D. Ferguson

REFERENCES

Abdellah, F. (1972). Evolution of nursing as a profession. *International Nursing Review*, 19(3), pp. 219–238.

American Association of Colleges of Nursing. (1986, Feb.) Essentials of college and university education for nursing. A working document. Washington, DC.

Barringer, F. (1991, March 11). Census shows profound changes in social makeup of the nation. *The New York Times*, p. A1.

Beyond the melting pot. (1990, April 9). *Time*, p. 29.

Farson, R. (1969, Sept. 6). How could anything that feels so bad be so good? *Saturday Review of Literature*, pp. 20–21.

Ferguson, V. (1994). Chapter 1. The future of nursing. In Strickland, O. and Fishman, D. (eds.), *Nursing Issues in the 1990's*. Albany, New York: Delmar.

Hunt, A. (1997, March 14). Education is seen as essential ingredient for success. *Wall Street Journal*.

Lincoln, A. (1862, Dec.). Second Annual Message to Congress. Washington, DC.

Sabatino, F. (1991). Foundations' funding priorities shift from acute to primary care. *Hospitals*, 65(11), pp. 34, 36–37.

United States Department of Labor, Census Bureau (1997). The state of the nation. Washington, DC: U.S. Government Printing Office.

United States Department of Health and Human Services. Public Health Service. (1992). The registered nurse population. Washington, DC: U.S. Government Printing Office.

Part I

Guideposts in an Information Age

Changes are occurring at a phenomenal rate and forcing us to examine nursing's work in relation to the demands of the information age. The caring nurse and those preparing today's students for practice in the 21st century recognize that new competencies will be required in a new age marked by complexity and filled with temporary systems. An incredible amount of information is available to us which must be organized and mastered as health services are provided.

Guideposts are useful to chart a path for a relevant practice in the future amidst the changes which abound. Dr. McCormick offers three of them that challenge us to action—evidence- (science) based practice, informatics and unified language systems.

1

Nursing in the 21st Century— Guideposts in an Information Age

Kathleen A. McCormick

Everywhere the old order changeth, and happy those who can change with it.

Sir William Osler, 1895

In the 20th century, nurses developed the role of comforter and assistant to the physician. The nurse took temperatures, measured pulses, read blood pressure, and held patients' hands—and in emergency rooms, and during wartime across the globe, nurses got their hands bloody as they nursed (Alliance for Health Reform, 1996). Nurses of the past decade defined the scope of nursing practice and focused on the assessment and process of delivering care. That nurse moved in the latter part of the century into defining and using information systems to improve care. The nurse of the 20th century is noted for being knowledgeable, competent and prepared to care for highly complex patients.

That nurse, though nobly remembered, is far removed from the nurse that we see ahead in the 21st century as we approach a new health care environment that is complex, conflicting, and ever changing. It is an environment driven by different models of financing and delivery often-

This paper is based upon the Patricia Chomley Oration, delivered May, 1996 at the Royal College of Nursing, Australia, Annual Meeting, Parliament House, Canberra, Australia.

5

times using telecommunication. It is a system that focuses on outcomes, performance measures, and the use of technology to deliver care to wider audiences than previously covered. It includes a vision of the advanced prepared nurse as an expert consultant to nurses in environments with few resources and large geographic areas to traverse, and vast patient conditions to include. The advanced nurse specialist serves as consultant to the nurse generalist, and to those with little formal training through telecommunications. It is an environment where distance learning is common in health care. The turn of the century nurse then needs new guideposts in forging ahead. These guideposts are evidence- (science) based practice, informatics, and unified language systems. But first, what is the evidence that these forces are needed?

NURSING—THE CARING PROFESSION

The experiences we have in common bond us together. We are nurses, we belong to a caring profession that has consumer advocacy, healing, nurturing and caring as our code of ethics. The differences between us, as specialist or generalist, community-based, hospital-based, or academic are forces that can also tear us apart. For the next century we need to focus on forces that unify us because we are nurses. We need one place that the government looks to for decisions about nurses and nursing, the professional organization that sets policy, and guides and conducts research on the major forces affecting the nursing profession.

The Workforce

Hospitals will remain vitally important in our delivery of health care to those who are critically ill and require high-intensity, high-tech nursing care. The PEW Health Professionals Commission recently concluded that we will have as many as 200,000 to 300,000 nursing jobs lost "with the eclipsing of the role of the acute care hospital" (Pew, Critical Challenges, 1995).

The United States Bureau of Labor Statistics, however, relies on more historical data, and they are predicting significant growth in nursing employment over the next decade, with employment in hospitals expected to grow, however, more slowly than elsewhere (U.S. Bureau of Labor Statistics, 1995). In the United States, the balance between supply and demand will be related to the education of nurses and the number of employment opportunities created. Distribution of nurses between rural, remote areas, inner city, and urban areas will enter heavily into this formula.

The Increase of Older Persons

In the United States, the number of elderly persons is expected to increase. Currently, the percent of the population who are 65 years and older is between 8-13 percent (U.S. Dept. of Commerce, 1993). By the year 2025 the percentage of those aged 65 years and older will be as high as 20 percent. For the United States that represents a 101 percent increase. In 1990 the life expectancy in the United States was 75.6.

Because of the increased number of aged persons at the turn of the century, Bureau of Health Professions' Reports and another Pew Health Professions Commission on the "Primary Care Workforce 2000" recommend that more nurse practitioners be prepared who can work not only with the elderly, but also the larger minority population. These reports echo the recommendations of the National Institute on Aging for "Personnel For Health Needs of the Elderly through the Year 2020." This report predicts that health care will be focused on preventive, rehabilitative, and primary care to adequately assist the elderly in maintaining their function in the community.

Expanded Nursing Practice

Advanced practice models in health prevention and treatment require more high-tech and computerized decision support. The definition of advanced practice nurses includes certified nurse midwives, nurse practitioners, clinical nurse specialists, and certified registered nurse anesthetists.

Much of nursing will be delivered in isolated environments, including rural or remote areas and inner cities where doctors are scarce, and in frontier regions where the nurse is often the first to evaluate patients, provide early diagnosis and triage, and promote health. The places where nursing care is practiced that will become more dominant at the turn of the century are outpatient, ambulatory, primary, community, and long-term care settings. In those environments case management responsibility will fall upon the nursing profession. As this trend increases, the role of managing health risks, detecting and diagnosing common symptoms, understanding the health needs of the entire population, and working well as part of a large team of several professionals communicating with patients will be required.

Achieving Nursing Outcomes

Nursing will demonstrate its stake in *curing* patients' symptoms, like pain management, incontinence, pressure ulcers, mucositis, fatigue, and nausea and vomiting. Report cards will be issued on nursing performance in these areas as well as on preventing patient injuries such as falls, preventing staff injuries like back problems, preventing nosocomial infections, for example, urinary tract infections and pneumonia, and preventing deep vein thrombosis. Nurses will become better equipped for predicting unanticipated complications and iatrogenic events as well as infections. Reduced medication errors, returns to surgery, and readmissions to hospital after discharge will be more closely scrutinized to investigate failure of nursing care to achieve desired patient outcomes. The mental and emotional status of the patient at the time of discharge, and acceptance and coping with diagnosis in the ambulatory and community setting, will be independently managed by nurses.

In the community and ambulatory care settings, the psychiatric and psychological consults will be handled by advanced practice nurses. Our role in patient compliance with medications and treatments, exercise, and diet will become more clearly explicated. The unexpected death and unplanned entry of patients into nursing homes shortly after discharge, will be blamed on poor nursing judgment in the acute care environment. In the nursing home and for care at home, the nutritional status of the patient becomes more of a role for nursing since, unlike the acute care environment, dieticians are often not available in the home or nursing home for consultation.

Nurse-managed programs of care in normal pediatrics, in diabetes compliance, in cardiovascular rehabilitation, and in geriatric continence care will be more prominent during the next century. Already in some countries, nurses are primary coordinators of wards for patients with eating disorders. High-risk infant management is another area where nurses have responsibility for statewide screening, tracking, and referring high risk infants for development, neurological, and physician examinations. In specialized diabetes care, nurses run programs for foot care and for teaching patients to prevent eye complications. As the cost impacts of these programs are revealed, with the quality profiles maintained, these nurse-managed programs will expand during the first half of the 21st century. They will provide demonstrated quality care, satisfaction to patients, and efficient and effective care at a cost that is justified.

In all the preceding domains, nurses will assume more roles currently delivered by other health providers. In lean and mean times, the nurse will assume those roles as the costs of additional health providers cannot be justified. The nurse practitioner with skills in drug management, diet counseling, diagnostic and treatment management will be required in rural areas. Registered nurses are already moving from direct care to managing, coordinating, and supervising care in hospitals, functioning as *case managers* for the entire episode of a patient's illness. This trend is expected to continue and expand at the turn of the century.

Nursing's role in assuring a patient's return to homeostasis with normal vital signs will be more rigorously monitored. The return of patients to functional status and health status such as mobility at time of discharge, or achieved later in community and long-term care settings, will be described as goals of nursing outcomes.

The patient and family, or significant other's satisfaction with care will be reclaimed by nursing. Even if the patient's status at discharge was deceased, the outcome of achieving family satisfaction will become important to measure and claim. During the dying process, the nurse's treatment of pain and delivery of comfort measures will provide quality care and family satisfaction that needs to be measured and attributed to positive nursing outcomes. Appropriate grief counseling of family members will yield higher satisfaction with care delivered to their dying loved ones.

Expanded Practice vs. Mix of Nursing Personnel

In some areas of health care, expanded practice is not necessary, however, the appropriate mix of nursing personnel is required. Measurement of this in long-term care and nursing homes has been the hallmark of nurse researchers. In a recent report issued in the United States from the Institute of Medicine, the United States Congress has been urged to mandate around-the-clock registered nursing coverage in nursing homes by the year 2000 (IOM, 1996). The report further stated that the mix of different types of nursing personnel, the quality of patient care in nursing homes, as well as the incidence of work-related injuries and stress among nursing staff could be reduced with higher numbers of registered nurses. The current mix of RNs is not enough to meet the future demands of a rapidly changing health care system. Related to the cost and quality impact, the report notes that if more RNs were in nursing home environments, fewer elders would be transferred to high cost hospital care for complications, iatrogenic consequences of care, and serious conditions. The potential impact of keeping the acutely ill aged in nursing homes was predicted to reduce costs significantly. Greater RN presence on all shifts in the nursing home should lead to higher rates of patient survival, improved ability of residents to function independently, fewer hospitalizations, and earlier discharges from nursing homes.

Unlike the decline in work related injuries in the private sector, the rate of work related injuries for hospital and nursing home staff has increased by 52 percent and 62 percent respectively in the United States. These are primarily back injuries and needle wounds.

THREE NEW GUIDEPOSTS

Three guideposts that will move us closer to patient quality and accountability with the consumer for our role in health care are: evidence-(science) based practice, informatics, and unified language systems.

Evidence-Based Practice.   Evidence-based practice means basing nursing care on scientific principles. It may be protocol generated, guideline derived, pathway-based, or algorithm-based. The next 100 years promise unimaginable progress in science and technology, genetics, and biochemical treatments at the cell level. The science of genetics alone holds promising keys to the diagnosis and treatment of many diseases. On the other hand, the development and collection of enormous masses of information on individuals and families will create serious new issues of confidentiality and appropriateness of use. These explosions of information and knowledge will require nurses to have access to information that comes in synthesized products in order to keep pace, minimize, or manage the problems that could arise. Nurses will be challenged to demonstrate why 150 different treatments of pressure ulcers are delivered within 20 hospitals in a network. They will be equally challenged to define the science behind common nursing interventions, such as the treatment of mucositis in patients receiving chemotherapy. Clinical practice guidelines are such products; however, in the 21st century the private sector will be challenged to develop the guidelines based upon evidence accumulated by professional organizations and government agencies.

In the global medical literature, the National Library of Medicine processes 1,700 new citations a day. This volume of information is daunting to health care deliverers. Who has time to read it? Staff need synthesized information or knowledge at the point of decision making. Guidelines, protocols, algorithms, best practice methods, critical pathways, and other tools are to be integrated into computerized decision support systems. An educational challenge is to educate nurses to search information. As Desrochers and Detmer (1990) put it, we need to change the concept of the *university* to the *unisearchity*.

The Agency for Health Care Policy and Research (AHCPR) in the United States has produced three products to support evidence-based practice: 1) clinical practice guidelines, 2) indicators (review criteria) to measure quality of care, and 3) performance measures. To date, 20 clinical practice guidelines have been published and disseminated from AHCPR. They are available for the health provider and the consumer on a variety of topics. To date over 48 million copies have been disseminated internationally. CD-roms have been sent to many sites nationally and internationally. But by far, the most useful link is through the Internet where the guidelines are available from the AHCPR home page: http://www.ahcpr.gov.

Recently, over 750,000 guidelines per month were downloaded to the United States and 70 other countries. Early in 1996, United States nurses and doctors were the fifth largest group to access the guidelines. Still higher usage was found among health professionals from Canada, the United Kingdom, Australia, and Japan.

A guideline can be translated into specific indicators to measure quality of care. These are review criteria which are: "systematically developed statements that can be used to assess the appropriateness of specific health care decisions, services, and outcomes" (IOM 1990, pg. 44). Further guidelines, translated to review criteria can be used to monitor benchmarks of care. The third product is called performance measures.

Performance measures are "methods or instruments used to estimate or monitor the extent to which the actions of a health care practitioner or provider conform to practice guidelines, medical review criteria, or standards of quality" (IOM 1990, pg. 49). These new tools are also available on the AHCPR home page under CONQUEST. The products of the review criteria and performance measures close the quality loop and demonstrate accountability in health care delivery.

Guideline development involves an analysis of the evidence. Much of the evidence in nursing effectiveness has related to pain management, pressure ulcers, and incontinence. Beyond that the evidence is scanty in the areas of functional assessment before and after surgery or medical procedures. There are many health conditions (e.g., cataract surgery, benign prostatic hypertrophy) that are billion dollar health conditions and have no nursing study findings. To participate in outcome studies and guideline development in the future, the research base for nursing must be solidly linked to the major health conditions of the country.

When sufficient evidence related to patient symptom management exists in the nursing literature, it will be timely in the 21st century for the nursing profession to develop guidelines. For example, after acquiring ample evidence on the nursing treatment of mucositis in cancer patients, or the prolongation of the symptom-free state in patients receiving chemotherapy, nursing could write its own guidelines for recommended best practice in health care.

Informatics

When the entire medical record is an electronic medical record, the use of guidelines will be outmoded. Only the algorithms that drive the protocols of best practice, the match to review criteria, and performance measures will be needed. When best practice can be tracked on an electronic medical record, the hospital, health department, state, region, or national organizations can retrieve information on what positive outcomes are being achieved in health care.

The documentation of nursing on the computer-based patient record is a vision of the next century. However, this documentation does more than automate what we have done manually. This documentation interrelates with knowledge sources like guidelines, policies, and literature, to facilitate decision making. The development of expanded clinical decision support systems will facilitate the integration of advanced practice concepts where the lowest prepared health professional can deliver and improve care. For example, protocols for assessing and treating urinary incontinence in long-term care facilities have been written by a nurse gerontologist with a PhD in informatics. This product, called UNIS (the Urological Nursing Information System), demonstrated that the lowest prepared health provider in the US, an aide in a nursing home, could provide better quality and improved outcomes by following the protocol of an expert nurse (Petrucci, et al., 1992; Johnston, et al., 1994).

Petrucci's model is unique to nursing. However, in our future, nurses in academic or regional health areas can design the knowledge synthesis and implement it in decision support systems, to be utilized by health providers in remote, rural, and frontier areas. These systems need to be built, implemented, evaluated for outcomes, quality, and cost impact in our near future. When these systems travel distances, the systems are part of telenursing networks.

Nurses have begun to communicate in telenursing networks from around the world. The applications being addressed are distance learning, licensure requirements, and examples of telecommunication use within the nursing profession. Expanded practice nurses are grasping the potential advantages of their participation in these new technologies. What seem like science fiction applications of telecommunications now will be common clinical practice during the first quarter of the next century. The nurse in specialty settings will be provided consultations via communication networks to nurses in inner city, remote and frontier environments. The nurse in those environments will have rich resources, knowledge acquisition skills, and search capabilities to be in touch with information that was only within the purview of the specialized academic-based hospital or university in the 20th century.

Expert informatics nurses will be certified in knowledge of information science. Already the US has led and continues to participate in international leadership in nursing informatics. The nurse at the turn of the century who is illiterate about information systems will be akin to being illiterate at the turn of the last century. It is the challenge of educators and leaders in the nursing profession to prevent this from occurring in the nursing profession in the US.

Unified Nursing Languages.   Abraham Lincoln had a vision to understand that national policies are unfinished masterpieces—great works in perpetual progress. When he said "A house divided against itself cannot stand," he was telling us that nations have to remain united to complete their work. The same goes for health professions. There are many wedges that the new health care delivery systems may try to place between the nurse and the patient. That is why nurses at the turn of this century and well into the 21st century will be challenged to demonstrate the most cost-effective means to offer quality care to those they serve. That will require that we can name what we do with uniform precision in our vocabulary, and measure it in terms of effectiveness and efficiency in our delivery.

The use of unified languages for nurses is moving from local to national to international levels. Locally, nurses are developing the vocabulary to use in practice and research. There amongst the other countries in the International Council of Nurses (ICN), the US has placed the North American Nursing Diagnosis vocabulary (NANDA), the OMAHA Visiting Nursing Association vocabulary, the Georgetown Home Health Care Project Vocabulary, and the Nursing Intervention Classification from the University of Iowa (McCormick, et al. 1994). These vocabularies have been added to the Unified Medical Language System of the National Library of Medicine to begin to link the words through semantic networks, and a metathesaurus to the nursing vocabularies in the Read Code from the United Kingdom. In that way, the utilization of the words can be studied, words can be recommended for addition or deletion from the list, and eventually, words may be harmonized into a common vocabulary of use nationally and internationally.

This is not a new concept in nursing. In 1909, Hampton-Robb said at an ICN meeting:

> "While attending a special meeting of the ICN in Paris, I was naturally at once struck by the fact . . . that the methods and ways of regarding nursing problems, were, in many respects as foreign to the various delegations as were the actual languages, and the thought occurred to me that if . . . we hoped ever to realize the aims of the International Council, one of which is: to confer upon questions relating to the welfare of their patients, sooner or later we must put ourselves upon a common basis, and work out what may be called a 'Nursing Esperanto' which would, in the course of time, give us a universal nursing language, and methods for all of our affiliated countries."

Issues and Barriers

What will the educational needs be for this nurse in the 21st century? What will be the skills necessary for nurses working in nontraditional roles in the future? In global nursing areas, distance education will become the more utilized process of acquiring nursing education. Because of the large number of aged persons, gerontological content will have to be examined. In the US, by the year 2000, 46 percent of registered nurses will be giving care to the elderly (Wells, 1993).

National efforts relating to nursing education should focus on assuring that the workforce is appropriate for the changing health care models emphasizing community-based health care.

The needs of the growing elderly population will include not only rehabilitative and physical needs, but mental health needs. Predicted to be areas of unmet needs in the next century are cognitive, psychiatric, and substance abuse disorders. New methods for research need to include the unique measurement techniques to deal with these cognitively impaired populations.

How then will content on gerontology, primary care, expanded public health and community health, telehealth and informatics be handled to meet the increasing demands?

National resources and program initiatives need to be strategically targeted to assure the development of an adequate nursing workforce prepared to meet the demands for services in a changing health care environment.

Barriers to practice should be removed to enable health workers to function in their maximum scope of practice.

Development and monitoring of the nursing workforce should be supported by targeted national analytic efforts (Desrochers & Detmer, 1990).

Summary

There are strong forces changing the way that we will practice and behave as nurses in the future. Those forces include cost effectiveness, efficiencies, and reform. Whether here or in other countries, the need for new guideposts for nursing will be needed. This author suggests that three new guideposts that will articulate our way in the future are evidence-based practice, informatics, and unified nursing languages. The evidence for these guideposts come from the expansion of information and knowledge, changes in health delivery, changes in the age of the recipient of nursing care, and expanded practices in rural and frontier areas.

REFERENCES AND BIBLIOGRAPHY

Alliance for Health Reform (February, 1996). *The Twenty-First Century Nurse.* 1900 L. Street, NW, Suite 512, Washington, DC 20036.

Desrochers, L., & Detmer, D. E. (1990). From the Ivory Tower to the Unisearchity. *The Educational Record*, 71, pp. 8–14.

Duggar, B., & Palmer, H. et al. (1995). *Understanding and Choosing Clinical Performance Measures to Quality Improvement: Development of a Typology and Attachments*. Rockville, MD: Agency for Health Care Policy and Research, 2101 East Jefferson St., Suite 501. Publication No. 95-N001; 95-N002.

Grady, M. L., & Weis, K. A. (1995). *Cost Analysis Methodology for Clinical Practice Guidelines*. Rockville, MD: Agency for Health Care Policy and Research, 2101 East Jefferson St., Suite 501, Publication No. 95-001.

Hampton-Robb, I. (1909). *Reports of the Third Regular Meeting of the International Council of Nurses*. Geneva: International Council of Nurses.

Institute of Medicine (1996). *Nursing Staff in Hospitals and Nursing Homes: Is It Adequate?* Washington, DC: National Academy Press, 2101 Constitution Avenue, NW, Lock Box 285, ISBN 0-309-05431-1.

Institute of Medicine (1992). *Guidelines for Clinical Practice: From Development to Use*. Washington, DC: National Academy Press, 2101 Constitution Avenue, NW, Lock Box 285.

Institute of Medicine (1990). *Clinical Practice Guidelines: Directors for a New Program*. Washington, DC: National Academy Press, 2101 Constitution Avenue, NW, Lock Box 285.

Johnston, M., Langton, K., et al. (1994). Effects of computer-based decision support systems on clinician performance and patient outcome: A critical appraisal. *Annals of Internal Medicine*, 120, pp. 135–142.

McCormick, K. A., Lang, N., Zielstorff, R., Milholland, D. K., Saba, V., & Jacox, A. (1994). Toward standard classification schemes for nursing language: Recommendations of the American Nurses Association Steering Committee on Databases to Support Clinical Nursing Practice. *Journal of the American Medical Informatics Association* (JAMIA), 1, pp. 421–427.

McCormick, K. A., Moore, S. R., & Siegel, R. (eds.) (1995). *Clinical Practice Guideline Development: Methodology Perspectives*. Rockville, MD: Agency for Health Care Policy and Research, 2101 East Jefferson St., Suite 501, Publication No. 95-0009.

National Institute on Aging (1987). *Personnel for Health Needs of the Elderly through the Year 2020*. Bethesda, MD: U.S. Department of Health and Human Services, Public Health Service.

PEW Health Professions Commission (1994). *Primary Care Workforce 2000: Federal Policy Paper*. San Francisco: PEW Charitable Trust/UCSF Center for Health Professions.

PEW Health Professions Commission (November, 1995). *Critical Challenges*. San Francisco: PEW Charitable Trust/UCSF Center for Health Professions.

Petrucci, K. A., Jacox, A., McCormick, K. A., Parks, P., Kjerulff, K., Baldwin, B., & Petrucci, P. (1992). Evaluating the appropriateness of a nurse expert system's patient assessment. *Computers in Nursing*, 10(6), pp. 243–249.

Schoenbaum, S. C., Sundwall, D. N., and Bergman, D., et al. (1995). *Using Clinical Practice Guidelines to Evaluate Quality of Care.* Vol 1. Issues. Vol 2. Methods. Rockville, MD: Agency for Health Care Policy and Research, 2101 East Jefferson St., Suite 501. Publication No. 95-0045; 95-0046.

U.S. Bureau of the Census (February 1992). International Population Reports: An Aging World II. Washington, DC: US Government Printing Office, Publication No. P25/92-3.

U.S. Labor Bureau of Labor Statistics (1995). *Occupational Outlook Handbook.*

Wells, T. J. (1993). Setting the agenda for gerontological education. In C. Heine (ed.). *Determining the Future of Gerontological Nursing Education: Partnerships between Education and Practice*, Publication No. 14-2508. New York: National League for Nursing Press.

Wykle, M., & Musil, C. (1995). Psychogeriatric mental health content in gerontological nursing education. In T. Fulmer & M. Matzo (eds.) *Strengthening Gerontological Nursing Education*. New York: Springer Publishing Co.

Part II

A Cycle of Culturally Sensitive Care

Nursing has a long and illustrious history of responding creatively to the realities that confront people in need of nursing services at any given time. Dr. Dickason, Ms. McNeal and her colleagues provide examples of nursing's challenging work as individuals, families and communities in great need of health care services are served by nurses.

At the turn of the 20th century school nurses emerged in New York City. They provided services to the new immigrants living in poverty in crowded tenements and lacking the language facility required for their new environment. School nurses focused on the control of communicable diseases thereby reducing absenteeism as children returned to school. As school nurses respond to today's challenges they serve as consultants, coordinators and health managers. Among their major initiatives are facilitating personal responsibility for behavior to assure healthier life-styles and the assurance of safe environments as violence is controlled.

Then as now, nurses are providing culturally sensitive services to at-risk populations in their communities where significant barriers to a healthy lifestyle exist. The mobile health program of MercyCARE is yet another creative example of nursing's work in response to the public's need.

Nurse educators can learn much from nursing's history as the 21st century nurse is prepared for the presenting challenges and opportunities as they practice in a new age.

2

Culturally Sensitive Care in the Community—School Nurses

Elizabeth L. Dickason

Historically, the need for nurses in schools was recognized in New York City in the early 1900s by Lillian Wald (Woodfill & Beyrer, 1991). While providing care to immigrants in crowded tenements in New York City, she became aware that children were being sent home from school because they had contagious diseases. Many of the adverse health conditions could have been treated successfully with simple measures at home, thus allowing the child to return to school in a short time. However, because the parents were often poor, uneducated and did not speak or read the English language they were unable to comprehend why the children were denied access to school. When Wald realized that very large numbers of poor immigrant children were denied access to public schools on a daily basis, she requested that the school board allow a nurse to be assigned to one school to teach prevention and treatment of contagious diseases (Zurek & Hunt, 1997).

In 1902 Wald assigned Lina Rogers, a Public Health Nurse, to a school setting as an experiment to determine the effectiveness of nursing care in improving the health of children and reducing the number of daily absentees (Igoe & Speer, 1996). She worked with students and teachers and also made follow-up home visits to instruct students and parents in the principles of good hygiene. As a result of this experiment absenteeism for health reasons was significantly reduced. Following this successful demonstration of the effectiveness of nursing interventions, school boards across the country began to hire nurses for the purposes of disease control. However, the nurses faced a considerable challenge in accomplishing their mission, even for simple health measures, due to the formidable barriers presented by communication with the children and their parents. While cultural differences were not addressed directly they certainly must have had an impact on the immigrant's compliance with the nursing plan.

EDUCATION

Currently, the educational preparation of a school nurse ranges from diploma or associate degree, through the master's level (Rea, 1996). The majority of school nurses are prepared at the baccalaureate level with a small number (~400) prepared at the School Nurse Practitioner level (Igoe & Speer, 1996). The National Association of School Nurses recommends the baccalaureate in nursing as the appropriate entry level degree for school nurses (Proctor, 1990).

For nurses prepared at the baccalaureate or higher level, it can be assumed that they have had relevant courses in Community Health and Health and Physical Assessment that would enhance their ability to provide care to individuals and groups. Community Health Nursing (CHN) practice is general and comprehensive with the dominant responsibility being to the population as a whole. The focus of CHN is on the prevention of illness and the promotion and maintenance of health in individuals, families and the population as a whole. Nursing activities to attain these goals include education, counseling, advocacy and management of care (Lancaster, Lowry & Martin, 1996). These activities should be an integral part of any comprehensive health program for the school population, therefore, nurses with a background in CHN will be better prepared to execute such programs. A Health and Physical Assessment course provides the theory and skills necessary to complete a comprehensive health history and perform a complete physical examination. The information obtained from this activity can be used to plan interventions to promote, maintain or restore the health of individual students. School nurses prepared at less than the baccalaureate level should pursue the relevant courses necessary to obtain the appropriate education and skills.

School nurses may also seek certification as a school nurse, school nurse practitioner, community health nurse or other clinical nurse specialist through their national nursing organizations. In some states the State Department of Education requires an additional state certification for school nurses (Igoe & Speer, 1996).

Role

The role of the school nurse has evolved over the years from the primary focus of disease control to the current role of consultant/coordinator. A newer role as health manager or coordinator as described by Igoe and Speer (1996) includes: (a) involvement in activities that influence policy decisions for comprehensive and integrated health programs, (b) case management to assist families to find the resources necessary to meet their unique needs, (c) development of a system of school health activities as an integral part of the school and community health system, and (d) health promotion and health protection activities which include health education within the school curriculum, health screening, follow up and referral for health problems. The school nurse is also responsible for assessing the environment within the school setting regarding safety for the children and the staff.

Health Programs

A major point to remember in any discussion of school health is that the states are free to develop their own health programs (Kub & Steel, 1995). National standards do not exist for mandatory inclusion of specific health program content for the general student body. This results in variation of programs across the country. Although the programs vary from state to state, there are areas of concern that are common to the majority of programs offered for the health of school age children. These areas of concern which include health services, health education, and a safe environment, have guided the development of school health programs (Kub & Steel, 1995).

Health services consist of screening, referrals, record keeping regarding state laws and special needs, first aid, counseling and education for individual students, parents and teachers. Some schools have school nurse practitioners providing care in clinics within their schools (Kub & Steel, 1995).

In the past, the focus of health education was on hygiene and communicable disease control. Currently, the focus is on health promotion and the influence of personal behavior on health status. Many school districts have a comprehensive planned health program in place for students in kindergarten through high school which includes information, skills and positive attitudes toward health (Kub & Steel, 1995).

A safe and healthy school environment includes both physical and psychosocial aspects. The evaluation of a safe physical environment includes assessing for proper sanitation, presence of asbestos or lead, playground safety, proper lighting in stairwells and fire safety (Kub & Steel, 1995). The school nurse is responsible for bringing these matters to the attention of the administrators for resolution.

A psychosocial safety issue that is increasingly important to students of any age and to the school nurse is violence in the schools. Violence is described as non-accidental acts that result in physical or psychological injury to one or more persons (Campbell & Landenberger, 1996). Schools are often the places where everyday stressors and frustrations can lead to violence. For example, during adolescence, students are often self conscious and vulnerable to verbal attacks which may lead to a physical altercation (Prothow-Stith & Weissman, 1991). The school nurse could be very instrumental in reducing the incidence of violence in the student body. The nurse could collect data regarding reported events of stress or injury due to violence and develop and implement a program within her school to prevent further incidents. With the cooperation of other school nurses it would be possible to extend this program throughout the district. The factors that contribute to violence often originate in the community from problems of over-crowding, poverty, and unemployment. When these factors are present the incidence of violence will be increased in the general population. The violent behavior seen in the community will be reflected in the behaviors of school age children (Prothrow-Stith & Weissman, 1991). The school nurse could act as facilitator in a structured program where students learn the skills of conflict management. Students can be led to identify and discuss sources of stress and the effect of violent behavior on individuals and groups.

Student Demographics

In schools today the problems resulting from a diverse population who are often poor and who do not speak English are not dissimilar to those faced by school nurses in the 1900s. Such diversity however, is no longer found exclusively in cities; it has extended to the suburbs, small towns and rural areas. In the 1900s the nurses were challenged to aid the student in assimilating into the new world's culture. Today, however, the primary goal is not to assimilate but to understand and value our cultural differences and similarities by providing culturally sensitive care to all school children.

In many schools today an array of people from different racial, ethnic, social and geographic backgrounds make up the student body. This culturally diverse population exposes the heterogeneous group to multiple world views and the new arrivals must adjust to a different cultural perspective (Strasser, Maurer & Kavanaugh, 1995). In order for the school nurse to function in a therapeutic manner with all of the students, the nurse must be willing to gain knowledge of multiple cultures and develop an understanding and sensitivity to the influence of cultural beliefs on the health of the school population.

In the past, new members of the group wanted to assimilate themselves into the native culture and the term *melting pot* was assigned to this process. Today, however, the new description for this process of adapting to a new culture is *salad bowl*, which implies that people want to be a part of the whole but still retain their unique identities. A further implication of this new description is that members of the population have to understand the cultural beliefs of their own group as well as the beliefs of the other groups. This understanding then helps individuals with different cultural beliefs develop a sensitivity to the values of these beliefs. This process is known as cultural accommodation.

For school nurses to be successful in the salad bowl environment, they must be willing to develop a level of cultural sensitivity which Orlandi (1992) suggests is a process that precedes and leads to the development of cultural competence. This process begins with nurses' analyses of their own cultural beliefs and culminates in the acceptance of the cultural beliefs of others. A school nurse who is sensitive to a client's cultural needs and has developed cultural competence will be able to develop a nursing plan that is congruent with the client's belief system. The nurse will also be able to establish a nurse-client relationship based on trust that will in turn help facilitate improved health for the client.

Cultural Sensitivity

The process of developing cultural sensitivity includes overcoming the barriers of ethnocentrism, cultural imposition and stereotyping which may be so ingrained in the nurse's own belief system as to be accepted as truth. Ethnocentrism as described by Leininger (1978) is the tendency of an individual or group to believe that one's own lifeways are the most desirable, acceptable or best and to act in a superior manner regarding the lifeways of other cultures. All members of society belong to various groups which provide traditions which in turn provide guidance to life's problems (Leininger, 1991). These traditions or cultural beliefs are learned at an early age through contact with members of that culture. When a school nurse exhibits ethnocentric behavior, the students and their families become aware that their values are not respected and will resist the advice of the nurse. For example, a school nurse has arranged a meeting with an Asian mother to discuss immunization requirements that the children must have prior to entering school. The school nurse wants to make the mother feel comfortable in this new setting and greets her by her first name not realizing that this behavior is a sign of disrespect to the Asian mother. This feeling of not being respected by the nurse may cause the Asian mother to resist the nurse's advice. This resistance could result in the children not being immunized and therefore, not being allowed to attend school.

Another barrier to cultural sensitivity is cultural imposition, which is defined as the tendency of individuals to impose their beliefs, values and patterns of behavior upon others for varied reasons (Leininger, 1991). A school nurse who has been educated in a scientifically based health care system may assume that this is the best type of health care for all students to receive. If the nurses impose their scientific methods on the student without acknowledging the value of the student's health beliefs the nurses will be unable to intervene effectively.

For example, when providing care to African American students in the rural south the nurse must be cognizant of the use of folk healers by this group. Many African Americans seek advice from a *Granny* who is knowledgeable about home remedies such as spices, herbs and roots, for a wide range of maladies (Cherry & Giger, 1995). When school nurses attempt to provide scientific care to an African American student with conjunctivitis who has visited a folk healer or *granny*, the nurses must be careful not to impose their values on the student. The nurse needs to assess what cultural home remedies have been used to alleviate the symptoms of this problem. The nurse can then determine if the home remedies will interfere with scientific health measures. If the nurse discounts the value of the *granny* it is likely that the student will still seek the advice of the *granny* but will be reluctant to share that information with the school nurse. The best approach for the nurse to follow would be to include the folk medicine advice with scientific measures whenever possible, thus reinforcing that both the dominant culture and the student's culture have value.

Stereotyping is the assumption that all people in a similar, cultural, racial or ethnic group share the same values and beliefs. Stereotyping students based on beliefs about their perceived behavior can create problems for both the student and the nurse. A school nurse who believes that all Hispanic males are lazy might overlook a Hispanic student with a health problem who has a history of absenteeism or lateness due to oversleeping and who complains of being tired. If the nurse assumes that the student is lazy and doesn't want to attend school because he would rather stay home, the nurse might not follow through with a thorough health assessment to determine whether or not his tiredness is symptomatic of a health related problem.

Developing Cultural Sensitivity

Hosang (1996) described a five step task oriented program for developing cultural sensitivity. The first four steps are designed to facilitate cultural awareness in the learner and overcome the barriers of ethnocentrism, cultural imposition, and stereotyping. The goal of the final step is the acceptance and respect of another's cultural needs. Participation in this program allows school nurses to recognize the influence of their own values on their behavior and to accept the variation of culture in others.

Anderson and McFarlane (1996) state that the goal of providing culturally sensitive care can only be achieved through conscious efforts of gaining knowledge about how various diverse cultures explain, understand, and treat their own health problems. It has been suggested that the best time to gain this knowledge of diverse populations is during the student education process (Zurek, 1997). The American Association of Colleges of Nursing document, *Essentials of College and University Education for Professional Nursing* offers support for the position that this process should occur during the academic preparation of professional nurses (1986). The document recommends that the education of nurses ensure the ability to understand other cultural traditions in order to gain a perspective on personal values and differences among individuals and groups (p. 4). The National League for Nursing also values the placement of cultural education for meeting the needs of diverse populations in basic nursing programs (1996). This addition of knowledge of diverse populations to the nursing curricula is relatively new, having occurred over the past ten years. Therefore, many nurses practicing today may not have received education in their basic programs regarding diverse cultures. School nurses who did not have the opportunity to participate in these programs, may choose to attend continuing education courses to aid them in developing cultural sensitivity.

The need to acquire an understanding of other cultures is made evident by the current demographic distribution of the United States. The United States Census (1993) data indicate that the majority of citizens are white (75.4%) with African Americans (12.2%) and Hispanics (9.0%) representing the largest minority groups. Other minority groups include Asian/Pacific Islanders (3.0%) and Native Americans (1.0%). It is interesting to note that professional nurses represent a different profile, with 90 percent of the nurses representing the white population followed by African American (4.0%), Asian/Pacific Islanders (3.0%), Hispanics (1.4%) and Native Americans (.04%) (United States Department of Health and Human Services, 1994). It is evident from the demographic data that the majority of school age children will receive health care from a white school nurse. Until recently the education of many school nurses was based on the biopsychosocial characteristics of the dominant white culture. Therefore, in addition to acquiring cultural sensitivity, it is essential that the school nurse acquire knowledge of physical and biological variances in diverse groups in order to provide appropriate nursing care. These variations occur in the areas of skin color, growth and development, enzymatic differences and susceptibility to disease (Giger & Davidhizar, 1995). The need to have nurses who are prepared to provide culturally sensitive nursing care in today's school health setting is evident. It is important that each school nurse assess the unique biopsychosocial needs of the school population and develop a program that will provide culturally sensitive care.

Biological Variations

The most significant biological variation in the initial physical assessment of diverse populations is skin color. School nurses must be able to make an accurate assessment of all students and it is more difficult to assess for color changes in darker skinned children. For African American and Hispanic American children, the school nurse would have to assess skin color changes by observing skin surfaces which have the least skin pigmentation such as the palms of the hands or the soles of the feet. The nurse may observe keloids at sites of minor or major trauma in students with dark skin since their skin is more susceptible than white skin to the overgrowth of connective tissue as a result of injury (Overfield, 1981).

Assessing for pallor, jaundice or cyanosis in children of color might present a problem for a school nurse who has not participated in a health assessment course that includes assessment skills for biological variations in skin color. The nurse should assess the conjunctiva, oral mucosa, and the nail beds for signs of pallor, jaundice or cyanosis (Roach, 1981).

School age children often present to the health office with bruises that they have received while playing on the school ground. In order to determine the extent of injury to a non-white student, the nurse may not be able to assess the skin for redness that would indicate the severity of the trauma. Therefore, the nurse should place the dorsal surface of her hand lightly over the area of trauma to determine areas of warmth and tenderness (Roach, 1981).

Nurses in the high school setting would need to have knowledge regarding the development of lactose intolerance in the teen years. Many African Americans (75%), Hispanic Americans (66%), American Indians and Asian Americans lack the enzyme to convert lactose to glucose and galactose which results in gastrointestinal symptoms of bloating and diarrhea. The problems of embarrassment and discomfort associated with this health problem may only intensify the difficulty some teens experience as they make the transition to young adults. The school nurse would have to be aware of their physical and emotional developmental needs while providing a nutritional program that addresses the students' cultural needs (Giger & Davidhizar, 1995).

School nurses must always assess the needs of their assigned population which includes a knowledge of biological variations in stages of physical development. For example, African American female children often reach puberty at an early age. A school nurse in an elementary school with a population of African American students would need to be aware of the need to provide puberty education to students as young as nine or ten years of age in fourth grade (Overfield, 1985).

Many Hispanic children are smaller in stature which could make it appear that this is an abnormality when they are compared to standard growth charts for the white population. The school nurse would need to have knowledge of the deviations within different groups and growth charts that are appropriate for the diverse populations in the nurse's school setting (Giger & Davidhizar, 1995).

Communication

An additional barrier to cultural sensitivity between students and the school nurse may emerge as a response to differences in communication styles and accents. This response may make it difficult for the school nurse to make an accurate assessment of the student's needs and to provide information regarding appropriate interventions. This barrier may be a two sided issue; for example, foreign born students often are not yet fluent in English and conversely, the school nurse may not speak or understand the student's native language. Also, many minority students have communication patterns and dialects that are dissimiliar to those of the school nurse. These communication issues may result in feelings of anger, alienation, helplessness, or frustration which can lead to non-compliance, withdrawal, hostility, lack of patience and other negative reactions on the part of both the student and the school nurse (Giger & Davidhizar, 1995). In order to provide culturally sensitive care to school children, the school nurse must be willing to develop a sensitivity and understanding of various communication styles, accents and dialects. This could be accomplished through continuing education courses or seminars sponsored by the School Nurse Association.

FUTURE OF SCHOOL NURSING

In the beginning of the 20th century when Lina Rogers provided nursing care to inner-city school children the importance of this care was measured by the single outcome of decreased absenteeism. The hospital based training in the early 1900s was adequate at that time, however, the role of the school nurse has expanded over the years requiring a broader education. Today, the school nurse has a wide range of activities in health services, health education and in providing a safe school environment for all students which results in multiple measurable outcomes in regard to the health of school children.

The increasing complexity of social and health related problems, such as poverty, drugs, HIV infection, violence, single parent homes, homelessness and chronic health conditions is broadening the negative effect on the well being of school children. Therefore, the role of the school nurse in the 21st century will require educational standards to prepare the nurse with knowledge and skills necessary to effectively meet these increasingly complex challenges.

It is expected that early in the 21st century the dilemma of the educational requirement for an entry level position as a school nurse will be resolved. National standards for educational preparation will likely include the baccalaureate degree with some positions in school health requiring the skills of a master's prepared advanced practice nurse.

A new model for health care which is emerging in the United States includes a focus on wellness and disease prevention and community-based care with services provided in the home, work site and schools. This is an area where school nurses could be a major force in implementing this model. The majority of children are healthy and by focusing on ways to promote and maintain health during their formative years, one may expect to see improved health in their early and middle adult years when compared to past generations.

In the 21st century the percentage of the population representing diverse populations will increase. The impact of this increase will be to facilitate the acceptance of cultural differences. Also, school nurses will graduate from baccalaureate programs where they have received appropriate education in the care of multicultural clients in all settings. In addition, school nurse certification programs will focus on the biopsychosocial needs of diverse school age children. Therefore, the school nurses will be adequately prepared to meet the challenges of the next century in the same confident manner as did Lina Rogers all those years ago.

REFERENCES

American Association of Colleges of Nurses. (1986). *Essentials of college and university education for professional nursing.* Washington, DC: Author.

Anderson, E. T., & McFarlane, J. M. (1996). *Community as partner: Theory and practice in nursing.* Philadelphia: Lippincott.

Campbell, J., & Landenberger, K. (1996). Violence and human abuse. In M. Stanhope & J. Lancaster (Eds.), *Community health nursing,* (4th ed. pp. 731–753). St. Louis: Mosby.

Cherry, B., & Giger, J. M. (1995). African Americans. In J. M. Giger and R. E. Davidhizar (Eds.). *Transcultural nursing,* (pp. 165–203). St. Louis: Mosby.

Giger, J. M., & Davidhizar, R. E. (1995). Biological variations. In J. M. Giger & R. E. Davidhizar (Eds.), *Transcultural nursing*, (pp. 127–161). Mosby: St. Louis.

Hosang, M. R. (1996). Community Health nursing in a multi-cultural society. In J. M. Cookfair (Ed.), *Nursing care in the community*, (pp. 39–64). St. Louis: Mosby.

Igoe, J. B., & Speer, S. (1997). Community health nurse in the schools. In M. Stanhope & J. Lancaster (Eds.), *Community health nursing*, (4th ed. pp. 879–906). St. Louis: Mosby.

Kub, J., & Steel, S. (1995). School health. In C. Smith & F. Maurer (Eds.), *Community health nursing*, (pp. 747–771). W. B. Saunders: Philadelphia.

Lancaster, J., Lowry, L., & Martin, K. (1996). Organizing frameworks applied to community nursing. In Stanhope, M. and Lancaster, J. (Eds.). *Community health nursing*, (pp. 179–205). St. Louis: Mosby.

Leininger, M. (1978). *Transcultural nursing concepts, theories, and practices*. New York: Wiley.

Leininger, M. (1991). Becoming aware of types of health practitioners and cultural imposition. *Journal of Transcultural Nursing, 2*(2), 32–39.

National League For Nursing. (1996). *Criteria and guidelines for the evaluation of baccalaureate and higher degree programs in nursing*. New York: Author.

Orlandi, M. A. (Ed.). (1992). *Cultural competence for evaluators*. Washington, DC: U.S. Department of Health and Human Services.

Overfield, R. T. (1985). *Biological variations in health and illness: Race, age and sex differences*. Reading, MA: Addison-Wesley.

Overfield, R. T. (1981). Biological variation: Concept from physical anthropology. In G. Henderson & M. Primeaux (Eds.) *Transcultural health care*, (pp. 279–286). Menlo, CA: Addison-Wesley.

Proctor, S. (1990). *Guidelines for a model school nursing program*. Scarborough, ME: National Association of School Nursing.

Prothrow-Stith, D., & Weissman, M. (1991). *Deadly consequences*. New York: HarperCollins.

Rea, M. (1996). School health nursing. In J. M. Cookfair (Ed.), *Nursing care of the community*, (pp. 747–771). St. Louis: Mosby.

Roach, L. B. (1981). Color changes in the skin. In G. Henderson & M. Primeaux (Eds.), *Transcultural health care*, (pp. 287–292). Menlo Park, CA: Addison-Wesley.

Strasser, J., Maurer, F. A., & Kavanaugh, K. H. (1995). The relevance of culture and values for community health nurses. In C. M. Smith & F. A. Maurer (Eds.), *Community health nursing theory and practice*, (pp. 139–167). Philadelphia: W. B. Saunders.

U.S. Bureau of Census. (1993). *Population profiles of the United States 1993*. (CPR series p-23, no. 185). Washington, DC: U.S. Government Printing Office.

U.S. Department of Health and Human Services. (1994). *The registered nurse population: 1992*. Washington, DC: U.S. Government Printing Office.

Woodfill, M., & Beyrer, M. (1991). *The role of the nurse in the school setting: An historical view as reflected in the literature*. Kent, Ohio: American School Health Association.

Zurek, E. L. (1997). Cultural considerations. In R. Hunt & E. L. Zurek (Eds.), *Introduction to community based nursing*, (pp. 79–118). Philadelphia: Lippincott.

Zurek, E. L., & Hunt, R. (1997). Practice settings and specialties. In R. Hunt & E. L. Zurek (Eds.), *Introduction to community based nursing*, (pp. 30–56). Philadelphia: Lippincott.

3

Culturally Sensitive Mobile Health Services for At-Risk Populations

*Gloria J. McNeal, Ann Doherty,
Donna Gentile O'Donnell, and Barbara Mallory*

W*ith the inception of* the Health Care Reform movement and the progressively spiralling costs of health care delivery, affordability and access have recently become hotly debated topics at all levels of government. The current health care dollar overwhelmingly commands almost 15 percent of the gross national product, an emergent situation that has forced acute care institutions to diligently search for more cost effective, alternative modes of care delivery, or face closure. Compounding the problem of affordability, the recent move from a retrospective to a prospective reimbursement payment system has significantly added to the growing numbers of under- and uninsured Americans. Unfortunately, the populations most severely affected tend to be those minority groups that currently reside in the nation's hardcore urban and suburban communities. With the continuing increase in hospital mergers and consolidation of health care conglomerates, efforts to serve the poor and the needy are becoming ever increasing challenges.

Recognizing the trend toward delivery of community-based care (Aldana, Jacobson, Harris, & Kelley, 1993; Cunnane, Wyman, Rotermund, & Murray, 1995; McGee, Morgan, McNamee, Bartek, 1995; McGovern, 1996; Paine, 1994; Paris & Porter-O'Grady, 1994; Wilson, Crupi, Greene,

Gaulin-Jones, Dehoux, and Korol, 1995), multi-facility health science centers have refocused their mission statements to include a need to consider the health care concerns of their adjoining neighborhoods. To address those issues surrounding access and affordability, medical science centers have taken the lead in the development of innovative community-based initiatives designed to decrease length of stay, reduce utilization of the more costly tertiary care facilities, and meet the health care needs of indigent populations.

One such community-based program was conceptualized over one year ago through a collaborative venture that joined The City of Philadelphia, SmithKline Beecham and the Mercy Health System in the development and implementation of the MercyCARE Mobile Health Program. A one-million dollar corporate grant provided the initial funding that operation-alized the construction and staffing of a small fleet of mobile vehicles, designed to bring comprehensive health care directly to the neighbor-hoods of the medically underserved. Grounded in the theoretical con-structs supporting public health nursing and sociolinguistic theory, the MercyCARE Mobile Health Program applies concepts related to those principals governing use of epidemiological approaches and communica-tion models in the implementation of its mission. Servicing an array of needs for multicultural populations, MercyCARE strives to provide culturally and linguistically sensitive approaches to care delivery.

The purposes of this chapter are to:

1. Identify those factors that currently limit access to care delivery;

2. Present the theoretical frameworks supporting the design of the MercyCARE Mobile Health Program;

3. Identify the components of the MercyCARE Culturological Assessment Guide, which was designed to serve as an aid in the gathering of culture-specific information; and,

4. Describe MercyCARE's approach to community-based care de-livery for culturally diverse populations.

BARRIERS TO ACCESS

It has been well documented (Department of Health and Human Services, 1990; McNeal, 1996) that individuals living in the nation's blighted urban and suburban areas experience significant barriers to health care delivery. As a result of these barriers, cohorts of such at-risk populations tend to postpone health care until advanced stages of disease progression have been reached (Spector, 1991), and tend to inappropriately utilize the emergency departments of tertiary care facilities for conditions that are not urgent in nature. Such practices are directly related to the increasing costs of health care. Despite an existing network of community-based health centers, federally-funded health agencies, and hospital-based clinics, the need is not being met. Underutilization of existing health services has been attributed to some of the following barriers to access:

1. Transportation Barriers—When location of clinic sites exceeds a two-mile radius from the client's home, transportation becomes particularly problematic, especially for those with ambulatory difficulties secondary to aging or physical disability. Additionally, for those living at or below the poverty level, costs for public transportation are prohibitive (Department of Health and Human Services, 1990).

2. Cultural Barriers—The health seeking behaviors of diverse populations are often different from those of the dominant society, and are more likely to be guided by folkways and customs. As well, cultural perceptions regarding western health care practices may be negative in orientation, especially for those whose health beliefs are grounded in magicoreligious or holistic theories of illness causation (Spector, 1991).

3. Financial Barriers—With the move from retrospective to prospective payment plans and capitated payor fee schedules, there is little incentive for health care providers to offer services for low-income minorities. Under our current system, under- and uninsured populations lack third-party reimbursement mechanisms. Given that a major shift to disease prevention has yet to occur within the present disease-oriented health care delivery focus, national health promotion initiatives have not attained priority status. Out-of-pocket costs for preventative health maintenance in this country remain the largest in the world (Department of Health and Human Services, 1990).

4. Language Barriers—English is a second language for 14 percent of the nation's diverse populations. Non-English speaking cli-

ents are often unable to understand either the spoken or written English word. Adding to the challenging array of linguistic diversity found throughout the nation is the recent increase in some of the fastest growing languages: Tagalog, Mon-Khmer, Vietnamese, French, Spanish, Creole, Hindi and Gujarathi (Epstein, 1994).

MercyCARE Mobile Program Mission

As the rapidly changing demographics of the American society produce a more culturally diverse population, a resounding clarion call for a more global health care perspective has been directed toward the nation's health professionals. Given the holistic, spiritual, and psychosocial orientation of the discipline of nursing, nursing health professionals must stand ready to be positioned at the forefront of a reformed health care delivery system, designed to implement culturally congruent care (American Academy of Nursing, 1992; Leininger, 1994). Consistent with that philosophical orientation is the mission of the MercyCARE Mobile Health Program, a health care ministry of the Sisters of Mercy. The Program strives to provide mobile health services that enhance access to health care delivery and that ensure a continuum of care for persons in need. MercyCARE focuses on primary and secondary health promotion and disease prevention, state-of-the art health screenings, and access to tertiary care. The primary goal of the initiative is to link resources and caregivers with residents of the culturally diverse communities served by the program.

THEORETICAL FRAMEWORKS

Public Health Nursing Theory

The operational design of this comprehensive mobile health program is based on the Conceptual Model of Public Health Nursing's Preferred Future (Clarke, Beddome, & Whyte, 1993). Themes central to this model include:

Multidisciplinary collaboration as a process for more integrated community systems. The infrastructure that drives the daily operations of the Mercy-

CARE Team consists of health care professionals representing nursing, radiology, religion, social work, and educational psychology. Information systems, medicine, mental health, pharmacy, and nutrition provide consulting services for the team's operations. The foundational support for the MercyCARE Team is composed of the three entities that formed the collaborative venture: City of Philadelphia, SmithKline Beecham and Mercy Health Corporation. The City of Philadelphia facilitates programmatic linkages with the Department of Public Health, Streets Department, Department of Recreation, Philadelphia Police Department, and the Partners for Progress Initiative. SmithKline Beecham serves as a corporate funder for the program. The Mercy Health System is a multi-facility health care entity that provides acute/tertiary care facilities, home health services, health professional consultancies, and spiritual direction.

Principal of empowerment in a client-driven system.   Recognized community leaders interface with MercyCARE Team Outreach coordinators to facilitate the establishment of linkages between the team and the various communities served. It is well understood that to ensure the success of the program, community receptivity and support are vital components. Through educational programs and outreach initiatives in the form of community volunteerism, clients are assisted to achieve self sufficiency in the establishment of appropriate health care practices. Educational materials are translated into the language of the community served, and, when possible, translators are available on site to facilitate communication.

Utilization of socio-ecological approaches that concentrate on the health needs of clients within the context of their home/community environment.   Three mobile health units travel throughout the city and its surrounding counties targeting low-income minority populations in medically-underserved neighborhoods. The units set up on site to deliver comprehensive health care services at the client's place of work, home, or community center. Telecommunication capabilities enable the team to transmit and receive data from remote access sites, and to electronically interface with health care providers as the need arises.

Population focused perspective of public health nursing practice.   Newer conceptual models of public health nursing practice identify health of the public initiatives as functions of collaborative health promotion efforts that focus on specific client populations (Rothman, 1990). With this concept in mind MercyCARE has targeted the homeless, underserved pediatric and adult clients, the elderly, HIV clients, and those in need of obstetric and gynecologic services, as specific client populations in need of care.

Sociolinguistic Theory

Given that the cultural context within which the client is situated is of fundamental importance in the delivery of culturally congruent care, sociolinguistic theory was used to serve as the organizing theoretical framework supporting use of the MercyCARE Culturological Assessment Guide. The guide was devised to gather information regarding the client's sociocultural relationships and to incorporate those findings into the plan of care.

The theory of sociolinguistics is derived from a variety of disciplines: linguistics, anthropology, sociology, psychology and education. The theoretical construct of sociolinguistics is primarily concerned with the manner by which language, and other communicative strategies and techniques, maintain and govern the underlying meanings associated with social rules and behavior found within and among cultural groups. The act of communication is influenced by such factors as age, sex, education, occupation, race, ethnic identity, customs, beliefs and practices (Gumperz & Hymes, 1986; Shulz, Florio, & Erickson, 1982). These influencing sociocultural factors were selected to form the categories supporting the process of inquiry used to elicit relevant client information included under each heading of the MercyCARE Culturological Assessment Guide (see Table 3.1). Given the magnitude of diversity in the typical community-based setting, it is suggested that in using the guide a flexible approach be assumed by the interviewer, to maximize the rendering of culturally sensitive care.

Culturally competent care delivery begins with the first component of the assessment phase of the nursing process, the client history. In the community-based setting, the health professional and client, or significant other, begin this phase with the interview, a planned dialogue in which very personal and intimate findings are shared. The interviewing process sets the stage for the gathering of culture-specific data in the establishment of the culturological assessment, and must be conducted in a setting which allows for unbiased and open social encounter.

Table 3.1
The MercyCARE Culturological Assessment Guide

Ethnicity and Ancestral Heritage

• How does the client identify his racial affiliation? _____
• To what ethnic group does the client assign his membership? _____

Birthplace and Place of Residence

• In which country was the client born? _____
• In which country has the client resided? _____ Years _____

Communicative Competence

• Is there a written form of the client's language? Y _____ N _____
• What is the client's native language? _____
• Are health-related materials available in the client's native language?
  Y _____ N _____
  if yes, specify _____
• What is the client's English fluency level?
  Mild _____ Moderate _____ Extreme difficulty _____
  No difficulty with use of English _____
• Does the client require an interpreter? Y _____ N _____
  if yes, specify _____
• List any nonverbal cues by the provider that facilitate or hinder
  communication _____
• List any nonverbal cues by the client that facilitate or hinder
  communication _____

Food Sanctions/Restrictions

• Are religious beliefs and practices influencing factors in the client's daily
  diet? Y _____ N _____
  if yes, specify _____
• Does the client's religion mandate fasting during certain times? Y _____
  N _____
  if yes, specify _____
• May certain foods be consumed during the fasting period? Y _____ N _____
  if yes, specify _____
• Can the client identify any food sanctions or restrictions? Y _____ N _____
  if yes, specify _____

Table 3.1 (*continued*)

- Are foods specially prepared? Y _____ N _____
  if yes, specify _____
- Are any cultural meanings associated with the act of eating? Y _____ N _____
  if yes, specify _____

Religious and Spiritual Beliefs and Practices

- What is the client's religious affiliation?
- What are the client's perceptions regarding death and dying and the grieving process?
- What is the role of the client's religious representative?
- Do the client's religious practices include inhalation/ingestion of substances used for sensory enhancement? Y _____ N _____
  if yes, specify _____

Health Beliefs and Folk Practices

- What is the role of the client's beliefs and practices during health and illness?

  _____

- List any folk medical/home remedies practiced by the client

  _____

- Does the client rely on lay/cultural healers? Y _____ N _____
  if yes, specify _____

Socioeconomic Considerations

- List the client's health insurance coverage
- Is the client employed? Y _____ N _____
  if yes, specify _____
- What are the client's sources of financial support?

  _____

- What is the client's socioeconomic level?
  Upper _____ Middle _____ Lower _____ Below Poverty Level _____
- Is there a need to consult social services? Y _____ N _____
  if yes, specify _____

Family Structure/Role and Social Network

- What constitutes the client's family composition?
- Which members of the family serve as caregivers?

Table 3.1 (*continued*)

- Decision making in matters of health is the primary responsibility of the client _____ his family _____ his social support network _____
- What is the composition of the client's social support network?

Educational Consideration

- What is the client's highest level of schooling completed?
  1–6 years _____ 7–12 years _____ 13–16 years _____ 16+ years _____ None _____
- If applicable, list the country(ies) of residence in which school was attended

---

- Based on the client's learning needs, behavioral learning objectives should be written in which of the following domains?
  Psychomotor _____ Cognitive _____ Affective _____
- If the client has a learning deficit, indicate the type of deficiency and specify alternative approaches
  Cognitive _____ Perceptual _____ Sensory _____ Motor _____

Explanatory Model of Illness Causation

- From which perspective does the client view the cause of illness?
  Scientific _____ Holistic _____ Magicoreligious _____ Combination _____

CULTUROLOGICAL ASSESSMENT GUIDE

The MercyCARE Culturological Assessment Guide addresses the health care customs, beliefs, and practices specific to the sociocultural orientation of the client-family-community triad. The primary aim of this assessment is to establish a baseline of value-free information in the delivery of culturally congruent nursing care. Such information provides the framework which grounds the bio-psychosocial-spiritual and cultural dimensions of nursing practice (Leininger, 1991; Villaire, 1994), and supports those holistic considerations germane to the establishment of culturally relevant nursing diagnoses and interventions (Geissler, 1991).

The guide (Table 3.1) utilizes an open-ended format as the mode of inquiry to facilitate use of broad opening statements during the interviewing process. To most who effectively utilize the tool, the following guidelines serve to provide the supporting rationale for the guide's format and inquiring statements designed to facilitate the social exchange in a multicultural environment.

Ethnicity and Ancestral Heritage

Many members of ethnically diverse populations residing in the United States prefer to maintain strong linkages with their cultural heritage. By having the client identify his racial and ethnic group affiliations, the interviewer gains a better understanding of the degree to which the client chooses to maintain his cultural orientation. While once believed to be a valued goal of all foreign-born and indigenous ethnic groups residing in this country, the process of acculturation has not been successful in the establishment of a homogeneous mix of the dominant society. Indeed, the *melting pot* concept has failed, largely owing to the extent of variance found throughout the nation's cultural subpopulations and the recent increase in rates of immigration, especially among ethnic people of color (McNeal, Gonzalez, Petit de Mange, & Perez, 1996).

The variances associated with language, religion, country of origin, and health care practices found among the nation's four federally-defined minority people of color have been well documented (Department of Health and Human Services, 1990; Spector, 1991). Among the Native American and Alaskan Natives there are currently over 500 federally recognized tribes. Throughout each of these tribes are spoken languages and dialects that are not universally comprehended within and among the many tribal groups (Cook & Petit de Mange, 1995). Asian Americans and Pacific Islanders represent a host of subgroups with differing languages and dialects, as in Vietnamese, Chinese, Korean and Japanese; and, with societies of origin ranging from China to Japan to the Philippines and Southeast Asia. The Black American communities consist of groups emanating from Africa, South America, and the Caribbean Islands, with languages ranging from Swahili to French to Spanish to Dutch and English. Hispanic Americans are composed of Spanish-speaking subgroups, with countries of origin ranging from Spain to Mexico to Cuba to Puerto Rico and the Caribbean Islands (McNeal, et al., 1996).

When identifying ethnic and racial affililation, it is important to remember that ethnic group categories are as much sociopolitically appointed as self selected, and, as such, are devoid of the scientific rigor associated with anthropologic racial designations. Given the intent to render culturally sensitive care, assumptions regarding classification ought not to be made without the client's corroboration.

Birthplace and Place of Residence

The client's country of origin, duration and place of residence are important data to be obtained during the interview. Such information provides the interviewer with a richer appreciation for the client's level of cultural orientation, and degree of association with the dominant society's values and practices. More recently arriving ethnic groups and socially isolated cultural communities of more long-standing residence, may have a limited understanding of the nation's health care practices. Again, with the client's corroboration, information regarding birthplace and residence allows the interviewer to make a general assessment of the client's orientation and knowledge of western health care treatment methodologies, and potential willingness to accept same.

Communicative Competence

Communicative competence refers to the kinds of communication skills that members of cultural groups need in order to interface in ways that are socially acceptable, and that employ effective strategies in the processing of social exchange. The term consists of three components: 1) knowledge of the assumptions supporting socially correct behavior, 2) possession of verbal and nonverbal performance skills, and 3) possession of those interpretive skills which facilitate the comprehension of underlying meaning (Shulz, et al., 1982).

Knowledge. The first component of communicative competence, the extent to which different cultures have knowledge of the socially correct behaviors of the larger society, is indeed difficult to measure, and may be arrived at by indicating the duration of residence and degree of cultural identity documented under the guide's first two headings. The length of time one lives within and is exposed to the dominant society determines, to some degree, the extent to which the client may have developed knowledge of the social behaviors of the majority culture.

Skills. The second component of communicative competence, possession of verbal and nonverbal performance skills, concerns those aspects of communication that assist in the establishment of meaning ascribed to the spoken word via related body language and speech patterns, and to the written word via characters, punctuation, and accentuation. Some 32 million Americans speak languages other than English in the home, and in some five states (New York, California, Texas, New Mexico, and Arizona), the number of non-English speaking domiciles is at or greater than 20 percent (Epstein, 1994). Further, even in those instances in which English is the native tongue, the rhythm and intensity of the spoken language may be foreign to the interviewer (Villaire, 1994). Speech prosody, intonation, syntax, and lexicographic selection are all culture-specific linguistic styles of communication (Gumperz & Hymes, 1986), and may significantly differ from that used by the dominant society, making it incumbent upon the interviewer to become familiar with varying speech styles.

To further challenge effective communication, a written form of the language may not currently be in existence. Even if present in written form, the language may use an unfamiliar, non-alphanumeric code, consisting of characters with elaborate forms of punctuation and accentuation. Formatting for the written word may also pose challenges, as some languages are designed to be written and read horizontally, from right to left (Hebrew); others have a vertical orientation (Chinese); while, still others are presented in elegant styles of calligraphy (Sanskrit).

Knowledge of the client's written and spoken language will be helpful to the interviewer in determining the existence of health-related materials that may be available in the client's native tongue. When such materials are not available, the interviewer may need to seek the assistance of an interpreter. However, care will need to be taken in selecting an appropriate interpreter as age, gender, specific ethnic group affiliation, and knowledge of health care terminology will have to be factored in to the final selection. It may be culturally insensitive to choose interpreters who, while able to correctly speak the language, may be too young, a member of the opposite sex, of a different cultural subgroup, unfamiliar with medical terms and vocabulary (Haffner, 1992), or unwilling to share sensitive information (Villaire, 1994).

In those instances in which the client does speak English, the interviewer will need to assess the client's English fluency level. Levels of difficulty with use of the English language will have to be taken into consideration in planning care, and appropriate strategies developed that address problems associated with English speech and literacy. For example, the interviewer may need to develop pictorial guidelines and learning packets as teaching methodologies, for those who acquired English reading skills may not support reading levels at or above a primary school education. For those who may not speak English fluently, the interviewer may need to use simple sentence structures and to refrain from use of idiomatic, expressions, slang, and complex medical vernacular.

Interpretation.   The third component of communicative competence, possession of those interpretative skills which facilitate the comprehension of underlying meaning, underscores the importance of understanding the communicative relevance of nonverbal cues (Gumperz & Hymes, 1986; Erickson, 1982), i.e., those cues that may require the interviewer to use some level of interpretation, in order to arrive at the correct meaning associated with the social interchange. The discipline of sociolinguistics identifies the need to possess both interpretive skills, and knowledge of those culture-specific contextual cues that facilitate communication. There now are methodologies, developed within the last several decades, to augment the study of communication within and among culturally diverse populations: sociolinguistic analysis of sound-image recording or microethnography (Erickson, 1982); speech transcription; and gestural mapping, a method used to schematically depict body language associated with the spoken word. Such techniques assist the sociolinguistic theorist in the implementation of qualitative methodologies, used to derive the explanatory theories that define how communication is effected among and between groups (Gumperz & Hymes, 1986; Shulz, et al., 1982). Interpretive skills may need to be employed, for example, in those situations in which it may be culturally appropriate for the client to avoid direct eye gaze and to assume a deferential stance when addressing a health care provider, as in the case of some Asian American clients. The interviewer should be cautioned not to interpret such body language out of cultural context. From the perspectives of both the interviewer and the client, it is important to document those nonverbal communicative cues that may facilitate or hinder effective communication.

Food Sanctions and Restrictions

Food preference and avoidances are oftentimes inextricably bound to religious practices (Spector, 1991). In such instances, dietary observances will be dictated by the client's religious beliefs. Failure to honor such practices may render the client culturologically compromised. The interviewer must endeavor to ensure that dietary meals are mutually planned in observance of such religious teachings. Under this category, as well, the interviewer will need to document social meanings ascribed to the act of eating, to obtain the client's definition of food, and to ascertain methods of food preparation. A nutritionist may need to be consulted to assist in the planning of culturally sensitive therapeutic diets.

Religious and Spiritual Beliefs and Practices

Religious and spiritual practices vary across all cultural groups. The interviewer may need to identify the degree to which the culturally diverse client relies upon the use of religious and spiritual healing arts. The role of the religious leader may be a very important one, necessitating the need to have such persons present in the health care environment (Spector, 1991). Because religious practice is a basic right in this country, it is incumbent upon the interviewer to facilitate religious observances. When considering the client's religious affiliation, it is important to remember that both known and unknown religious doctrine must be honored; for, it is not within the purview of the interviewer to discount religious orientations that may be unfamiliar to the general populace. Additionally, it is important to recognize that some religions may sanction the use of mood altering substances to effect incorporeal transcendence. Again, the interviewer must remember that such practices are protected rights of the client.

Under this category the interviewer may appropriately explore the client's concepts related to death and dying and the grieving process. The client's expression of loss may have a cultural orientation that is vastly different from that expressed by the dominant society (Spector, 1991). In assisting the client to relate his feelings regarding these concepts, the interviewer will gain invaluable insight and understanding necessary for the rendering of culturally congruent care.

Health Beliefs and Folk Practices

Recent works of nurse authors (Leininger, 1994; Leininger, 1991; Spector, 1991) have been instrumental in assisting the profession to understand the importance that folk practices and health beliefs hold for members of culturally diverse groups. Western health care practices may be unfamiliar concepts for some culturally diverse populations that may heavily rely upon the practice of folk medicine. Clients may feel the need to employ traditional cultural healers and to use home remedies, to achieve a state of balance within the mind-body-spirit triad. Where such practice does not conflict with western health care methodologies, the interviewer should endeavor to support the client's beliefs. Where the two concepts may not be compatible, the interviewer must be comfortable with assisting the client to arrive at a decision consistent with the client's health beliefs.

Socioeconomic Considerations

Many factors contribute to the client's socioeconomic situation. The interviewer must consider the impact health care will have upon the client's lifestyle, occupation, living conditions, and emotional orientation. The sources of financial support, the type of health care insurance coverage, and the socioeconomic level of the client and his family are all determinants in the client's access to health care delivery options (Department of Health and Human Services, 1990).

Family Structure/Role and Social Network

As sperm banking, in vitro fertilization, surrogate mothering and adoption bring the possibility of parenting to childless couples of all sexual orientations, the traditional definition of family has been forced to undergo evolution. While these more recent methodologies currently drive the change in family composition for the dominant society, members of diverse populations have consisted of nontraditional family structures for decades. Such nontraditional familial associations have been found to be fluid in nature, multigenerational, or composed of multiple households (McGoldrick, Pearce, & Giordana, 1982), unmarried cohabitants (Skolnick & Skolnick, 1989), or single parents. Nontraditional family units demonstrate an array of possible orientations: matriarchal, patriarchal, monogamous, polygamous, or homosexual.

Under this category, particularly with regard to parenting and decision-making, the interviewer may note a marked variance from the traditional family structure. For some families, the parenting role may be assumed by grandparents, siblings, or gay and lesbian couples with biological or adopted offspring. In some cultures all family decisions are made by one person in authority, while in others, decisions regarding health care considerations are matters that must be deliberated by the whole family; and, in still others, all decisions are made by an entire subcultural community. In the latter cases, the client must abide by the decisions made by the family or community acting as a single entity. Indeed, Leininger (1991) challenges the use of nursing's metaparadigmatic framework (person-health-environment-nursing), especially for those cultures in which the concept of person is nonexistent; for the preservation of the family and community may well supercede all other concerns oriented toward the needs of the individual.

In those instances in which the family structure is nontraditional, the importance of the client's social network cannot be underestimated. The interviewer will need to have the client identify all significant others, including the health care role each is to assume during times of illness. In some cultures, health caring behaviors are performed by members of both the client's family and sociocultural network (Gonzalez, 1995).

Educational Considerations

The client's level of educational attainment is another important assessment. Knowledge of the client's educational background helps to guide the interviewer in the selection of appropriate teaching and learning methodologies. Here, it is important for the interviewer to assess the educational training acquired both in this country and abroad. It is culturally insensitive for the interviewer to assume a lack of educational attainment based on the client's inability to communicate in the English language. The interviewer should seek to ascertain both the level of formal schooling completed and the country in which the education was acquired. Such information can assist the interviewer in the provision of health care instruction that is oriented toward, and recognizes the level of sophistication that might be employed in the construction of learning materials. More and more, health care institutions are recognizing the need to use interpreters to translate written English materials to the language of choice, while, in the translation, sensitively maintaining appropriate reading levels.

The style of learning which best suits the needs of the client is another consideration to be addressed. The interviewer may need to creatively design instructional modalities that utilize objectives, leveled according to the needs of the learner and written within one or all of the following domains: psychomotor (hands-on presentation), cognitive (verbal presentation), and affective (attitudinal presentation).

The client's capacity to learn is another assessment that will be helpful to the interviewer in developing educational approaches. The client may demonstrate the presence of a learning deficit, either acquired secondary to a disease state or previously existing. Whatever the cause of the deficiency, the interviewer will need to assess both the type of deficit (cognitive, perceptual, sensory, or motor) and the extent to which the condition impacts upon the client's learning capacity. In some instances, occupational and physical therapy may need to be consulted for more indepth assessment and intervention.

Explanatory Model of Illness Causation

Diseases of the body may be viewed from three different perspectives, according to the client's cultural orientation: scientific, holistic and/or magicoreligious (Spector, 1991). Western medical practices are based on the scientific explanatory model of illness causation, which states that all conditions of health and illness have a measurable cause and effect. American nursing practice is based on principles supporting the scientific explanatory model. The other two perspectives, to date, have not been widely addressed in the nursing literature.

The holistic explanatory model posits the existence of a natural world order in which human beings are both composites of the mind-body-spirit triad (Dossey, Guzzetta, & Kenner, 1992), and an integral part of the overall cosmos. Health is maintained by keeping the triad in a state of balance with the universe. Many Asian subcultures refer to that balance as the Yin-Yang Theory; while, in many Hispanic subcultures that balance is referred to as the Hot-Cold Theory.

The magicoreligious perspective credits the supernatural forces of good and evil with the ability to maintain or disrupt the health status of the individual. Most organized religions believe in the presence of spiritual beings, who possess the power to bring about states of health. Some Black American subcultures may practice voodoo or faith healing, and may use root doctors and religious representatives to bring about a return to homeostasis. Some Native American tribes employ the medicine man, who uses, among other things, herbs and plants to combat illness states (Spector, 1991).

It is important for the interviewer to recognize that a combination of beliefs may be held by the client. As well, medical science has begun to incorporate some of the treatment methodologies of the two lesser known explanatory models. The following list of interventions identifies some of the more common holistic and magicoreligious therapies that are now an integral part of scientific nursing and medical practice: acupuncture, therapeutic touch, relaxation techniques, hypnosis, biofeedback, guided imagery, foxglove (digoxin), erythroxylon coca shrub (cocaine), and cannabis sativa (marijuana), to name a few. Indeed, contemporary pharmaceutical agents are derived from the roots and herbs that comprise the tools of the trade of medicine men, root doctors, and the early twentieth-century apothecarist.

The culturally competent nursing health professional is one who is able to obtain value-free culturological information, and who is prepared to utilize that information in the design of care delivery models that meet the needs of diverse populations. With cultural sensitivity and awareness as a primary focus of the MercyCARE Mobile Health Program, the last section of this chapter describes the multidisciplinary design of this innovative community-based program and its multicultural approach to care delivery.

Multicultural Approaches to Care Delivery

To better address the health care needs of the culturally diverse populations that visit MercyCARE, a Volunteer Program was developed. Translators, health care professionals, students, and retired persons have been recruited to assist the program to achieve its mission to provide culturally and linguistically sensitive approaches to health care delivery. Bilingual members of the Volunteer Program translate all client health related materials, and serve as translators in the clinical field as the need arises.

The interiors of the health vans contain attractively displayed educational materials and posters written in the languages of the clients served. Care is taken to select toys and games that demonstrate sensitivity. Several members of the MercyCARE Team are multilingual and its full complement represents many cultural backgrounds.

To ensure community receptivity, the Program Director regularly meets with community representatives of churches; schools; recreation, daycare and senior centers; homeless shelters, and public housing units. Through attendance at community meetings, members of the community can directly address questions and concerns to MercyCARE personnel, to effect the development of mutually determined solutions.

To provide a continuum of care, clients are encouraged to identify primary care providers. The MercyCARE Team facilitates the establishment of linkages with health professionals throughout the city. In those instances in which clients prefer to utilize the services of a mobile program, clients are referred to appropriate governmental entities for submission of all necessary forms to complete the process.

DESCRIPTION OF THE MercyCARE MOBILE HEALTH PROGRAM

The MercyCARE Mobile Health Program consists of two mobile health clinics and one mobile educational unit that travel around Philadelphia and surrounding counties bringing comprehensive health care directly to the communities. Each of the two mobile clinics contains an examination room, a mammography suite with darkroom, a waiting area, a bathroom, and a nurses' station. The clinics are staffed by a team of five: one master's prepared social worker, two family nurse practitioners, one mammography technologist, and one community outreach coordinator/driver. The educational unit, equipped to perform routine screenings and to conduct community-based educational programs, is staffed by a team of part-time registered nurses, drivers and volunteers.

Three days per week the mobile units travel to several neighborhoods and set up on site, in collaboration with community leaders, to provide: screenings for cholesterol, cancer, lead, diabetes, and hypertension; adult and pediatric immunization; physical examinations; mammography; electrocardiography; vision and hearing assessment; dental assessment and referral; HIV/STD testing and counseling; obstetric and gynecologic care and referral; substance abuse counseling and referral; nutrition assessment and teaching; social services; and, health education. The services are provided at no out-of-pocket expense to the client. The units are credentialled as primary care provider sites and seek to annually maintain 2,000 covered lives. To augment client revenues, additional funding is being sought through grant requests made to philanthropic and governmental agencies.

One stipulation of the credentialling process mandates that the larger units maintain permanent location at a fixed site 20 hours per week, a necessary requirement to facilitate visits by the capitated clientele. The Philadelphia fixed site is located on the grounds of a local public school, and serves as the school-based clinic for approximately 180 children, their families, and members of the surrounding communities. The suburban county fixed site for the second mobile unit is located in close proximity to two shelters for women and children, where the unit serves as the primary care provider for the residents of the shelters. The third smaller unit, designed to perform screenings and promote health maintenance through education, does not have a fixed location requirement.

Service Delivery

MercyCARE sees an average of thirty clients per day. At four-hour intervals and in collaboration with the City of Philadelphia Partners for Progress Initiative, the unit has been positioned throughout the city's most medically underserved neighborhoods. Clients have been screened, treated or referred for various acute and chronic conditions. Clients representing the following age groups have visited MercyCARE: pediatric, adolescent, young adult, middle-aged adult and geriatric. The program has delivered care to a representative sample of clients belonging to each of the four federally-defined minority populations: Native American and Alaskan Native, Asian American, Hispanic American, and Black American.

Clinical Practica

Four schools of nursing currently utilize the Mobile Program as a clinical site for senior level student nurses: Gwynedd Mercy College, West Chester, Neumann College, and Widener University. During the Fall 1996 semester, a total of 11 nursing students assisted the Mobile Team in the provision of health care services. Beginning with the Spring 1997 semester, master's level graduate students will be preceptored by the Mobile Program's FNPs, and the Team will be joined by nursing students and faculty at Eastern College, LaSalle University, and the University of Pennsylvania. Faculty have expressed their delight with this "invaluable clinical experience." In the future, the program will serve as a clinical rotation for medical residents.

Referral Mechanisms

Lead Poisoning. In those instances in which children are screened and found to have elevated lead levels, arrangements have been made with the City of Philadelphia Department of Public Health to follow up all reported cases.

Mammography.   All mammograms are currently being read by the Radiology Department of the Mercy Hospitals. Clients having any evidence of abnormality are contacted by letter and follow-up is provided by the Office of Radiology. For all necessary surgical/medical intervention, clients are admitted to the Mercy Health System.

Uninsureds.   All clients currently without health insurance and in need of follow-up care are given information regarding the state's various plans for insurance coverage. The Mercy Health Plan is one of the options provided by the Commonwealth offering a continuum of care.

Social Services.   Social service needs are addressed on a case-by-case basis. The program's MSW identifies the nature of problems encountered and initiates a plan of action with evaluation.

Family Planning.   In accordance with the religious teachings of the Sisters of Mercy, family planning services are not provided by the MercyCARE Program. All clients in need of counseling for family planning are referred to one of three organizations, as appropriate, to provide this service: Healthy Cities, Planned Parenthood or the Philadelphia Department of Public Health District Centers.

Reimbursement

Grants.   In the next quarter, philanthropic grant funding organizations will be identified and grant applications submitted to offset operating expenses. The Linda Creed Foundation has agreed to reimburse all mammograms meeting criteria at $50.00 each. The Mercy Health System and SmithKline Beecham have agreed to establish a five-year financial commitment to the program.

American Cancer Society.   The Program Director has met with representatives of the American Cancer Society for both the counties of Philadelphia and Montgomery. Discussions were initiated regarding use of the mobile units as subcontracted entities for large scale cancer screening programs. MercyCARE staff will work in collaboration with the American Cancer Society to provide breast, cervical and prostatic cancer screening.

Capitation. The credentialling process has been executed to appoint the Family Nurse Practitioners (FNPs) to the Medical Staff of the Mercy Health System. Upon certification, each FNP will be granted full medical privileges and afforded the opportunity to work collaboratively with private primary care physician practices. Current state reimbursement mechanisms require that clients capitate to a primary health care provider. With credentialled FNPs aboard the mobile health vehicles, plans are to have MercyCARE certified as primary health care provider sites, either as extensions of Mercy Health System ambulatory care clinics or of Mercy Health System private physician practices.

Fee for Service. In addition to capitated per member per month (PMPM) rates, the program will be able to bill for certain fee-for-service options: mammography, Early Periodic Screening Detection and Treatment (EPSDT) and vaccine administration. Revenue estimates have been calculated for 2,000 covered lives, and other billable services.

Telecommunication Technologies

Consistent with the national trend to computerize the patient care record (Hagland, 1966; Snow, 1996), the MercyCARE Program electronically links data from the mobile units with clinical laboratories, tertiary facilities, and physician offices. Multiple laptop computers aboard the vehicles, conveniently located in treatment rooms at the nurses' station, permit data entry, and remote transmission and retrieval of all clinical information. The program utilizes Dr. Chart, a totally computerized patient care record system, to manage all information systems. Dr. Chart supports the remote transmission of patient information, trending prognostications, and hard copy documentation. Electrocardiographic data are obtained on board the vehicles and transmitted to the physician's office for analysis. Cellular mobile telephone lines afford clinicians opportunity to talk directly with consulting health professionals as the need arises. Beepers keep all members of the team in close communication. In the planning stages are telecommunication capabilities for transtelephonic monitoring, pacemaker surveillance, and interactive video transmission.

MercyCARE Team Members' Roles and Responsibilities

Team Composition. The MercyCARE Mobile Team consists of fourteen culturally diverse health professionals: three doctorally prepared advanced practice nurses, one of whom is a family nurse practitioner and two of whom are certified nurse midwives; a master's prepared social worker; a master's prepared educational psychologist; three additional family nurse practitioners; two mammography technologists; an information systems specialist; and, a community health educator. A deputy commissioner and an administrative liaison from the Department of Public Health each devote 20 percent of their time with MercyCARE. The team represents a variety of religious orientations, age groups, and ethnic backgrounds. While women comprise the majority of the team, two members are men.

Director.   The Program Director provides the coordination and direction of MercyCARE in all phases of program development, implementation and maintenance; monitors quality assurance mechanisms; implements standards of care; facilitates the development of a viable network in the provision of a continuum of care; secures funding through external sources; and meets regularly with an advisory team consisting of members representing the diverse communities served.

The Program Director designs and maintains the suprastructure of the MercyCARE Program, establishes collaborative initiatives with the subsidiaries of the Mercy Health System, and with governmental and private agencies, and promotes linkages with academic institutions.

Coordinator.   The Program Coordinator works collaboratively with the Director to provide the direction of the program, networks with regional health providers, and identifies and pursues financial support to expand services.

The Program Coordinator maintains the infrastructure of the program and handles the daily operations. She meets on an ongoing basis with the maintenance crew, dialogues directly with the van manufacturers to ensure daily operations of the units, and works with the staff and nursing students in making community assessments and identifying community needs.

Nurse Practitioners.   The Family Nurse Practitioners (FNPs) are responsible for providing care to both well and ill clients, educating clients and their families with regard to health promotion and disease prevention, and maintaining professional growth through attendance at continuing education and staff development programs.

The FNPs meet regularly with the medical staff to discuss client interventions and related protocol and procedures. Working as a subgroup of the team, the FNPs have established guidelines for standards of practice and related policies.

Mammography Technologists.   The Mammography Technologists perform diagnostic and screening mammography procedures as directed by the physician, to ensure the highest quality of care in an economically sound and efficient manner. They work closely with the radiologist and staff in the processing and evaluation of mammograms. One of the technologists serves as the Volunteer Coordinator for the Team.

Outreach Counselor/Driver.   The Community Outreach Counselor/ Driver maintains a positive relationship between MercyCARE and the communities served; facilitates community linkages with community leaders; appropriately conducts counseling sessions to meet the needs of those suffering from substance abuse, HIV infection, and psychosocial illnesses; and, demonstrates ability to maintain vehicular safety in the driving of the mobile units.

Social Worker/Driver.   The Social Worker is the health professional who identifies high-risk clients; coordinates comprehensive planning; addresses the medical, social and environmental factors which affect the client; and, through counseling intervention, provides comprehensive health care follow-up. Additionally, she demonstrates ability to maintain vehicular safety in the driving of the mobile units.

The Social Worker meets with clients in the field to address social service needs on a case-by-case basis, and establishes a network of resources for related social service needs and follow-up.

Information Systems Specialist/Driver.   The Information Specialist assists in the development and implementation of the medical and nursing information systems; provides training for all team members; ensures proficient use of all telecommunication and computer systems; works collaboratively with systems analyst consultants and outside vendors in the establishment and efficient operation of the computerized patient care record; and demonstrates ability to maintain vehicular safety in the driving of the mobile units.

Community Health Educator.   The Community Health Educator oversees a team of registered nurses, drivers and volunteers in the development and implementation of health screenings and educational programs; maintains all appropriate accreditation standards and records; schedules all educational programs; and procures all related supplies and equipment.

Deputy Health Commissioner.   The Philadelphia Department of Health Deputy Commissioner for Policy and Planning serves as the consultant to MercyCARE in all matters related to public health initiatives, assists in the establishment of policy and procedure in the delivery of care, and coordinates linkages between MercyCARE and various city departments.

Administrative Liaison.   The Administrative Liaison works out of the office of the Deputy Commissioner for Policy and Planning to assist in the development of positive relationships with communities served by MercyCARE, works with regional health care provideres and the City to ensure development of a viable network for the provision of a continuum of care, and assists with data collection and report writing for grant funding initiatives.

Conclusion

With the current move to offer more community-based health care services, especially to meet the needs of culturally diverse populations, it has become a national imperative to provide innovative programs that address health care issues while maintaining cultural sensitivity. In order to obtain culture-specific client information, the health care professional must recognize the need to establish a supportive social environment that promotes the exchange of diverse values and beliefs. This chapter has described one community-based program that grounds its philosophical orientation in theoretical constructs that support the implementation of culturally sensitive health care delivery.

REFERENCES

Aldana, S. G., Jacobson, B. H., Harris, C. J., & Kelley, P. L. (1993). Mobile work site work health promotion programs can reduce selected employee health risks. *Journal of Occupational Medicine, 35*(9), 922–928.

American Academy of Nursing. (1992). Expert panel report: culturally competent health care. *Nursing Outlook, 40*(5), 277–283.

Clarke, H., Beddome, G. & Whyte, N. (1993). Public health nurses' vision of their future reflects changing paradigms. *Image: Journal of Nursing Scholarship, 25*(4), 305–310.

Cook, L., & Petit de Mange, B. (1995). Gaining access to Native American cultures by non-Native American nursing researchers. *Nursing Forum*, 30(1), 5–10.

Cunnane, E., Wyman, W., Rotermund, A. & Murray, R. (1995). Brief report: innovative programming in a community service center. *Community Mental Health Journal*, 31(2), 153–161.

Department of Health and Human Services (1990). *Health status of minority and low-income groups*, 3rd Edition. Washington, DC: US Government Printing Office.

Dossey, B., Guzzetta, C., & Kenner, C. (1992). *Critical care nursing: Body-mind-spirit*. Philadelphia: J. B. Lippincott Company.

Epstein, A. (1994, June 5). "English only" can be fighting words. *The Philadelphia Inquirer*, p. C4.

Erickson, F. (1982). Audiovisual records as a primary data source. In A. Grimshar (Ed.). *Sociological methods and research*, (special issue on sound-image records in social interaction research), 11(2), 213–232.

Geissler, E. M. (1991). Transcultural nursing and nursing diagnoses. *Nursing & Health Care*, 12(4), 190–92; 203.

Gonzalez, E. W. (1995). Mental health of culturally diverse clients. *Journal of Cultural Diversity*, 2(2), 39.

Gumperz, J. J., & Hymes, D. (1986). *Directions in sociolinguistics: The ethnography of communication*. New York: Basil Blackwell, Inc.

Haffner, L. (1992). Translation is not enough: Interpreting in a medical setting. *The Western Journal of Medicine*, 157(3), 255–259.

Hagland, M. (1996, November). Making patient records meaningful to patients. *Health Management Technology*, 16–20.

Leininger, M. M. (1991). *Culture care diversity and universality: A theory of nursing*. New York: National League for Nursing Press.

Leininger, M. M. (1994). Transcultural nursing education: A worldwide impera-tive. *Nursing & Health Care*, 15(5), 254–257.

McGee, D., Morgan, M., McNamee, M. J., & Bartek, J. K. (1995). Use of a mobile health van by a vulnerable population: homeless sheltered women. *Health Care for Women International*, 16, 451–461.

McGoldrick, M., Pearce, J., & Giordano, J. (1982). *Ethnicity and family therapy*. New York: Guilford Press.

McGovern, B. (1996). Taking stock of community-based care. *Case Review*, 90–92.

McNeal, G. J. (1996). Mobile health care for those at risk. *N&HC: Perspectives on Community*, 17(3), 134–140.

McNeal, G. J., Gonzalez, E. W., Petit de Mange, E., & Perez, I. (1996). Multicul-turally diverse clients. In J. Rothrock (Ed.). *Perioperative nursing care planning*, 2nd Edition. St. Louis: CV Mosby Company.

Paine, B. (1994). A kids "care van". *Health Progress*, 54–55.

Paris, N., & Porter-O'Grady, T. (1994). Health on wheels. *Health Progress*, 34–41.

Rothman, N. (1990). Toward description: Public health nursing and community health nursing are different. *Nursing and Health Care*, *11*(9), 481–483.

Shulz, J. J., Florio, S. & Erickson, F. (1982). Where's the floor? Aspects of the cultural organization of social relationships in communication at home and in school. In P. Gilmore & A. Glatthorn (Eds.), *Children in and out of school*. (Language and Ethnography Series #2). Washington, DC: Center for Applied Linguistics.

Skolnick, A. S., & Skolnick, J. H. (1989). Family in transition. Glenview: Scott Foresman Company.

Snow, C. (1996, August 5). Mobile telemedicine clinic eases care in Oklahoma. *Modern Healthcare*, 100–102.

Spector, R. (1991). *Cultural diversity in health and illness*. Norwalk, CT: Appleton and Lange.

Villaire, M. (June, 1994). Interview: Toni Tripp-Reimer: Crossing over the boundaries. *Critical Care Nurse*, *14*(3), 134–141.

Wilson, K. G., Crupi, C. D., Greene, G., Gaulin-Jones, B., Dehoux, E., & Korol, C. T. (1995). Consumer satisfaction with a rehabilitation mobile outreach program. *Archives of Physical Medicine and Rehabilitation*, *76*, 899–904.

Part III

Education, Inquiry and Inclusion

Some observers of the rapidly changing demography of the United States have labeled it the first universal nation, a truly multicultural society marked by unparalleled diversity.[1] It is expected that the face of this nation will change markedly as the *browning* of America becomes more apparent.[2] Now one in four Americans claims African, Asian, Hispanic, or Native American ancestry with striking growth in the non-white population expected in the next century. It is predicted that by the year 2000, 50 percent of the population or more than 135 million people will be people of color.

Accompanying these profound population shifts is the need for using language and labels with greater clarity. All too often, *culture, race* and *ethnicity* are used interchangeably. On too many occasions as well, are those who assign *culture* to those not like themselves, most often using the term when referring to members of minority groups.

As the number of people of color increases a better understanding of *culture, race* and *ethnicity* is required. Dr. Outlaw calls for a commitment to the provision of competent care to diverse groups of people as a priority for the profession in the 21st century. To move this agenda forward she challenges nurse scholars to develop the concepts that drive the theories which will assure the competent care required as culture, race and ethnicity are better understood and the interrelationship clarified.

Despite the rising number of racially and ethnically diverse members of society, no concomitant increase in the number of registered nurses is evident. The Department of Health and Human Services in its national sample survey of registered nurses of March 1992 revealed no significant increase in the number of racial and ethnic minority nurses when compared with the surveys of 1984 and 1988. Out of an estimated 2.2 million nurses, about 9 percent of the registered nurse population, or 203,835 RNs were racial/ethnic minorities.[3]

---

[1] Barringer, F. (March 11, 1991). Census shows profound changes in social makeup of the nation. *The New York Times*, p. A1.

[2] Beyond the melting pot. (April 9, 1990). *Time*, p. 29.

[3] United States Department of Health and Human Services. Public Health Service. (1992). The registered nurse population. Washington, DC: U.S. Government Printing Office.

The School of Nursing at Temple University has responded to a major challenge of the times with a model of inclusion for underrepresented minority groups and economically disadvantaged students in a city whose population mirrors the new look of this nation. Ms. Patrinos describes some successful initiatives through the Nursing Career Opportunity Program (NCOP) which are useful to replicate in other settings as the number of students who succeed in nursing programs increases.

Diversity also characterizes the higher education system. At a time in our national life when there is general agreement that education is at the heart of the economic agenda, increasing access to higher education resonates well with the American people. Peter Hart, the pollster, states that concerns about education are at the top of the national agenda in a way the pollsters have not seen in over a generation.

Dr. Mengel and Ms. Sherman have clearly addressed the role of associate degree nursing within community colleges. The diversity of age, gender, race, academic ability and socioeconomic status, a hallmark of community college students, can serve us well as increased opportunities are afforded this nation's diverse population. Grounded in the community, which continues to take on a more dominant role in our lives, community college graduates can contribute a great deal to our understanding of communities, their needs and how best to meet them.

4

A Call for Scholarly Inquiry on Human Diversity

Freida Outlaw

The beginning of a new century will require that the nursing profession embrace and foster a scholarly interest in human diversity. Although many nurses have been engaged for at least three decades in the study and practice of culturally sensitive care, the concepts used to discuss human diversity are defined in the nursing literature in a variety of ways. The lack of mutually agreed upon definitions of the terms used to describe diversity is validation that the scholarly work clarifying these concepts has to be enhanced. For example, common explanatory terms such as *race, culture,* and *ethnicity* are often used interchangeably by nurses (Habayeb, 1995; Outlaw, 1994) exemplifying that nurses have not become *self-conscious* (Avant, 1993, 52) about how these words are being used and what they are intended to describe. Lack of clarity about the nomenclature used to describe phenomena has been called a deterrent to clear thinking and communication (Avant, 1993).

According to Walker and Avant (1988), although concept development is an essential element in theory development, nursing, like many other disciplines, often neglects this process. Therefore, when nurses use *culture, race,* and *ethnicity* to describe, explain, or predict patient phenomena, often they are not using the terms in a consistent, generally accepted manner. When concepts are present in the nursing literature but are not clearly defined, Walker and Avant (1988) suggest that concept analysis be implemented as a strategy to refine and clarify the concepts in question. The outcome of this clarification will enhance possibilities for clear communication and better understanding among nurses with regard to the diverse groups of patients for whom they are caring. Additionally, theory development in the area of the meaning of *race*, *ethnicity*, and *culture* for nurses who are caring for diverse groups of patients will not continue to progress until these concepts, vital to the practice of nursing in the 21st century, have been clarified.

The purpose of this chapter is to review the definitions of *culture* as they appear in several literary sources, including nursing literature. The concept of *culture* was chosen because a review of nursing literature demonstrated that this term is often used without being defined; or it is used interchangeably with other related terms; or *culture* is used as a form of shorthand to describe people of color (Barthwell, Hewitt, and Jilson, 1995; Germain, 1992; McGoldrick, Giordano, and Pearce, 1996; Outlaw, 1994). Further, the literature review and appropriate discussion will be used to propose strategies for moving the analysis of "culture" into nursing's agenda for the 21st century.

DEFINITIONS FROM THE LITERATURE

Culture is defined in the *American Heritage Dictionary* (1991) as "the totality of socially transmitted behavior patterns, arts, beliefs, institutions, and all other products of human work and thought characteristic of a community or population" (p. 348). The term has been closely identified with anthropological literature. Kroeber (cited in Berry, Poortinga, Segall, and Dasen (1992, p. 166), noted that although the word *culture* was first introduced to the lay public in a dictionary in the 1920s, it had been used in anthropological literature by Taylor as early as 1871. Taylor (cited in Berry, Poortinga, Segall, and Dasen, 1992, p. 165) defined *culture* as "that complex whole which includes knowledge, belief, art, morals, laws, customs and any other capabilities and habits acquired by man as a member of society." However, the most widely used definitions of culture were (cited in Berry et al., 1992, p. 165) defined by Linton and Herskovits, respectively. Linton defined culture as the "total social heredity of mankind" while Herskovits believed that culture is "a man-made part of the human environment" (cited in Berry, et al., 1992, p. 165). Another widely used definition of culture (cited in Berry, et al., 1992) was developed by Kroeber and Kluckhohn who stated that "culture consists of patterns, explicit and implicit, of and for behavior acquired and transmitted by symbols, which constitute the distinctive achievements of human groups, including their embodiments in artifacts: the essential core of culture consists of traditional (i.e., historically derived and selected) ideas and especially their attached values; cultural systems may on the one hand be considered as products of action, on the other as conditioning elements of further action" (p. 166).

Berry, Poortinga, Segall, and Dasen (1992), as part of their review of the widely used definitions of *culture*, suggested that because *culture* has become a commonly used concept in our society it is pertinent to discuss the difference between what it means in professional fields and the lay connotation of the concept. They noted that *culture* is not only reserved for describing what, in this society, has been labeled *high culture* (e.g., classical music and art), but, instead, is meant to describe all products of human life including such creations as comic books and pop music (Berry, et al., 1994). The point of this distinction is that culture is not synonymous with what is identified in society as *refinement*. Further, these authors also noted that *culture* is not a synonym for *civilized*. They stressed that all human groups have a culture.

This fact is noteworthy because there is a tendency for culture to sometimes become a metaphor that is used to denote what is thought to be inferior or primitive (Blank and Slipp, 1995; McAdoo, 1993; McGoldrick, 1996; Outlaw, 1994). Berry, et al. (1992) also caution us that *culture* is not to be confused with the term *society*. They posit that *culture* and *society* are often used interchangeably; however, they suggest that while the two concepts are linked, a society is made up of people, while their culture is the combination of beliefs, values and attitudes that they share.

A review of literature focused on cultural diversity and multiculturalism found similar definitions for *culture*. For example, Blank and Slipp (1995) defined *culture* as similar values, beliefs, behavior, background, and experiences shared by members of a group. They caution, however, that they avoid using the word *culture* in many instances and use, instead, *group tendencies* because, in the last few decades, culture has been used frequently and narrowly to describe ethnicity and race. Similarly, Kavanagh and Kennedy (1992) offered an eclectic definition of *culture* as "a learned system of symbols with shared values, meanings, and behavioral norms"

(p. 11). Both of these definitions emphasize that culture is learned and dynamic, and is shared over time by members of a group.

The uniqueness of culture as defined by Helman (1995) is that it provides a set of guidelines that directs the person's worldview, their emotional experience of the world, while directing how they are to behave in the world. He posits that symbols, language, art, and rituals are the means through which generations pass cultural guidelines to future genera- tions, and that growing up in a culture causes the individual to slowly acquire the orientation of the group. He calls this acquisition of a *cultural lens* a form of enculturation.

Helman's definition of culture is somewhat different, though the differ- ence is subtle. Previous definitions have described the combination of shared values, symbols, art, and language as the essence of culture, while Helman emphasizes that these are the means of transmission of a culture. He also emphasized that culture has to be considered not in isolation but as one component of a complex set of influences that condition to a significant extent what people believe, how they live their lives, and what they value. Again, Helman (1995) examines the complexity of how culture is to be conceptualized when trying to understand how culture influences patients' responses to health and illness.

Tanner (1986), in her work exploring the differences in conversational styles of men and women, defines *culture* as "simply a network of habits and patterns gleaned from past experience" (p. 133). She believes that boys and girls are treated differently from the time that they are born and, therefore, they grow up with different expectations of the role of conversation in relationships. She believes men and women develop divergent cultural lenses through which they view the meaning of conver- sation in a relationship.

In sum, the definitions of *culture* found in this body of literature were, for the most part, broad in their conceptualizations. They stated or implied that culture involves learned ways of being, transmitted through language, symbols, and rituals, that influence behavior.

Definitions of Culture in the Mental Health Literature

Hughes (1993) suggests that in psychiatry *culture* has been considered a peripheral concept. He based this observation on the manner in which culture is referenced in the standard diagnostic psychiatric manual (DSM IV). The references that are found describe unusual or non-Western culture-bound syndromes. Hughes (1993) defined culture as "a learned configuration of images and other symbolic elements (such as language) widely shared among members of a given society or social group which, for individuals, functions as an orientation framework for behavior; and, for the group, serves as the communicational matrix which tends to coordinate and sanction behavior" (p. 7). He believes that in the clinical setting it is critical to consider culture when working with patients, but it is equally important to do it well. To this end he advocates learning as much as possible about different cultural groups. However, he cautions that to learn the variances that might manifest themselves in an individual patient one must not assume that the patient possesses certain cultural characteristics, but must focus efforts on collecting from the patient information regarding her or his culture.

Moffic and Kinzie (1996) defined culture as "shared group values developed and preserved over time, often over generations" (1996, p. 582). Although this article chronicles the evaluations in organized psychiatry of awareness of the essential task of shifting from generic treatment, in which all patients are considered the same, to recognizing cultural differences among patients, they also demonstrated the lack of clarity that exists among professionals regarding the meaning of the terms *race, ethnicity,* and *culture.* For example, when they described the patterns among groups accessing psychiatric services, they spoke of Caucasians as one cultural group who exhibited the same behaviors relative to seeking treatment and responding with similar positive outcomes while implying that patients from minority and refugee groups were not accepted into treatment nor did they have the same positive treatment outcomes experienced by Caucasian patients. This article is a typical example of forward thinking about how to incorporate culturally-sensitive care into psychiatric services while demonstrating the lack of clarity that results from not creating a standard language among disciplines with which to discuss important cultural differences.

Chrisman (1991), a recognized medical anthropologist, defines culture as "a learned, shared, and symbolically transmitted design for living" (p. 45). Chrisman believes that it is culture that helps people make sense out of the world by assisting them with giving meaning to life events. He cautions, however, that human cultural needs are not as easily categorized, treated, or studied as the biological needs of patients; yet he believes that culture has to be taken into account when clinicians are providing care to diverse groups of people if providing optimal, humanistic care is the goal.

Kleinman (1978), a psychiatrist who has done extensive work in cross-cultural psychiatry, defined *culture* as "a system of symbolic meanings that shapes both social reality and personal experience" (p. 86). He advocates developing a more precise, quantifiable operational definition of the concept *culture* so that the field of health care can develop a valid model of care that is informed about and sensitive to cultural differences.

Definitions of Culture in Nursing Literature

Leininger (1991), the developer of the theory of transcultural nursing, defined culture as "the learned, shared, and transmitted values, beliefs, norms, and lifeways of a particular group that guides their thinking, decisions, and actions in patterned ways" (p. 47). This definition is congruent with definitions found in literature from other disciplines. She suggests that when nurses are working with patients that are of a different culture than their own, they have some knowledge of the patients' culture so that they (nurses) can make sense of what they see, hear, and experience during interactions.

A version of Leininger's definition of culture is used by several nurses (Douglas, 1995; Fong, 1985; Giger and Davidhizar, 1991). Giger and Davidhizar (1991) identified six cultural phenomena that they claim are present in all cultural groups: (1) communication, (2) space, (3) social organization, (4) time, (5) environmental control, and (6) biological variations (p. 4). These cultural phenomena are the areas that they believe need to be assessed when nurses are giving care to culturally diverse patients.

Kagawa-Singer (1996) calls culture a tool that is used by groups to translate their view of the world into concrete values, beliefs, and behaviors that they employ to solidify their world. According to Kagawa-Singer (1996), the two primary functions of culture are, first, integrative which provides the individual an identity and purpose in life by establishing mutually agreed upon values and beliefs; and second, the provision of rules of behavior for the individual that contribute to the person's self-worth and provide for the stability and welfare of the group.

Finally, Germain (1992) defined culture in broad terms as "the way of life of a particular group of people" (p. 1). She elaborated on the definition by including among the attributes of culture language, values, behavioral norms, type and style of dress, dietary patterns as well as other functional characteristics practiced by cultural groups. Germain (1992) elaborated specifically on the influence that culture exerts on individuals and groups with regard to sickness prevention, the attributions one ascribes to the reasons for an illness, the methods used by individuals to cope with illness, and, finally, the rituals surrounding death and dying practiced by cultural groups.

Critique of Definitions of Culture Found in Nursing Literature

A review of a cross-section of definitions from nursing literature reveals that there is general agreement among the writers about the definition of culture. However, the definitions most frequently used are broad and the meanings can be interpreted in many ways. In fact, according to Habayeb (1995), the definitions of culture found in nursing literature are very rarely explicit, but, instead, promote implicit interpretations of the meaning of the concept.

Swendson and Windsor (1996) believe that the conception of culture has changed over time and that the definition has changed because of current lay, popular use of the term. They also maintain that culture is historically and politically grounded (Swendson and Windsor, 1996). The notion that culture is something that is synonymous with minority status or race and ethnicity, and concurrently is an insidious short-hand for inferiority, is an example of how the meaning of the concept has been politicized. Swendson and Windsor (1996) take issue with Leininger's work on transculturalism asserting that her definition of culture, which they maintain is the center of her functional theory, is problematic because it is too simplistic and thus inadequate: it focuses on the attributes of a cultural group instead of involving an examination of the process of marginalization of selected groups of people under the purported neutral heading of culture. They are concerned that the focus of transculturalism and the driving, organizing concept of culture decontextualizes the influences of social and political changes on marginalized groups, which are traditionally immigrants and peoples of color.

Barbee (1993) developed a similar analysis of the use of culture. She maintains that in nursing there exists a type of denial of race and racism, so that discussions about racial differences are subsumed under the rubric of cultural diversity. She believes that the term *cultural diversity* is being used with increasing frequency because it allows nursing to avoid confronting the reality that individual as well as institutional racism exists in nursing. She further posits that when cultural diversity is substituted for racism, attention is diverted from the structural issues that contribute to and maintain inequity and reduces the problem to one of ethnocentrism which can simply be corrected by education.

Finally, Culley (1996) believes that the common theme dominating nursing literature at present, one that calls for nurses to understand cultural aspects of care obscures the way in which race and ethnicity have been ignored by health care providers. She believes that emphasis is placed on the notion that the predominant issue in health care with diverse populations is being sensitive to differences, including problems of communication. Culley (1996) believes that what is ignored in the discussion about culturally sensitive health care is that this society is structured by inequalities resulting from invidious discrimination against persons identified by race, gender, and class. As a result, she maintains, the assumption of the multiculturalist is that knowledge is the key to improving health care that is delivered to diverse groups of people. She states that "the task of the professional educator is thus primarily one of increasing nurses' awareness of cultural differences in dress, diet, health beliefs, religious worship, rites and rituals, illness behavior, child rearing patterns, personal hygiene, naming systems, teaching the importance of respect for one's own and providing information on specific conditions which affect minority groups disproportionately" (p. 565). Education, then, is determined to be the key to help health care providers become tolerant of non-white groups of people so that persons in these groups can receive appropriate health care.

The flaw in this type of culturalist agenda, which dominates nursing literature, is that it is one dimensional. That is, the focus is on teaching health workers about other cultures so that they can be more tolerant of difference thus making them more able to provide appropriate health care to individuals who are racially, ethnically, or culturally different from the health care worker. Concomitantly, the notion that institutional racism is the greatest influence on how care is delivered is usually ignored.

The challenge for nursing scholars interested in creating paradigms to guide nurses in providing care that is competent, sensitive, and appropriate to culturally diverse groups of people requires that concepts such as *culture* that are used to shape, organize, and influence nursing practice, research, and education be clearly defined and all of its complex dimensions identified and distinguished from other concepts.

CONCEPTS RELATED TO CULTURE

Two concepts related to *culture* that are often used interchangeably are *race* and *ethnicity*. In fact, the terms *race, ethnicity, socioeconomic status*, and *minority group* have come to be closely associated with culture (Barthwell, Hewitt, and Jilson, 1995; McAdoo, 1993; Outlaw, 1994). One manifestation of this association is the frequent tendency on the part of many white people to think that the terms *ethnicity* and *culture* refer only to people of color who are often viewed as peripheral to the normal, dominant social group(s). For example, in nursing it is rare to have ethnicity or culture considered as a variable when care is planned if the patient is from the dominant (white) racial group.

Spott (1993) supports the definition of *ethnicity* as "a consciousness of group belonging that is differentiated from others by symbolic markers (culture, biology, territory), that is rooted in bonds of a shared past and perceived ethnic interest" (p. 190).

Berry et al. (1992) posits that ethnicity is hard to define in specific terms; therefore common characteristics have to be identified from the definitions that appear most often in the literature. They maintain that the two aspects that appear in most definitions are the objective facet and the subjective aspect. The *objective facet* refers to people who are biological and cultural offsprings who can be identified by objective criteria such as name and genealogy. Groups constituted by these facets maintain versions of food preference, language, religion, and other cultural phenomena generation after generation although there is moderation of the facets over time (Berry et al., 1994). The *subjective aspect* involves an identification and attachment to the group that fosters a sense of belonging and a need to maintain membership in the group. Berry et al. (1994) believe that both the objective facets and the subjective aspects are necessary in order for an ethnocultural group to exist.

It is common to find the term *ethnic group* used to describe the concept *ethnicity*. For example, McGoldrick (1982) speaks of an ethnic group as "those who conceive of themselves as alike by virtue of their common ancestry, real or fictitious and who are so regarded by others" (p. 4). Ethnicity has been identified as a powerful determinant of identity, which is an essential psychological need (McGoldrick, 1982). She also believes that ethnicity, the root of which is group identity and has as its smallest unit the family of origin, shapes our thinking, feelings, and behavior in ways that are often outside of our awareness (McGoldrick, 1982).

Barthwell et al. (1995) defined ethnicity by describing the commonalities of ethnic groups. They describe an ethnic group as "a collection of people who conceive of themselves as being alike by virtue of their presumed common ancestry and cultural heritage (i.e., race, religion, or national origin) and who are regarded by others to be part of such a group" (p. 433). They use the term *ethnic groups of color* to describe groups that are diverse and whose differences, historically, have placed them at risk for being less accepted in American society and who, because of invidious discrimination, tend to experience more poverty than many other ethnic groups.

Yancey, Ericksen, and Juliani (1976) maintain that many of the attributes that we use to define an ethnic group need to be tested. They believe, for example, that the monolithic treatment of ethnicity in research does not take into account the very important differences found within an ethnic group. They are persuaded that much of specific ethnic behavior has been determined not by heritage passed on from one group to another, but rather is a manifestation of the structural situations in which groups have found themselves. To illustrate this point Yancey et al. (1976) suggest that the Irish domination of city governments in the nineteenth century had more to do with the fact that city governments were expanding at the time when there was an insurgence of Irish immigrants migrating to cities and not their cultural aptitude for coping with bureaucracies.

Illustrating that certain factors that have been recently attributed to ethnic behavior of the black urban poor may be a function of the structural and occupational conditions in which they find themselves, Wilson (1996a, 1996b) explains what has happened to urban, primarily poor black residents of America's inner cities. He describes the elimination of many manufacturing jobs throughout America as the catalyst that created jobless communities in urban areas. As a result, he maintains, the black urban poor, who lost their jobs as a result of the *suburbanization* of employment, began living in racially (and economically) isolated neighborhoods where cultural changes occurred because of the high jobless rates, not because of ethnic group values, heritage, or beliefs. Further, Wilson believes that the high rates of joblessness found in inner-city neighborhoods serve to undermine social organization. When social organization is destroyed among groups of people, problems such as family disorganization, crime, violence, drug addiction, and hopelessness weaken the "social processes that regulate behavior" (Wilson, 1996a, p. 29). He cites research on the relationship between joblessness and violent crime as an example of how social disorganization—not ethnic group cultural beliefs and values—influences the behavior of urban poor people. According to Wilson (1996a), reporting research by Elliott "the black-white differential in the proportion of males involved in serious violent crime, although almost even at age 11, increases to 3:2 over the remaining years of adolescence, and reaches a differential of nearly 4:1 during the late twenties" (p. 22). When the researcher "compared only employed black and white males, he found no significant differences in violent behavior patterns among the two groups by age 21" (p. 22).

When nurses are taught that *ethnicity*, *culture*, and *race* are shorthand terms for predictable, fixed behaviors of certain groups, a concise formula for providing care can be developed based on the list of characteristics that they develop (Tripp-Reimer & Fox 1990). Swendson and Windsor (1996) call the list approach to understanding diverse people a decontextualized and mechanistic way of conceptualizing diversity. However, this approach to understanding cultural diversity does not explain the way political, economic, and social changes have impacted the lives of diverse groups of people, especially those of color, and influenced their responses to health and illness.

Race in nursing literature is not defined but is explained as associated with biology or phenotypically identified groups (Giger and Davidhizar, 1991; Kagawa-Singer, 1996). According to Outlaw (1996) *race* can be thought of as a "cluster concept which draws together under a single word references to biological, cultural, and geographical factors thought characteristic of a population" (1996, p. 20). Additionally, in order to understand race, he believes that all the features that make up a proposed racial type do not have to be shared equally by all the individuals or groups who have been defined as members of a particular race. He maintains that race refers to "heterogeneous complexes of socially normed biological and cultural characteristics. And the biological features referred to when making racial distinctions are always conscripted into projects of cultural, political, and social construction" (Outlaw, 1996, p. 21). What is advocated by Outlaw (1996) is the formulation of a "cogent and viable concept of race" that can serve to describe phenomena without the invidious characterizations that often are attached to the concepts of race and ethnicity.

Review of definitions of the related concepts of ethnicity and race reveal that the meaning of these definitions, like those for *culture*, are dynamic and complex and still need to be explored to determine how they are to be conceptualized to enhance the everyday life experiences of patients in the care of nurses.

The recent debate regarding Ebonics sparked by the Oakland (California) School Board is an example of how invalid perceptions of the attributes of a particular racial group, in this case black Americans, can influence public policy. The School Board decision to have Ebonics taught to teachers as a way to enhance their understanding of African American students and thus to promote better teacher-student relations and more productive and successful teaching and learning sparked a national debate about whether Ebonics was the spoken language of black Americans. Race became the variable that was highly associated with the speaking of non-standard English, instead of class and geographic location. The speaking of non-standard English is a form of behavior that can be observed across races among most poor, undereducated people in this country in both urban and rural settings.

In sum, *culture* in nursing literature is vague, for the most part, and does not include in its definitions any reference to the political, economic, or social contexts that influence the cultural adaptations of diverse groups. It is also important to note that the patterned behaviors that are demonstrated by groups that are attributed to culture are learned, not genetically transmitted. Therefore, people who share a common racial or ethnic connection are not necessarily going to have all of the same cultural orientations. Many of their cultural experiences will be related to other complex variables such as whether they are acculturated or assimilated into what has been defined as *American culture*.

The historical context(s) of members of the same racial group have to be considered since they may not have the same experiences. For example, black West Indians and African Americans can trace their genealogies to Africa. However, their historical experiences have been very different, in important respects. For example, most African Americans began their lives in this country as slaves, a beginning that has had tremendous social, political, and economic impacts on them, while most black West Indians migrated to this country with all the expectations that have come to be associated with most immigrants who come to America. Therefore, an assumption that the beliefs, values, and other cultural interests are the same for persons in both groups is erroneous. As Tripp-Reimer and Fox (1990) suggest, narrowly conscripted functional approaches to the treatment of individuals and groups is both a-theoretical and fragmented. As a consequence, nurses who believe they are providing culturally competent care using a functionalistic framework are often basing their approach on simplistic, and often stereotypic, characterizations of diverse groups of persons, especially those of color.

MOVING NURSING'S DIVERSITY AGENDA
INTO THE 21st CENTURY

Several authors have described the dramatic demographic changes presently occurring and predicted to continue into the 21st century in America
(Andrews, 1992; Blank and Slipp, 1995; Tucker-Allen, 1994). By the
year 2000, Andrews (1992), reporting on the predictions of the U.S.
Bureau of the Census, suggests that people of color—among them people
of African descent, Hispanics, Asians, and Native Americans—will comprise more than half of the racial, ethnic, and cultural diversity in this
country. Andrews (1992) reports that by the year 2080 people of color will
comprise 51.1 percent of the total American population. The changing
demographics will require that nursing prepare its practitioners, researchers, and educators to meet the health care needs of a racially, ethnically,
and culturally diverse population whom they will be called upon to serve.

The American Nurses Association (ANA) has encouraged the inclusion and integration throughout the entire nursing curricula of well
thought-out conceptions of cultural diversity (Andrews, 1992). Contro-
versy continues, however, about how the concepts are defined and used
by nurses in practice, education, and research. For example, Kikuchi
(1996) urged nurse educators to "critically examine what is being taught
with regard to the place of judgment in nursing practice amidst cultural
diversity" (p. 164). She suggests that after examining the nursing literature
as well as listening to selected nursing educators speak, it is evident
that respecting the patient's cultural values and beliefs is a tenet of
"multicultural ethics that is becoming considered 'sacrosanct' in nursing"
(Kikuchi, 1996, p. 159). While she believes that nurses have embraced
multiculturalism because of a genuine desire to meet the needs of diverse
groups of patients, she is nevertheless concerned that the tenets and
moral injunctions placed on nurses have instructed them to respect the
patient's cultural values to the point that it has become apparent that
responsible nursing practice may be hindered. She has called for nurse
educators to develop strong transcultural ethics that are based on realism
to guide student nurses through situations in which they are challenged
to deal with the conflicting desires of cultural groups. Simply put, she
cautions nurses to rethink how they are going to practice nursing when
their interventions meet resistance from patients because of what has
been loosely determined as a conflict with the patient's cultural health
values and beliefs.

Culley (1996) calls upon nurse educators to disavow themselves of the notion that educating health professionals about culture will reduce ignorance, overcome prejudice, and develop tolerance of racial, ethnic, and cultural differences among health care providers who are mostly persons of dominant racial and ethnic groups. She maintains that infusing nurses with information about other cultures as the primary mechanism for creating culturally sensitive health care providers avoids the discussion of the manner in which racism and invidious prejudice permeate institutional and professional organizations and influence how diverse groups receive health care. She suggests that though nursing literature is heavily endowed with prescriptive notions regarding the cultures of different groups, very little scholarly work has been done on the ways in which health care providers internalize cultural understanding (Culley, 1996).

Culley's (1996) argument parallels one made by Outlaw (1994); both authors urge rethinking in nursing of how culture, race, and ethnicity are conceptualized in the literature of nursing. They both have argued for examining the concepts and their complexities in a more scholarly fashion so that the welfare of culturally diverse groups who will be served by this knowledge are not damaged. For example, the notion of simplifying and sweeping attributions of negative or static behaviors and values to groups, especially peoples of color, have been noted in much of the literature on cultural diversity (Culley, 1996; McAdoo, 1993; McGoldrick, 1982; Outlaw, 1994; Spott, 1993; Tripp-Reimer & Fox, 1990). It is not unusual to hear in research or clinical discussions such statements as "when talking about sexual behaviors you can frankly discuss this subject with black women because they are used to it, while Hispanic women would be upset if you introduced the subject of sex to them." Other statements such as "black women raise their daughters, but they love their sons" is another example of an attribution of an erroneous generalization to a particular group of people that has far reaching implications for the type of clinical interventions engaged in or research implications that might be drawn. Both these statements were made by clinicians and researchers in a meeting of research scholars and psychiatric clinicians. Statements like these are based on reductionist, simplistic, fixed generalizations about particular cultural, racial, and ethnic groups, generalizations which are based, in many cases, on anecdotal data, but more frequently on inconsistencies in how conceptualizations of culture, race, and ethnicity are operationalized in nursing. Culley (1996) cautions nurses that strict adherence to racial, cultural, and ethnic categories in such a way as to perpetuate racial stereotypes in which statements such as "African Americans will . . ." or "Hispanics believe . . ." creates the idea that members of particular groups, especially those of color, are homogenous and can all be expected to have the same needs, beliefs, values, and behaviors.

Porter and Villarruel (1993) questioned whether the conceptualization of culture in nursing is comprehensive enough to guide nurse researchers in understanding how race and ethnicity, and the concomitant variables of racism and invidious discrimination, influence the phenomena they are interested in i.e., the health behaviors and the health outcomes of diverse groups of people, especially people of color. For instance, they suggest that theoretical knowledge and empirical data about the influences of race (and racism), culture, and ethnicity have not been included in the formulation of nursing frameworks through which diverse groups of people are viewed. They believe that lack of courage is the primary reason that the majority of nurses avoid the issue of race when discussing the health behaviors and outcomes of patients who are members of divergent cultural groups.

It has been suggested that race and its invidious social dimension, racism, have been extricated from the cultural diversity discussion in nursing because to admit that racism in nursing exists would to be to acknowledge the violation of one of the primary principles of nursing— caring (Barbee, 1993). To this end, then, nursing has avoided bringing to the table dimensions of the discussions about how to conceptualize the more social and political term *race*, substituting, instead, *culture* as a euphemism thereby avoiding the social, historical, and political contexts that the term *race* invokes. The result of this avoidance behavior in nursing has been the creation of approaches to working with culturally divergent patients that supports attributing over-generalizations of characteristics and behaviors to people of color that have interfered with the quality of health care that they receive.

The most problematic outcome is the creation in nursing of flawed conceptualizations used to provide the direction for understanding the meaning of race, culture, and ethnicity. These flawed approaches have served to assure nursing that there is a legitimate body of knowledge about how to provide culturally competent care to divergent people thereby promoting placid complacency in some circles and benign neglect in others of the importance of the issue.

PARADIGMS FOR THE FUTURE:
CULTURE AND NURSING

The review of nursing literature supports the assessment that *culture* and related concepts such as *race* and *ethnicity* have not been clearly defined in a way to "shape, organize, and implement theory, practice, and research in a logical and focused manner" (Habayeb, 1995, p. 224.). As a result the quest for clarity which influences clear thinking and communication about how to provide culturally competent care is lacking. With the change in demographics in this country, changes projected into the 21st century, pressures will continue to fall on the profession of nursing to be more responsive to the racially, ethnically, and culturally diverse populations it serves. Additionally, in order to fully actualize caring as one of the core principles of nursing, nurses are being compelled to provide culturally competent and appropriate care to the patients that they serve.

The first step in moving the agenda for providing culturally competent care to diverse populations into the 21st century is to recognize that in nursing the concepts *culture, race,* and *ethnicity* are not articulated in a clear and concise manner; therefore, they cannot be used in a systematic way to provide direction for nursing research, practice, and education.

This discussion, although not well developed among nurse scholars, is beginning to take place. It is a discussion that must be supported and encouraged by nurses. Consequently, articles that critique the validity of the way concepts concerned with diversity are defined and used to form conceptual and theoretical approaches to providing care to diverse cultural groups need more rigorous examination. Support for this type of scholarship has to be provided by leaders in schools of nursing, in research arenas, and in agencies where clinical services are provided.

Andrews (1992), citing the ANA's (1986) four approaches for integrating cultural content into the curriculum, describes as the first approach the "integration of cultural concepts throughout the entire nursing curriculum" (p. 13). If concepts such as *culture, race,* and *ethnicity* are poorly defined, used interchangeably, and have not been standardized in a way that supports mutual understanding among nurses, then the cultural concepts that are the basis for the content that is integrated throughout the curriculum will not be describing the same phenomena in a consistent way.

Inconsistencies in the definitions of concepts contributes to the more virulent problem of prejudging patient's behaviors, thus facilitating treatment decisions based on incorrect data. For example, is it always the case that the patient is culturally diverse from the nurse if the nurse is white and the patient is a person of color? What if both white nurse and patient of color are the same age, from the same demographic region, are nurses, and are women? Would one need a cultural broker to work with this dyad around health care issues? Would this be an occasion when one would define their exchanges as an intercultural communication? Are models in nursing that were reported on by the ANA expert panel (1992) on culturally competent nursing care highlighting the work of several nurse theories in which they describe conclusions from their work with diverse sub-cultural groups within the United States such as the old order Amish, substantively different from a study of African Americans in the United States? Is it possible that many black and white Americans may hold similar cultural beliefs and values regarding many issues? What happens to populations identified in the Task Force Report (1992) as minority groups (African Americans, Hispanics, Asian/Pacific Islanders, and Native Americans) when, very shortly, they become the majority groups in this country? Will other groups that have received very little attention in the health care system, such as gays, lesbians, and the homeless, still be identified with the majority group? Can we create competent approaches to people identified as minorities if our underlying premise is that their cultures are uniform and static (Tripp-Reimer & Fox, 1990)?

While as a discipline we profess not to do this, evidence of nurses thinking that culture is static and uniform for particular racial or ethnic groups is often manifest when clinical discussions examine health care issues as if all members of the group that is the focus of discussion will have the same orientation to their health care. This venue of thinking is particularly evident when the behavior is maladaptive or dysfunctional.

The majority of nurses recognize that it is critical to nursing to be health care providers, researchers, and educators who are leaders in developing the theory, conducting the research, and educating future nurses to provide the competent care diverse groups of consumers will be demanding in the 21st century. In order to accomplish this goal definitive concepts, among them *race, ethnicity,* and *culture,* the building blocks of diversity theory, will have to be rigorously defined and their interrelationships clarified in order to develop a viable structure for the conceptual framework that will guide practice, research, and curriculum development in nursing (Porter & Villarruel, 1993).

The Dreyfus Model of Skill Acquisition used by Benner (1984) to describe the competency levels of nurses engaged in clinical practice is a framework that can be used to assist nursing to determine the state of nursing knowledge about how to conduct research, educate the next generation of nurses, and deliver clinical practice to racially, ethnically, and culturally diverse groups of patients. The Dreyfus Model of Skill Acquisition identifies five stages of performance characteristics that an individual must acquire in order to be accomplished at a given task. The skill levels range from the *novice stage* in which, as beginners, nurses are taught about "situations in terms of objective attributes such as weight, intake and output, temperature, blood pressure, pulse, and other such objectifiable, measurable parameters of a patient's condition—features of the task world that can be recognized without situational experience" (Benner, 1984, p. 20). Many would describe the status of the current nursing theory related to understanding diverse groups as focusing on components of culture instead of their interrelatedness as being at the novice level since there is a dearth of understanding about the interrelation between the components of race, ethnicity and culture, the structure of society, including an understanding of socio-economic influences and institutional racism on issues of health care delivery to diverse groups of patients (Culley, 1996; Outlaw, 1994; Porter & Villarruel, 1993; Tripp-Reimer & Fox, 1990).

Benner (1984) states that novices tend to be inflexible in their approaches to patients because their behavior tends to be rule-governed instead of experience based. Therefore, novices tend to depend on fixed ideas which prevent them from moving beyond their cookbook approaches to patients. A major flaw in transcultural nursing is that it stresses a cookbook or list approach to describing patterns of behaviors of ethnically, racially, culturally diverse patients which serve to teach novice nurses, many of whom have never had any exposure to persons of color, rigid, stereotypical ways of thinking about these patients thereby giving rise to nursing assessments and the implementation of interventions that are not therapeutic for the patient.

Using Benner's criteria as a yard-stick, nursing scholars, while not yet at the competent stage of providing multicultural care, are beginning to examine and call for contextual examinations of concepts such as culture used to communicate about culturally competent approaches to ethnically, racially, and culturally diverse patients. However, if the goal in nursing is to develop the knowledge about providing competent care to diverse groups of people, then nurses interested in developing this body of knowledge have to move the discipline toward understanding the complex interrelations involved in moving the science of caring for ethnically, racially, and culturally diverse groups to the expert level. Benner (1984) states that experts "operate from a deep understanding of the total situation" (p. 32). Nursing has primarily embraced the notion that in order to provide culturally appropriate care to diverse patients the caregivers need to learn about the cultural beliefs, values, and behaviors (for example, the food habits and religious practices) of the groups of people they serve. While learning about particular groups' rituals and preferences is a laudable goal, it is the task of organized nursing to develop a systemic body of knowledge that includes understandings of the total situation that influences patient's responses to health and illness. Defining concepts like *culture* and understanding the context in which they are used to describe and give appropriate meaning to people's health beliefs, values, and behaviors, the total situation of their lives, is the hallmark of an expert nurse.

In order to become experts in the delivery of nursing care to diverse groups of people, nursing will have to move beyond the discipline's present limitations of basing care on concepts which have not been defined in nursing in any clear, concise, and standardized manner. When the concepts are developed in a scholarly way, the theory emanating from the concepts might well direct nurses to look beyond the functional list approach as the key to delivering culturally competent care. Instead, an analysis of race, ethnicity and culture will direct nurses to investigate the complex ways in which social, economic, and institutional structures impact on the health beliefs, expectations, and behaviors of diverse groups of people.

To move the agenda for nursing of providing competent care to racially, ethnically, culturally diverse groups of people into the 21st century, nurse scholars must develop the concepts that drive the theorizing about these phenomena in a way that contextualizes and demonstrates the interrelationships of race, ethnicity, and culture in this society. To accomplish this progressive move, nurse leaders have to commit themselves to the proposition that the provision of competent care to diverse groups of people is a priority for nursing in the next century. Commitment to this agenda means allocating resources to support this endeavor. The solution for learning about ethnically, racially, and culturally diverse groups is not only for researchers required to include *minorities* in their research as subjects, as required by the federal government, or to include a minority person on the research team, since even when minorities have been included in research studies often the instruments and the research methods have not been culturally appropriate or sensitive to measure the phenomena of interest. Additionally, often the researchers are not well versed about the diverse groups they are studying and therefore their findings may be misinterpreted. Further, when concepts like *race, ethnicity*, and *culture* are not clearly defined and used in a consistent and standardized way the phenomena researched are not always consistent and the findings are not generalizable.

Scholars who are interested in developing nursing knowledge about providing the care to diverse groups of people that is needed will need support from their colleagues including the Deans of Schools of Nursing and administrators of service organizations. Creative funding mechanisms for supporting this work will have to be developed since it is not the kind of scholarship that traditional nursing funding sources have supported. Lastly, the nursing scholars who are engaged in developing the body of knowledge that will prepare nurses in all areas to contribute to this development will have to network with disciplines outside of nursing such as sociology, economics, philosophy, and others in which there is needed knowledge that can assist nursing in meeting its goal of moving the agenda of providing competent care to racially, ethnically, and culturally diverse groups into the next century.

REFERENCES

ANA Expert Panel Report (1992). Culturally competent health care. *Nursing Outlook, 40*(6), 277–283.

American Heritage Dictionary (2nd College Edition). (1991). Boston: Houghton Mifflin Company, p. 348.

Andrews, M. (1992). Cultural perspectives on nursing in the 21st century. *Journal of Professional Nursing, 8*(11), pp. 7–15.

Avant, K. (1993). The Wilson method of concept analysis. In B. Rogers & K. Knafl (Eds.), *Concept development in nursing: Foundations, techniques, and applications*, (pp. 3–41). Philadelphia: W.B. Saunders Company.

Barbee, E. (1993). Racism in U.S. nursing. *Medical Anthropology Quarterly, 7*(4), 346–362.

Barthwell, A., Hewitt, W., & Jilson, I. (1995). An introduction to ethnic and cultural diversity. *Pediatric Clinics of North America, 42*(2), 431–451.

Benner, P. (1984). *From novice to expert: Excellence and power in clinical nursing practice*. California: Addison-Wesley Publishing Co.

Berry, J., Poortinga, M., Segall, M., & Dasen, P. (1992). *Cross-cultural psychology*. New York: Cambridge University Press.

Blank, R., & Slipp, S. (1995). *Voices of diversity: Real people talk about problems and solutions in a workplace where everyone is not alike.* New York: American Management Association.

Chrisman, N. (1991). Cultural systems. In S. Baird, R. McCorkle, & M. Grant. (Eds.), *Cancer nursing: A comprehensive text book,* (pp. 45–55). Philadelphia: W.B. Saunders Co.

Culley, L. (1996). A critique of multiculturalism in health care: The challenge for nurse education. *Journal of Advanced Nursing, 23,* 564–570.

Douglas, C. (1995). Cultural consideration for the African-American population. *Imprint, 42*(5), 57–59.

Fong, C. (1985). Ethnicity and nursing practice. *Topics in Clinical Nursing, 7*(3), 1–10.

Germain, C. (1992). Cultural care: A bridge between sickness, illness, and disease. *Holistic Nurse Practice, 6*(3), 1–9.

Giger, J., & Davidhizar, R. (1991). *Transcultural nursing: Assessment and intervention.* St. Louis: Mosby Year Book.

Habayeb, G. (1995). Cultural diversity: A nursing concept not yet reliably defined. *Nursing Outlook, 43*(5), 224–227.

Helman, C. (1995). *Culture, health and illness,* (3rd ed.). London: Butterworld-Heinemann Ltd.

Hughes, C. (1993). Culture in clinical psychiatry in culture, ethnicity and mental illness. In A. Gaw (Ed.), *Culture, ethnicity & mental Illness,* (pp. 3–41). Washington: American Psychiatric Press, Inc.

Kagawa-Singer, M. (1996). Cultural systems. In R. McCorkle, M. Grant, M. Frank-Stromborg, & S. Baird (Eds.), *Cancer Nursing: A comprehensive text book,* (2nd edition, pp. 38–52). Philadelphia: W.B. Saunders Co.

Kavanagh, K., & Kennedy, P. (1992). *Promoting cultural diversity: Strategies for health care professionals.* California: Sage Publications, Inc.

Kikuchi, J. (1996). Multicultural ethics in nursing education. *Journal of Professional Nursing, 12*(3) pp. 159–165.

Kleinman, A. (1978). Concepts and a model for the comparison of medical systems as cultural systems. *Social Science & Medicine, 12,* pp. 85–93.

Leininger, M. (1991). The theory of culture care diversity and universality. In Leininger, M. (Ed.), *Culture care diversity and universality: A theory of nursing.* New York: NLN Press.

McAdoo, H. (1993). Ethnic families: Strengths that are found in diversity. In H. McAdoo (Ed.), *Family ethnicity: Strength in diversity,* (pp. 13–14). Beverly Hills, CA: Sage Publications, Inc.

McGoldrick, M., Giordano, J., & Pearce, J. (1996). (Eds.), *Ethnicity & family therapy,* (2nd ed.). New York: Guilford Press.

McGoldrick, M. (1982). Ethnicity and family therapy: An overview. In M. McGoldrick, J. Pearce, & J. Giordano (Eds.), *Ethnicity and family therapy,* (pp. 3–30). New York: Guilford Press.

Moffic, H., & Kinzie, J. (1996). The history and future of cross-cultural psychiatric services. *Community Mental Health Journal, 32*(6), pp. 581–592.

Outlaw, F. (1994). A reformulation of the meaning of culture and ethnicity for nurses delivering care. *MEDSURG Nursing, 3*(2), 108–111.

Outlaw, L. (1996). "Conserve" Race: In defense of W. E. B. DuBois. In B. Bell, E. Groshalz, & J. Stewart (Eds.), *W. E. B. DuBois on race and culture*, (pp. 15–37). New York: Routledge Press.

Porter, C., & Villarruel, A. (1993). Nursing research with African-American and Hispanic people: Guidelines for action. *Nursing Outlook, 41*(2), 59–97.

Spott, J. (1993). The black box in family assessment: Cultural diversity. In S. Feetham, S. Meister, J. Bell & C. Gilliss (Eds.). *The nursing of families: Theory, research, education, practice* (pp. 189–199). Beverly Hills, CA: Sage Publications, Inc.

Swendson, C., & Windsor, C. (1996). Response: Rethinking cultural sensitivity. *Nursing Inquiry, 3*, p. 118.

Tanner, D. (1986). *That's not what I meant: How conversational style makes or breaks relationships*. New York: Ballantine Books.

Tripp-Reimer, T., & Fox, S. (1990). Beyond the concept of culture: Or, how knowing the cultural formula does not predict clinical success. In J. C. McCloskey, and H. K. Grace (Eds.). *Current Issues in Nursing*, (3rd edition, pp. 542–546). St Louis: Mosby Books.

Tucker-Allen, S. (1994). Cultural diversity and nursing education: An organization approach. *Journal of Cultural Diversity, 1*(1), pp. 21–25.

Walker, L., & Avant, K. (1988). *Strategies for theory construction in nursing*. Connecticut: Appleton & Lange.

Wilson, W. J. (1996a). *When work disappears: The world of the new urban poor*. New York: Alfred A. Knopf.

Wilson, W. J. (1996b, August 18). Work. *The New York Times Magazine*, pp. 26–31, 40, 48, 52, 53, 54.

Yancey, W., Ericksen, E., & Juliani, R. (1976). Emergent ethnicity: A review and reformulation. *American Sociological Review, 41*(3), pp. 391–403.

5

A Model of Inclusion For Nursing in the 21st Century

Dolores S. Patrinos

At the closing of the 20th century, America has experienced both polarity and contradiction in its response to multiculturalism. On one hand we recognize that the essence of the American experience is not expressed within one cultural group; one kind of civilization; one religion, Christianity; or only one language, English. We know that many cultures have contributed to the pluralistic American experience and the complex and contradictory identities of its people (Marable, 1995). Yet at the same time, we hold strongly to the illusionary ideal of the melting pot; a national character which transcends origin or race, and extends equal access to opportunities based on merit.

The 21st century will see the influence of greater cultural diversity in the United States more than in any other period in American history. Immigration has sharply transformed the ethnic, cultural and social composition and character of thousands of urban working class neighborhoods and communities. Along this changing social background, our notions of the social categories which convey the day-to-day meaning of *black* and *white* have also begun to change (Marable, 1995).

The consequences of this diversity are already being felt in every sector of society including the workplace, the arts, the health care delivery system, and in institutions of higher learning. All institutions will have to address the problem of continuing to find creative solutions to the challenges of access and retention, economic, educational, and class inequities, linguistic differences, disproportionate representation in the morbidity and mortality health tables, and underrepresentation in the decision making systems in the context of a global economy, in which at present the only significant factor is the producing of services at the lowest unit cost. For issues of diversity are problems of human relations and social equality and they need to be explored in a manner which will expand the principles of fairness and opportunity to all members of society (Marable, 1995, p. 118). To paraphrase W. E. B. DuBois, besides ageism and the previously mentioned economic factor, the challenge of 21st Century America may well be the multicultural democracy (Marable, 1995).

This chapter will examine how Temple University and the Department of Nursing took on the challenges of expanding the boundaries of democracy and access by expanding the pipeline of underrepresented groups in nursing, and providing them with support to maximize retention and graduation. The chapter will then propose the roles of nursing and nursing education in creating a rich pluralistic, and diverse health care system through increasing minority leadership in education, research, primary health care, and management.

SOCIO-POLITICAL AND ECONOMIC ISSUES RELATED TO TEMPLE'S COMMITMENT TO EDUCATE A DIVERSE NURSE WORKFORCE

Philadelphia is typical of those older urban areas of the Northeast where poverty and segregation in the city grew more concentrated in the 1970s because of 1) the suburbanization of work; 2) the elimination of manufacturing jobs; and 3) proliferation of low-paying service occupations. The result was the rapid spread of new and uniquely disadvantaged social environments linked to joblessness, teenage pregnancy, and single-parent families (Rodriquez, 1994). Between 1973 and 1988, the proportion of United States children in poverty grew by one-third (Shalala, 1993).

Philadelphia is typical in the relationship between poverty and educational opportunities. "How schools address poverty is an important test of an educational system. Children from poor families are, generally speaking, the least successful by conventional measures and the hardest to teach by traditional methods. Modern schools have persistently failed children in poverty" (Connell, 1994, p. 127). Beside income, there are other types of resources where inequality is significant: for example, access to public institutions such as schools, public utilities, colleges, and hospitals, as well as access to *safety and community health*. Connell points out that the poor are the least powerful, and yet the population most dependent on public education to uplift their lives, including the promotion of health.

The department cited four reasons to support a proposal which was funded in 1990 to admit and increase the academic performance of underrepresented minority groups and economically disadvantaged students at Temple University in the Department of Nursing. These reasons were:

1. minority and/or disadvantaged students are more likely to practice in underserved areas;
2. an insufficient number of minority and disadvantaged nurses are in practice;
3. an insufficient number of minority and disadvantaged nurses are in leadership roles;
4. there are insufficient economic resources for minorities in Philadelphia.

Underserved Areas Remain

Despite considerable private and public expenditure for health care in the United States, significant portions of the population have limited access to the care that is available. As the population figures increase among all ethnic minority groups and specifically among blacks and Hispanics, the morbidity and mortality figures also increase. Today, according to the latest data available, blacks and Hispanics lead all other ethnic and minority groups in morbidity and mortality in almost all but three of the major disease categories (Tucker-Allen, 1994; Rosella, Regan-Kubinski, and Albrecht, 1994). *Nursing's Agenda for Health Care Reform* (1992) proposed a paradigm shift in the delivery of health care, the use of nurse manpower in a socially responsible manner, and changes in the nurse curriculum to accommodate the new role and responsibilities.

Health Manpower Shortage Areas (underserved areas) are heavily populated by ethnic and racial minority groups in urban areas (O'Hare,

1992). The number of such communities has in fact increased in recent years, raising concerns about racial differentials in health status, access to health care, and the staggering record of health care problems for a significant portion of the population. Should the inequality of access continue without appropriate health promotion, prevention and intervention strategies, the burden and costs of long-term care will rise significantly in the future (US Division of Nursing, Bureau of Health Professions, HRSA, 1992).

Minority health professionals are more likely to enter primary care specialties and to voluntarily practice in or near designated primary health manpower shortage areas. Sixty to eighty percent of the underrepresented minority students trained in the health professions practice in or close to shortage areas with overwhelmingly minority patients (US DHHS, 1992). Consequently, increasing the number of minority health professionals may offer a partial solution to economic and racial disparities in health status that define *a public health crisis* (Rosella, Regan-Kubinski, and Albrecht, 1994).

Insufficient Minorities in the Health Care Professions

Because we want nursing to look like the rest of America, we have the expectation of professional diversity as an ideal.

Twenty-five percent of the U.S. population is either African American, Hispanic, or Native American (Department of Commerce, Bureau of Census, 1992). The gap between minority and white students in earned high school diplomas has nearly closed, but postsecondary graduation rates have remained inordinately low for students of color (Davis, 1995). Minority nursing students are nowhere near 25 percent of the total nursing student population (US DHHS, 1992). Table 5.1 compares the percent of minorities in nursing and nursing programs to their number in the total population.

The best barometer of access to the profession is completion of a course of study, and not enrollment (Fleming, 1992). Schools of nursing may admit more minority students, but the graduation rate has remained flat. Although blacks lead all illness indices, they are graduating from schools of nursing and entering the profession in lower numbers than any other racial or ethnic group. This figure has not budged in well over a decade. Minority and/or disadvantaged students are less likely to graduate than traditional students. Latino Americans are less likely than other minority

Table 5.1
Minority Groups and Underrepresentation in Nursing Programs.

	Minority Groups	African American	Latino	Asian American
Enrolled in B.S.N. program	15.8%	9.5%	3.2%	3.1%
B.S.N. graduates	9.9%	9.5%	3.2%	3.1%
M.S.N. students	12%	5.3%	3.3%	2.6%
Nursing Faculty	3.6%			
U.S. Population	25%			
Population of Philadelphia	48%	39%	6%	3%

Sources: Statistical Abstract, 1994; Nursing Database, 1991 and 1992.

groups to attend or graduate from college (O'Hare, 1992). The Department of Nursing has actively sought out students from the special admission programs at Temple University.

As the number of students graduating from undergraduate and graduate programs remains low, so does the minority pool of potential nurse practitioners, managers, researchers, and potential nursing faculty. There is increasing concern over the potential decline in underrepresented minority student enrollment—African American, Hispanic, and American Indian in nursing undergraduate programs (US Division of Nursing, Bureau of Health Professions, HRSA, 1992). In all reporting there is a decline in graduation rates for both African Americans and Latinos, while the rates for Asian Americans and Native Americans increased slightly (McBay, 1992). Raising the retention rate of minority students, therefore, has been singled out as probably the most effective means for increasing the number of underrepresented racial minority groups among health professionals (Saucier, 1994). "This bodes ill for any future change in the already devastating health/illness picture" (Tucker-Allen, 1992, p. 37).

Insufficent Economic Resources for Minorities in Philadelphia

In Philadelphia, nearly 110,000 students—half the Philadelphia School district enrollment—are from families on welfare. The number has jumped sharply in recent years, mirroring a rise in poverty in the city (*Philadelphia Inquirer*, October 23, 1994). In the North Philadelphia area, 50 percent of the families residing in census tracts around Temple University have incomes below the federal poverty level. This area is considered the poorest in the Commonwealth of Pennsylvania. An even greater percentage of children in this area are poor. Sixty-eight percent of the families are headed by single women, with nearly 25 percent having children under six years of age (Vital Statistics Report, 1991).

Given the bleak economic picture, it is not surprising that the evaporation of student financial aid has been the greatest contributor to low enrollment and high attrition rates. Financial factors are more responsible for minority attrition than the way students are treated at institutions (Manzo, 1994). Yet minority-targeted scholarships make up only 4 percent of total award money available at American colleges (Powell, 1992).

DESCRIPTION OF NURSING CAREER OPPORTUNITY PROGRAM (NCOP)

The Temple University Department of Nursing received ongoing federal support for its Nursing Career Opportunity Program (NCOP) listed in the Catalog of Federal Domestic Assistance, No. 93.178 from 1990 to 1995. In the implementation of NCOP, the Department of Nursing sought the academic and personal support necessary to admit and graduate low-income students and/or those from racial groups underrepresented in professional nursing. The program was consistent with the mission of the Department of Nursing: educating working-class students and providing nursing services to inner-city populations.

The five objectives of NCOP were: 1) To identify a large applicant pool of pre-nursing students from racial minority groups and disadvantaged backgrounds; 2) To facilitate the annual entry of these students into the undergraduate upper-division curriculum of the Department of Nursing; 3) To provide stipends and help overcome financial disadvantage and to facilitate continued enrollment; 4) To extend the nursing curriculum by conducting a transitional summer program, and providing specialized summer support services after graduation for the successful passage of state board examination; and 5) To identify students at risk for failure and provide them with personal and academic support.

Students for the Program were recruited from the following populations:

1. Underrepresented ethnic/racial minority groups enrolled in the Department of Nursing.

2. Educationally disadvantaged. Students from low-income families, often the first college student in their family, and those with poor academic preparation in inner-city schools. Even if students have achieved an upper rank in their high school class, they may be ineligible for regular admission to Temple because of poor scores on standardized tests. They are admitted through special admissions programs in the university. A large portion of these students are of African American and Latino heritage.

3. Transfer students From Community College of Philadelphia (CCP) who very much fit the profile described in the second entry.

4. Economically Disadvantaged. Members of families whose low income and/or social circumstances present significant obstacles to obtaining a nursing education.

Approximately 45 percent of students admitted to the Department of Nursing in Fall, 1994 were from racial minority groups, including Asian Americans and other students for whom English is their second language (ESL). With each successive year, ESL students have increased, reflecting the influx from the Caribbean, Eastern Europe, and Asia.

The NCOP Program was successful in: 1) increasing the number of applicants, acceptances, and matriculants among economically disadvantaged students and/or minority groups underrepresented in professional nursing; 2) improving the retention rate for these students; and 3) improving the NCLEX-RN passing rate for trainees who are disproportionately represented among those who fail the examination.

A six-week intensive pre-matriculation program called *The Transitional Summer Program (TISP)* was conducted for accepted students perceived to be at risk academically. This program was designed to simulate major components of the first-year curriculum in the Department of Nursing. Students were exposed to content from the high-risk nursing courses taught by nursing faculty. Through early and realistic exposure to the rigors of the nursing curriculum, participants were assisted in making the transition from pre-nursing undergraduate courses to professional curriculum.

NCOP provided for a reduced course load during the academic year by scheduling a combination of low-risk and high-risk nursing courses during summer sessions. Students rated the summer courses as an important factor in completing the nursing program in a timely manner.

During the second summer of nursing courses, about 50 percent of NCOP students remained through an additional summer session taking Patho-physiology II, reducing their course load even further for the fall semester of their senior year. Many other nursing students have joined the NCOP students in the summer sessions. Prior to NCOP summer courses in the Department of Nursing were limited. Now summer school is busy and full of students. Academic support is provided for pathophysiology through use of peer and graduate tutors. However, this course continues to be problematic, and engenders a great deal of anxiety. The need for additional self paced teaching strategies is evident.

Nursing education is a stressor in the life of students that requires changes and readjustments in the individual routine. The faculty believe that it is critical to have support systems to foster the student ability to cope with the stressful situations engendered by the process of change and readjustments. The student's ability to cope, to view a threat as a challenge, to feel in control of life choices, and to develop a self defined commitment is referred to as hardiness (Kobasa, 1979). Activities to activate personal resistance resources were informal relations created by student contact with NCOP staff through the Transitional Summer Program, the Enrichment Seminars, study groups, and unscheduled office hours for immediate encounters to address problematic issues.

The *Enrichment Seminar,* a one-credit course offered each semester, helps students learn and apply study skills. It provided a non-threatening constructive framework for interaction between students with a focus concern, not with teaching course work, but with the skills and methods required to assimilate course material. The faculty, which consisted of an NCOP staff and an NCOP minority alumnae/i, were constantly talking with students outside of the seminar, and establishing strong, informal relations so that students came to see them as soon as there were problem-atic issues. We supported the belief that the intellectual and social quality of the educational experience for minority students could be enhanced by faculty (Davis, 1995; and Tucker-Allen, 1992).

We found that *mentoring* and nurturing are critical factors in the personal and professional growth of students. Students of color may miss this critical ingredient because many are educated in institutions where there are usually so few minority faculty that the probability of the development of faculty mentor/student of color protege dyads are rare (Tucker-Allen, Steele, and Baker, 1992). What students may lose is the opportunity to be socialized as scholars through relationships with mentors. Mentors may shape, encourage, and often bless the dreams of

Table 5.2
Class Officer Positions Filled by NCOP Students

Class Officers	Academic Year					
	1990	1991	1992	1993	1994	1995
President	1		1			
Vice President	1		1			
Secretary	1					1
Treasurer	1					1

a neophyte, and instill the value of being bonded to the life of the mind. NCOP found that its very presence and its activities seemed to foster a sense of belonging to the academic community.

The Transitional Summer Program provided both peer and faculty mentoring the summer before entry into the nursing program. The trainees experienced contact with the staff and the Health Sciences Campus, as well as exposure to the curriculum, which provided hardiness. The number of students who campaigned and won class offices increased dramatically over the past five years, and most of the minority officers attended the summer program and are in NCOP (see Table 5.2).

In addition to NCOP staff and faculty mentoring, students were supported and learned from each other through informal friendships and student study groups designed to help them solidify content areas as they worked together. Minority professionals who successfully completed nursing programs can provide educational support by *reaching-back* to facilitate retention of students. *Reaching back* activities include mentoring nursing students so that the cycle regenerates itself.

We found individual peer tutoring less effective during the academic year because of the time constraints for students in a busy, fast-paced curriculum. In place of peer tutors, NCOP became more invested in lectures on videotapes, audiocassettes, practice examinations, and limited Computer Assisted Instruction (CAI) tutorials.

Students returned after graduation to talk to the NCOP staff about work situations, plans for the future, and simply to maintain contact. It became apparent that the transitional period into professionalism was very difficult for some of NCOP alumnae/i as they struggled to create a professional role in institutional systems that are not accustomed to minorities as professionals, and therefore, offer limited mentoring opportunities. Some of the issues perceived by them included:

1. Automatic questioning of their competence and not knowing how to address the issue without defensiveness.

2. Feeling uncomfortable about the limits of their responsibility to the staff on the floor. As several students said to the Project Director of NCOP, "I am doing my work. Why should I be expected to socialize?"

3. Graduate education and preparation for entry into schools.

The summer of 1994 graduates of NCOP were given a variety of study options to prepare for the licensing examination. The options included: 1) textbook and computer-assisted instruction, pencil-paper practice test questions, 2) lectures on key topics by faculty, 3) viewing lecture content video tapes and 4) listening to NCLEX-review audiotapes. These resources were used by twenty-seven students. To date, about 90 percent of those who have taken the licensing examination have been successful. A survey of those who participated in this study review has revealed a wide range of personal preferences. The ability to review material repeatedly, particularly the review of videotapes, is a recurrent theme that graduates cite in their successful preparation for the licensing examination. Lectures by faculty were lightly attended and are not cited by students as key to their success.

Since NCOP's inception in 1990, 106 students have been admitted as trainees, and 24 more have joined because of academic difficulties. Three groups have succeeded with an average 85 percent graduation rate that contrasts markedly with the national average of 9.9 percent (see Tables 5.3 and 5.4).

Table 5.3
Ethnicity of NCOP Trainees, 1990–1991

| Group | 1990 | | 1991 | | |
	Male	Female	Male	Female	Subtotal
African American	2	14	1	15	31
Latinos					0
Asian American		2		2	4
Caucasian		2	2		4
Total	2	18	3	17	39

Table 5.4
Ethnicity of NCOP Trainees, 1992–1994

Group	1992 Male	1992 Female	1993 Male	1993 Female	1994 Male	1994 Female	Subtotal
African American	1	11	1	13	3	14	43
Latinos	2	1	2	1	1	5	12
Asian American		2	1	1		4	8
Caucasian	2	1		1			4
Total	5	15	4	16	4	23	67

NCOP consistently retained about 98 percent of its students with about 83 percent of students graduating on time. About 22 percent of NCOP graduates had a GPA of 3.0 or better upon graduation (see Table 5.5).

The number of scholars graduating will be defined as those students who are inducted into Sigma Theta Tau, nursing's honor society (see Table 5.6).

Trainees are the original students who are admitted to the nursing program under objectives 1, 2, 3, and 4, beginning with TISP.

Delayed students are those who failed one of the high-risk nursing courses, thereby, not graduating on time.

Support students are those at risk for failure under objective #5, and join NCOP during the academic year (see p. 96).

The track record for project trainees under NCOP was a passing rate that exceeded the national passing rate for minority/disadvantaged students who participated in the NCOP Program: 1990–1994 (see Table

Table 5.5
Percentage of NCOP Students Receiving
Graduating GPA of 3.0 or Better

Graduating Year	% With GPA of 3.0 or Above
1992	27%
1993	22%
1994	18%
Total (Average)	22%

Table 5.6
NCOP Student Members of Sigma Theta Tau: 1992–1994

Graduating Year	Trainees	Support Students	Delayed Students
1992	5	2	
1993	3	1	
1994	5	1	

5.7). In researching the relationship between entering grade point average, graduating grade point average, and passing the NCLEX-RN licensure examination, no significance was found (Coefficient correlation was .1621). In reviewing the sorted list of NCOP students graduating in 1992–1994, note that the student with the highest entering GPA failed NCLEX-RN licensure examination the first time, and the student with the lowest entering GPA in our program passed the first time. One implication of this specific effect appears to be that an individual can prepare vigorously for the examination, and pass.

As noted previously, the experimental offering of a variety of study options to the summer of 1994 graduates yielded a 90 percent success rate for those taking the licensing examination. This result continues to attest to the impact and wide range of personal preferences for licensure examination preparation.

The graduates had the freedom to choose the approaches to learning that best met their needs. This academic year NCOP has continued to

Table 5.7
NCOP Student Profile, 1990–1994

| | NCOP Students | | | | Graduation |
Year	Trainees	Support	Delayed/ Withdrew	Total Enrollment	Trainees
1990–1991	18	3		21	0
1991–1992	20	3	2/1	43	16 (85%)
1992–1993	20	5	5/0	45	16 (80%)
1993–1994	20	15	6/0	60	18 (85%)
1994–1995	25	19	5/0	64	17 (82%)
Total	103	42	19/1	233	83%

supply students with the videotapes, audiocassettes, and test practice sessions. As requests increased we realized how limited our resources were and yet, how beneficial they were for several students who have had to repeat high-risk nursing theory courses in the past.

For Fall, 1994, NCOP extended its lending library to students who were retaking N201 (Nursing Theory III) after having failed the course in Fall, 1993. (This move was based on the favorable outcomes of the Summer, 1994 experiment.) One of these senior students had one of the highest test scores in the first examination for Nursing III. She told the NCOP staff, "It is important that I am able to see the lecturer and listen to the tape as a part of my preparation in understanding the content." This was a student who has had to struggle to demonstrate marginal mastery of subject matter. Many of the students who, like her, have taken courses twice, usually drop out. The question raised by her motivation and present performance is, how do we use the technology available to personalize learning so that, instead of students having to take the same course twice, they can be exposed to the same content in multiple ways for the purpose of mastery the first time around?

The health care-for-all goal of *Healthy People 2000* requires that nurses not only provide highly specialized care at the secondary and tertiary levels, but also function at the primary level. Universities are called upon to educate a whole new generation of nurses who are concerned with the general health of people rather than being concerned only with the acutely ill in hospital environments (Aksayan, 1994). The nurse practitioner will emerge as a primary mover in this transformation of health care. The minority nurse has an important role to play in shaping this role as the nursing community defines culturally relevant health care. This proposal addresses the education of the critical mass of minority practitioners, managers, and faculty. Our department is committed to meeting this challenge.

NURSING EDUCATION AND THE 21st CENTURY

For the 21st century, nursing has an opportunity to educate a rich, varied and diverse group of nursing leaders—researchers, educators, and managers. The impact of this proposal is: 1) the inculcation of cross-cultural literacy to shift the perception of minority status in health care delivery, and 2) the redefinition of collaborative care.

CROSS-CULTURAL LITERACY TO SHIFT IN THE PERCEPTION OF MINORITY STATUS IN HEALTH CARE DELIVERY

Cross-cultural literacy and awareness are critical to understanding the essence of the American experience (Marable, 1995). Minority health workers will continue to supply a disproportionate amount of manpower in cities and metropolitan areas. Health care professionals from minority and economically disadvantaged backgrounds have shown a tendency to practice in communities where there is a high concentration of ethnic and minority racial groups, and where poor populations identified in *Healthy People 2000* live. Table 5.8 shows the employment pattern of NCOP trainees and support students over the past three graduating classes.

From this group of nurses will come those who will go on to graduate education and prepare for future leadership roles in nursing and the health care system. As national groups (*Healthy People 2000*, 1992), and nursing organizations (ANA, 1991) propose a model of autonomous nursing practice to deliver primary care to a multicultural, underserved population, NCOP and the Department of Nursing are aware that the pool of these perspective graduate students depends on continuing to graduate a large number of minority students from baccalaureate programs. In our first survey of NCOP graduates, 35 percent are interested in pursuing graduate studies. These results are reported in Table 5.9.

INSUFFICIENT NUMBER OF MINORITY NURSES IN LEADERSHIP ROLES

In the 1960s, the goal of the civil rights movement was a struggle for a more inclusive and humanistic definition of democracy (Marable, 1995).

Table 5.8
Employment Pattern of NCOP Graduates

Class	Urban Area	Suburbs	Rural	Armed Services	Nursing Homes
1992	11	0	0	1	2
1993	14	0	0	3	3
1994	5	0	0	4	4

Table 5.9
NCOP Trainees and Graduate Education

Class	Part-time	Full-time	Interested
1992	2	1	2
1993	3	1	2

The challenges were to expand the boundaries of democracy and to transcend race, gender, and class. A part of the representation of this struggle was to be the expansion of minorities and women in positions of leadership and power. Yet in the 1990s, Table 5.1 shows that the number of minority nurses diminish as they enter leadership positions. In 1989–90 of the 5,477 students graduating from master's programs in nursing, 231 (4.6 percent) were black. The provision of graduate preparation for minority nurses is among the most important and pressing educational issues facing nursing today if we are to prepare primary care practitioners and managers, researchers, and nursing faculty.

Primary Care Practitioners and Managers

One of the major aspects of the crisis in health care is the lack of an adequate number of nurse practitioners from economically and culturally diverse backgrounds to serve as a critical mass in changing the way health care is delivered to populations (Healthy People 2000, 1992). The literature on nursing administration also supports that there are few minority nurses at the administrative level (Schmieding, 1991). It is on this group of nurses that ever-growing numbers of black Americans, Latinos, Asian/Pacific Islanders, and American Indians must depend for shifting the paradigm in health care delivery (Weekes, 1989).

Researchers

Minorities are poorly represented in research subject populations, creating the possibility of insufficient data for optimal use of treatment intervention (Rosella, Regan-Kubinski, and Albrecht, 1994; Svensson, 1989). Yet it has been demonstrated that race, class, and ethnic issues are of central importance to our understanding of health and illness (Cooper, 1991; Kumanyika & Golden, 1991).

Nursing Faculty

Ethnic minority educators and administrators are underrepresented in higher educational institutions. Emphasis on consciousness raising must be a part of the agenda, as institutional barriers continue to exist. Often, information on scholarly opportunities is not readily shared with minority faculty. In addition, minority graduate students may be overlooked when faculty choose students to work closely with them on scientific projects. In some instances, this oversight helps to maintain the perception that minority students are academically deficient and destined to fail. Also, "People tend to mentor those who look like them" (Tucker-Allen, 1994, p. 90). In order to improve the educational experience of minority students, institutions of higher education must enhance the intellectual and social environment by increasing the numbers of minority faculty members (Campbell & Sigsby, 1994).

THE REDEFINITION OF COLLABORATION

The intense political debate about the universality of health care benefits is a primary agenda item for now and in the future. As Americans move toward some model of universal health care benefits, we must be careful that we avoid the mechanisms of privilege and exclusion which maintain a two-tier system of delivery, one of insured, middle and upper classes, and the other for the poor.

Health care must be extended to everyone since the interests of the poor and the disadvantaged are not isolated from the broader pattern of a costly, fragmented health care system which does not work well for most. We need a broad agenda and a representative dialogue to overcome the formidable combination of class interests, professional routines, and institutional hierarchies (Russell, 1992).

The traditional model in health care in which minorities are disproportionately represented on the paraprofessional level does not lend itself to developing a broad agenda for health care reform. The new collaborative model will have a more representative proportion of all groups in the health care professions at all levels, in order to shift the bases of what constitutes competent and humane care in the 21st century.

The nursing faculty contributes to the diversified leadership by educating and graduating students who reflect the society's composition (Fong,

1991). The faculty contributes to the new agenda by making competence in work with disadvantaged groups central to the idea of professionalism in nursing.

REFERENCES

Aksayan, S. (1994). Education of nurses for primary health care. *World Health Forum, 15*, 150–152.

Campbell, D. W., & Sigsby, L. M. (1994). Increasing minorities in higher education in nursing: Faculty consultation as a strategy. *Journal of Professional Nursing, 1*, 7–12.

———— Caring for the emerging majority: Creating a new diversity in nurse leadership: Proceedings of an invitational congress (1992). Washington, DC: US Division of Nursing, DHHS, HRSA, Office of Minority Health.

———— Author. (1991). Nursing's agenda for health care reform. Kansas City, MO: American Nurses Association.

Connell, R. W. (1994). Poverty and education. *Harvard Educational Review, 64*(2), 98–107.

Cooper, M. C. (1991). Principle-oriented ethics and the ethics of care: A creative tension. *American Nursing Science, 14*(6), 22–31.

Davis, S. P. (1995). A challenge to develop a new paradigm shift in nursing education. *Journal of Cultural Diversity. 2*(4), 124–130.

———— Department of Commerce, Bureau of the Census. Statistical abstract of the United States. Washington, DC: US Government Printing Office, 1992.

Fleming, J. W. (1992). Change: Both a reality and a challenge. *Journal of American Black Nursing Faculty, 3*(3), 58–62.

Fong, C. M. (1991). Nursing needs minorities. *Advanced Clinical Care, 6*(1), 19–21.

———— *Healthy people 2000: National health promotion and disease prevention objectives* (1992). Washington, DC: US Department of Health and Human Services. DHHS Publication PHS 91-50212.

Kobasa, S. (1979). Stressful life events, personality, and health: An inquiry into hardiness. *Journal of Personality and Social Psychology, 37*(1), 1–10.

Kumanyika, S. K., & Golden, P. M. (1991). Cross-sectional differences in health status in US racial/ethnic minority groups: Potential influence on temporal changes, disease, and life style transitions. *Ethnicity & Disease, 1*(4), 50–59.

Manzo, K. (1994). Priorities: Retention more visible after decades of neglect. *Black Issues in Higher Education.*

Marable, M. (1995). *Beyond black and white: Rethinking race in American politics and society.* Verso: New York.

McBay, S. M. (1992). Quality education for minorities: Myths, realities, and strategies. *Perspectives in Nursing, 1991–1993*, pp. 23–34. New York: NLN Press. Pub. No. 41-2472.

———— Nursing's agenda for health care reform (1992). New York: National League For Nursing.

O'Hare, W. P. (1992). America's minorities—The demographics of diversity. *Popular Bulletin*, 1–72.

Powell, D. L. (1992). The recruitment and retention of African American nurses: An analysis of the current data. *Journal of National Black Nurses Association*, 6(1), 3–12.

Rodriquez, R. (1994). HACU examines the status of Hispanic education. *Black Issues In Higher Education*, 11(24), p. 11.

Rosella, J. D., Regan-Kubinski, M. J., Albrecht, S.A. (1994). The need for multicultural diversity among health professionals. *Nursing and Health Care*, 15(5), 242–246.

Russell, K. (1992). Strengthening black and minority coalitions for health policy action. *Journal of National Black Nurses Association*, 6(1), 42–47.

Saucier, B. L. (1994). Retention of nursing students: Intervention strategies. *Review of Research in Nursing Education*, Vol. VI, pp. 107–126. New York: NLN Press. Pub. No. 19-2544.

Schmieding, N. J. (1991). A novel approach to recruitment, retention, and advancement of minority nurses in a health care organization. *Nursing Administration*, 15(4), 69–76.

Shalala, D. E. (1993). Nursing and society: The unfinished agenda for the 21st century. *Nursing and Health Care*, 14(6), 289–291.

Svensson, C. K. (1989). Representation of American blacks in clinical trials of new drugs. *Journal of American Medical Association*, 26(13), 263–265.

Tucker-Allen, S. (1992). Diversity in nursing faculty hinges on diversity in nursing students. *Perspectives in Nursing, 1991–1993*. New York: National League for Nursing, Publication No. 41-2472, 35–42.

Tucker-Allen, S., Steele, R., & Baker, S. (1992). Mentoring role of black nursing faculty members. *Association of Black Nursing Faculty Journal*, 3(4), 89–92.

Weekes, D. P. (1989). Mentor-protegé relationship: A critical element in affirmative action. *Nursing Outlook, 37*, 147–156.

6

Access to Higher Education for All Americans—The Role of Associate Degree Nursing

Andrea Mengel and Susan Sherman

Community colleges are a uniquely American form of education. They are old enough to be an established part of higher education, yet their contributions to society and their mission are often misunderstood or misinterpreted. The mission of community colleges generally reflects five basic responsibilities: a transfer function; student services such as counseling and developmental or remedial education; technical curricula for the student preparing for a career; general education courses to meet community needs for personal growth and civic responsibility; and service to the community (Phelan, 1994). Most students enroll at community colleges for one of three purposes. One group of students attends to prepare for college level work. These students didn't apply themselves in high school or came from secondary schools which did not adequately prepare them for college level work, a common situation in inner cities. A second group of students enrolls to attain credits for transfer to a college or university in pursuit of a baccalaureate degree. The lower cost of community colleges frequently attracts this group which also includes students with family responsibilities who need to commute to school while living at home. Also represented in this group are students who are not certain that college is for them, so they elect to remain close to their support systems while they try college work. The third group of students consists of people wanting to develop job skills. This group is made up of women returning to the job market after rearing children and workers who are displaced or want a different type of career. This group also includes college graduates, some from elite four-year institutions and some with graduate degrees, who either want a new career or find they need more marketable skills. Given these various groups, it is difficult to describe a typical community college student, except to say the student is a person who wants or needs what the community college has to offer.

Community colleges have a tradition of serving Americans who did not always find a welcoming, supportive environment in higher education. This is true of associate degree nursing programs (ADN) as well, which have always attracted non-traditional students: older, minority, lower socioeconomic class and many times unsure of their educational goals. And as America becomes more racially and ethnically diverse, the role of community colleges in providing access to higher education takes on new importance. Today, approximately one fourth of Americans represent minority groups, yet less than ten percent of American registered nurses represent minority groups, and only about one percent of minority nurses have graduate degrees. The promised land of higher education is not a reality for all Americans. This chapter will explore some of the issues associated with this concern.

THE RISE OF ASSOCIATE DEGREE NURSING

Associate degree nursing programs were the first educationally planned and systematically evaluated nursing programs. They began in the early 1950s in response to the building of hospitals, important advances in biomedical treatment of illness and the expansion of private health insurance (Haase, 1990). At about the same time, community colleges were responding to the needs of Americans during and after World War II. This response led to a period of rapid growth. During World War II, licensed practical nursing program graduates (LPN) had supplemented the work of registered nurses, since so many registered nurses were in military service. At that time, the need for nurses was so dramatic that diploma schools accelerated their programs by decreasing the time of study from three years to two years. Concurrently, the federally financed Cadet Corps began, providing free education to nurses. This dramatically increased the number of registered nurse graduates, at the same time illustrating that high quality nursing education could occur in a shorter time period. Following the war, there was a rapid expansion in the number of hospitals, leading to an even greater demand for more nurses. With the GI bill and other money available to veterans for higher education, a much larger group of Americans found college education affordable. For the first time, many Americans had access to a college education, something that had been available previously to only members of the wealthy and upper middle classes.

Community colleges began to grow in number, expanding program offerings and increasing enrollments. They provided access to new and different populations—the older, non-traditional, commuter student— and were comfortable places for these students. Diversity in age, gender, race, academic ability and socioeconomic status was, and is, the hallmark of community college students. This diverse population was found among associate degree nursing students as well, because at the time, married students, pregnant students and men were not usually permitted to enroll in diploma programs, still the predominant form of nursing education (Haase, 1990).

The Issue of Access

Nursing is a vivid example of all that happens in education to limit access to secondary and higher education for groups of individuals. Nursing typifies how minority and low income students are advised early in life that college is not realistic for them. Feedback and expectations from teachers and guidance counselors direct these students into vocational programs or directly to the job market without additional education or training. The demographics of LPNs in inner cities and rural areas illustrate this well. A very large percent of LPNs in these areas are members of minority groups, challenging the imagination to accept that all of them chose this path without guidance.

Recent sincere, coordinated efforts to increase minority participation in higher education have had some positive effects. Yet, while minority student college enrollment is up, minority students are at risk for not successfully completing college. Minority students consistently have lower retention and graduation rates than majority students. Unfortunately, a lot of minority students think college is not within their reach. Others are hampered by sub-par secondary education and need substantial developmental or pre-college work prior to enrolling in college courses. Increasingly, a large portion of the resources of community colleges are dedicated to providing developmental, remedial, or pre-college support to students.

And some minority students leave college because they are disappointed by college or because they run out of money. Existing subsidies for college education are diminishing. Loans are becoming the primary way of financing education for needy students. In addition, there are fewer direct grants to schools of nursing and less money for traineeships for nursing students. Once again, as before World War II, finances are fast becoming a powerful, real barrier to accessing higher education. Combined with sometimes sub-par secondary education in inner city schools, this is threatening to reduce substantially the number of minority students choosing a career in nursing. Those who do may be unable to commit to a four-year education because of cost or the belief that they can not achieve or do not belong. Instead, they begin as licensed practical nurses or enter an associate degree nursing program. The challenge for nursing educators is to find ways to support these students in their pursuit of a nursing career.

The Case for Community Colleges

Community colleges offer affordable, accessible, convenient educational opportunities. They have a history of successful partnerships with the communities which support them, responding in fast, innovative and flexible ways to meet the needs of the community and of business and industry (Phelan, 1994). As the health care industry undergoes rapid change, transforming itself in a short time period, there will continue to be rapid changes in the nursing job market. Community colleges are well positioned to respond quickly to the work force needs of the health care industry by offering basic nursing education, continuing education and training of unlicensed personnel. Community colleges were built "on the philosophy of shared vision and accountability to the community. In this sense, they have always had a comparative edge in the marketplace" (Lindeman, 1995, p. 26). In addition to being accountable to the local community which provides support, community colleges are accountable to the demands of four-year schools to which some students transfer. These three sources of accountability—community, business and industry and four-year schools—coalesce to create unique tensions and opportunities. Community colleges must respond to a changing health care industry while serving the needs of their local communities and maintaining the high quality education expected by their students and by the four-year schools to which the students transfer. While this sounds daunting, it is not, as evidenced by the successes of community colleges and their graduates.

Community college nursing students are like all community college students in that they are a diverse group in terms of age, ethnicity, academic ability and socioeconomic class. They are different from most other nursing students in that they live in the community where they study and usually have deep roots in that community. Very few leave the community after graduation. This provides a valuable work force resource in underserved areas. Most associate degree nursing students are adult learners, motivated to succeed and having learned a few valuable lessons about life, work and priorities as a result of their prior experiences.

Community college students often *zigzag* from high school to work to the community college to the four-year college (Griffin and Connor, 1994). Rather than entering college directly after high school, these students may work for a few years after high school, take a course at a community college, continue to work while attending an associate degree nursing program, work as a registered nurse following graduation, return to the community college to take prerequisite courses needed for a baccalaureate degree, then enroll in a bachelor's degree in nursing program. In addition to providing flexibility and opportunity, the community college allows students to live at home, providing quicker and more frequent access to the student's personal support system. As part of their mission, community colleges also provide a variety of academic and other student support services to enhance success.

Obviously, this zigzag career path is not traditional, and it was not efficient before articulation models became commonplace. It is, however, a proven path to success for students who are unsure of their career goals, uncertain of their academic abilities, or unable to finance a college education. The function of community colleges is to give a chance to people who wouldn't have a chance otherwise, and, if they need it, a second and third chance (Griffith and Connor, 1994).

Questions About the Role of Community Colleges

Community colleges have been criticized for providing inferior education and for not doing enough to provide social mobility to minorities, women and people from lower socioeconomic classes. It has been said that the curriculum, students and faculty of community colleges do not compare favorably with those found in four-year schools (Pincus, 1994). Community colleges have also been faulted for reproducing race, class and gender inequalities that are part of larger society (Pincus, 1994). Critics contend that community colleges perpetuate the class structure by educating minorities for low paying, mid-level jobs while more advantaged students are able to attend a four-year school and capture the higher paying, higher status jobs (Pincus, 1994).

It is true that less advantaged students are more likely to attend community colleges. It is also true, and troubling, that the percent of community college students who transfer to four-year colleges and earn a baccalaureate degree is decreasing while the non-completion rate for community college students is increasing. The economic benefit to the student of attending a community college is under question (Pincus, 1994). Currently, this question is not being asked of associate degree nursing graduates because these graduates have a history of performing exceptionally well on the registered nurse licensing examination, being successful in their work and transferring with advanced standing to four-year nursing programs.

Perhaps expectations of community colleges are too high and too far reaching. Eaton (1994) argues that the expectation that community colleges produce a major change in socioeconomic status for a demographic group within a short time is unreasonable, and not demanded of any other educational institution. The focus on upward mobility for a group may be unrealistic and should be tempered by the upward mobility opportunities for individuals who are members of less advantaged groups (Eaton, 1994). Community colleges face a unique dilemma which originates in their mission and highlights the tension which sometimes arises between opportunity and excellence. More than any other educational institutions, community colleges are expected to provide both inclusion through open access and exclusion through curricular excellence (Eaton, 1994). It is a difficult balancing act which requires an ongoing commitment to access while strengthening transfer curricula and general education offerings which will, in turn, increase access to the baccalaureate degree. This will benefit all students who attend community colleges and expand an achievement agenda for minorities (Eaton, 1994).

THE ROLE OF ASSOCIATE DEGREE NURSING IN THE 21st CENTURY

Community colleges, with their multi-faceted missions, are uniquely positioned to respond to changes in the health care industry. At the same time, they are challenged to do more with fewer resources, as is all of higher education. As a result, their commitment to maintaining their multiple missions and flexibility in the twenty-first century will be tested (Griffith and Connor, 1994). The tension beween opportunity and excellence is sometimes evidenced in the student population of associate degree nursing programs. As a result of the meritocratic selection process, the nursing student body does not always mirror the demographics of the community college student population. Because community college students have the widest range of academic abilities, not all students are able to enter nursing, one of the most selective and challenging curricula found in community colleges. Meritocracy does not run counter to the mission of community colleges, but it does need to be balanced with the opportunity for students to develop their academic potential so they can enter the nursing curriculum based on merit.

Changes are occurring so rapidly in the health care industry that it is difficult to predict what work force is needed and how that work force can be best educated. Other industries have taught us that technology does not eliminate jobs; rather it creates a need for stronger basic skills (Griffith and Connor, 1994). We have also learned that fewer industries are offering their own training, placing that responsibility on workers or forming partnerships with educational institutions, especially community colleges. In addition, industry now seems to favor multi-skilled employees.

All of these factors bode well for the future of community colleges and lead to the question: what is the role of the associate degree graduate in the reconfigured health care industry? Nurses in the twenty-first century will need new skills to work in community settings and integrated health care. Continuing education will be needed to remain current and nursing education programs must be designed to accommodate and adapt to change (Canavan, 1996). As ADN programs incorporate community-based care in their curricula, the differences between ADN and baccalaureate nurses become less clear and baccalaureate nursing educators must demonstrate how their graduate differs from the ADN (Conway-Welch, 1996). While the Pew Health Professions Committee predicted an oversupply of registered nurses, it did not suggest closing associate degree programs. In fact, it endorsed multiple entry points for students wishing to become registered nurses (Pew, 1995).

In some ways, the entry into practice debate is an artifact of the late twentieth century. The new health care system demands a worker who can prove effectiveness of both cost and quality through outcomes research. Much of the work done by nurses will remain the same, regardless of the setting. Associate degree nursing graduates have a long history of being well qualified, valuable, effective employees. As associate degree curricula evolve to prepare graduates for new settings, they will compete with graduates of other types of programs for the same job. Since diploma, associate degree and baccalaureate nursing graduates have the same licensing credential, employers will choose based on what their organization needs. In a community-based care system, it makes sense for employers to hire associate degree nursing graduates, people of and committed to the community. The clearest differences in practice occur between associate degree and master's prepared nurses. When associate degree programs began, founders carved out the technical piece of nursing but did not define it in relation to professional nursing. At that time, the diploma was the professional nursing credential. Until the mid-1960s, associate degree programs were a subgroup of the diploma council of the National League for Nursing. Our history suggests that internal debates about entry into practice at the undergraduate level have been divisive and counterproductive. Now is the time for nursing to consolidate its efforts to advance nursing in a rapidly changing system by supporting multiple entry and exit points for nursing education.

Continuing the Tradition of Opportunity

Community colleges, a uniquely American endeavor, have done much to increase access to higher education for Americans, regardless of race, gender or class. In fact, they have done an admirable job of educating minority students, women and people from lower socioeconomic classes. While there is more to be done, changes in funding for students participating in higher education make it imperative that the opportunities provided by community colleges be maintained and strengthened. Whether preparing to transfer into a baccalaureate nursing program, catching up on basic skills before beginning college level courses, or completing an associate degree nursing program, the student attending a community college needs the enthusiastic support of the entire nursing profession. This is the route that will continue to provide a culturally and ethnically diverse nursing work force and supply nurses committed to working in underserved communities in the twenty-first century. With a seamless articulation model in place, community colleges undoubtedly will continue to launch nursing leaders of the twenty-first century.

REFERENCES

Canavan, K. (1996). Nursing Education on Cusp of Shift in Focus. *American Nurse*, September 1996.

Conway-Welch, C. (1996). Who is Tomorrow's Nurse and Where will Tomorrow's Nurse be Educated? *Nursing and Health Care: Perspectives on Community*, *17*(6), 287–290, November–December 1996.

Eaton, J. S. (1994). *Strengthening Collegiate Education in Community Colleges*. San Francisco: Jossey-Bass.

Griffith, M., & Connor, A. (1994). *Democracy's Open Door: The Community College in America's Future*. Portsmouth, NH: Boynton/Cook.

Haase, P. T. (1990). *The Origins and Rise of Associate Degree Nursing Education*. Durham, NC: Duke University Press.

Lindeman, C. (1995). Vision for Nursing Education Reform. In P. Bayles and J. Parks-Doyle, *The Web of Inclusion: Faculty Helping Faculty*. New York: NLN Press.

Pew Health Professions Commissions (1995). *Critical Challenges: Revitalizing the Health Professions for the Twenty-First Century*. San Francisco: Pew Health Professions Commissions.

Phelan, D. J. (1994). The Challenges and Obligations Facing Community Colleges in the Twentieth Century: A Community-Based Perspective (603–614). In G. A. Baker III, *A Handbook on the Community College in America: Its History, Mission and Management*. Westport, CT: Greenwood Press.

Pincus, F. L. (1994). How Critics View the Community College's Role in the Twenty-First Century (624–636). In G. A. Baker III, *A Handbook on the Community College in America: Its History, Mission and Management*. Westport, CT: Greenwood Press.

Part IV

Creating the Climate for Competent Response

Developing cultural competence is a requirement for the profession if we are to be responsive to the needs of an increasingly diverse population. It is encouraging to note the attention that many nurse educators are paying to preparing nurses to provide appropriate care.

Dr. Adderley-Kelly captures what can occur when the classroom serves as a laboratory for helping students who represent a widely diverse cultural mix. In such an environment students are challenged to become comfortable with their own culture following which they are able to share more readily with each other in a supportive environment. When the educator captures these *teachable moments* there is greater assurance that more culturally competent care results.

Dr. Drayton-Hargrove joins in the debate and believes that higher education must engage multiculturalism as a phenomenon to be seriously enhanced. She acknowledges that the concept is in direct opposition to assimilation. In addition, there is recognition of the need for support of the entire faculty for nurse educators who facilitate learning about multiculturalism, often an uncomfortable arena. Sharing the development of a two credit graduate course, Dr. Drayton-Hargrove provides a prototype which should prove useful to many.

Just as it is encouraging to note the strides being made to enhance student preparation in providing culturally competent care through course development, it is likewise encouraging to note the added dimension which minority students bring when asked about their experiences as students. We can learn a great deal from them regarding what is helpful to assure their completion of the nursing program. Student voices, as shared with us by Dr. Brennan, are instructive in enhancing the educational experience of selected minority students. Listening to others becomes a useful strategy in providing culturally competent care as well.

7

Developing Cultural Competence for Health Care in the 21st Century

Beatrice Adderley-Kelly

W*e are living in* a culturally diverse society which is becoming increasingly diverse everyday. We must accept the fact that cultural diversity in the United States is a reality which has far reaching economic, social and political implications. The cultural differences that exist among the various cultural groups must be addressed if we are to be considered a society of inclusion rather than one of exclusion. Providing culturally competent care to this diverse population will be a challenge for nurses and other health care providers and nurses will need to develop an understanding of culture and culturally competent care to be effective caregivers in this changing society.

This chapter focuses on the concepts of culture and culturally competent care and is organized in subsections. It begins with a discussion of the changing demographics followed by relevant definitions and characteristics of culture and the dimensions of culturally competent care. It provides a brief overview of an approach for developing cultural competence and ends with a discussion of how to develop cultural competence in beginning undergraduate nursing students. Culture is viewed as a common influencing stimulus and as such has an affect on all behavior (Roy & Andrews, 1991).

CHANGING DEMOGRAPHICS

By the year 2000 the racial and ethnic composition of the American population will be quite different from what it was just 50 years ago. People of color will be the majority in 53 of the largest cities in the United States. White, not including Hispanic, Americans will represent a smaller proportion of the population. Hispanics, the fastest growing population, will rise from 8 to 11.3 percent. The African American population will increase in proportion from 12.4 to 13.1 percent. Other racial groups, American Indians, Alaskan Natives and Asian Pacific Islanders, will increase from 3.5 to 4.3 percent of the total (Healthy People 2000). It has been predicted that by the end of the 21st century there will be no majority population, only minority groups. Other experts predict that by the year 2030 people of color will make up more than half of the U.S. population (Nestor, 1991 cited in Unity Through Diversity, Healthy Mothers, Healthy Babies Coalition, 1993). These demographics will have a definite impact on the health of the nation, particularly since among the different cultural groups experiencing rapid growth, many face worsening health problems. Nurses and other health care personnel will be interacting with clients, families and other health care consumers from virtually every place in the world. This will require that health care providers have knowledge and skills to meet the health care needs of this culturally diverse population.

There must be commitment at all levels to address the health care needs of this culturally diverse society, as well as understanding that cultural differences exist, not only among but within each cultural group. The health care system must recognize and respect cultural diversity and provide culturally competent services to the communities being served. Nursing education must recognize the impact that cultural diversity has on the profession, education, and health care. Curricula must embrace culturalism as a conceptual thread to enable nursing to provide culturally competent care (Alpers & Zoucha, 1996; Compinha-Bacote, Yahle & Langenkamp, 1996; Rosella, Regan-Kubinski & Albrecht, 1994).

Leininger (1994) states that providing culturally congruent care should be one of the highest priorities of nursing organizations and educational institutions as they plan for health care reform and to function in a multicultural world. Practicing nurses and nursing students must integrate the concepts of cultural diversity and culturally competent care into practice. This requires prerequisite knowledge of culture and its relevant concepts, cultural competence, culturally competent care, and the relationships that exist among these phenomena (Clinton, 1996).

CULTURE DEFINED

Culture is a complex and universal phenomenon with no single definition. There are many definitions of culture cited in the literature. A few which seem to encompass the salient points will be noted. Broadly defined, culture is a set of values, beliefs and traditions that are held by a specific social group and handed down from generation to generation. Values are personal perceptions of what is good or useful and values guide the differentiation of desirable from undesirable states of affairs (Taylor, Lillis & Lemone, 1993; Edelman & Mandle, 1994). Culture represents a way of perceiving, behaving, and evaluating one's world. It provides the blueprint or guide for determining one's values, beliefs, and practices (Andrews & Boyle, 1995). Leininger (1991) defines culture as including all human activities taking material and nonmaterial forms and expression. The American Academy of Nursing (AAN) defines culture as a socially transmitted design for living which includes traditional values, beliefs, rituals, and behaviors, prejudices, idiosyncrasies, and transmitted memory of a particular people, as well as changes that evolve over time through social exchanges and adaptations (Lenburg et al., 1995).

According to Roy and Andrews (1991) culture, along with family and developmental stage, are common influencing stimuli that affect a person's ability to adapt. Stimuli are defined as that which provoke a response. Sato (cited in Roy & Andrews, 1991) described culture as involving socioeconomic status, ethnicity and belief systems. Within this view, socioeconomic status provides an indication of the person's style of living and the material resources upon which the person has to draw. Different stimuli are evident in situations of different socioeconomic status. Ethnicity is viewed as including language, practices, philosophies, and associated values.

A belief system, as a component of culture, is viewed as involving spiritual beliefs, practices, and philosophies and may influence all aspects of a person's life. All facets of human behavior, according to Spector (1996) can be interpreted as being influenced by culture. These influences may be so subtle that people are rarely aware of their effect. Culture thus can be viewed as a contextual stimulus having an affect on all behavior.

Culture has several characteristics. Andrews and Boyle (1995) and Hamilton (1996) identify four basic characteristics: 1) It is learned from birth through the process of language acquisition and socialization, 2) It is shared by all members of the same cultural group, 3) It is adapted to specific conditions related to environmental and technical factors and to the availability of natural resources, and 4) It is a dynamic and ever-changing process.

Spector (1996) identifies six characteristics of culture to include the following: 1) Culture is the medium of present and social relationships, 2) Only a part of culture is conscious, 3) Culture is an extension of biological capabilities, 4) Culture is an interlinked web of symbols, 5) Culture is a device for creating and limiting human choices, and 6) Culture exists in two places at the same time, in a person's mind and in the environment. Nurses need to take these characteristics into consideration as they consider the effects of culture on nursing care.

In addition to the basic characteristics of culture, Giger and Davidhizar (1990, 1995) have identified six cultural phenomena that vary between cultural groups and are affected by culture. These include communication, time orientation, environmental control, biological variations, space and social organization. An understanding of these cultural phenomena and their implications for nursing care will enhance the nurse's ability to provide culturally competent care when working with clients from multicultural populations. These phenomena have been discussed in depth in other sources and only a brief overview will be presented here.

Communication

Communication and culture are closely intertwined. Communication, which involves verbal, nonverbal and body language, is the means by which culture is transmitted and preserved. Culture influences how feelings are expressed and what verbal and nonverbal expressions are appropriate. Communication patterns differ among cultural groups and among subcultures of a group. The nurse must develop a sensitivity to communication variances as a prerequisite for accurate assessment and intervention in multicultural situations. In all nursing situations the potential for misunderstanding the client is accentuated when the nurse and the client are from different ethnic groups. The most significant and obvious barrier occurs when the nurse and the client speak different languages (Kirkpatrick & Deloughery, 1995). However, the nurse must be aware of the fact that barriers to communication exist even when individuals speak the same language. The nurse must develop a familiarity with the language of the client, because this is the best way to gain insight into the culture (Baldonado, 1996).

Biological Variations

The ways in which people from one cultural group differ biologically from members of other cultural groups constitute their biological variations. Significant biological variations include body structure and build; skin color, enzymatic and genetic variations; susceptibility to disease, and nutritional variations. The biological differences evident among people in various racial groups must be considered when administering nursing care. Knowledge of these biological differences is necessary in order to provide culturally competent care (Giger, Davidhizar & Wieczorek, 1994).

Social Organization

Cultural behavior, or how one acts in certain situations, is socially acquired. Patterns of cultural behaviors are learned through a process called enculturation, also referred to as socialization. Enculturation involves acquiring knowledge and internalizing values. The social environment in which people grow up and live plays an essential role in their cultural development and identification. Patterns of cultural behavior are important to the nurse because they provide explanations for behavior related to life events.

Environmental Control

Environmental control is the ability of members of a particular cultural group to plan activities that control nature. Environmental control also refers to the individual's perception of ability to direct factors in the environment. Environment encompasses relevant systems and processes that affect individuals. Environmental control plays an important role in the way clients respond to health-related experiences, that is, the way in which they define health and illness and the way in which they use health care resources and supports. The systems of traditional health and illness beliefs, the practice of folk medicine, and the use of traditional healers are also included in the concept (Giger & Davidhizar, 1995; Specter, 1996).

Personal Space

Personal space is the area surrounding a person that is regarded as part of the person. This area, which is individualized to each person and to different cultures and ethnic groups, is the distance maintained from others during communications. Territoriality, a concept of the space and things that an individual considers as belonging to the self, connotes the pattern of behavior arising from an individual's feeling that certain spaces and objects belong to that person. When one's personal space is disregarded, one may become uncomfortable or even angry. Personal space as well as territoriality are influenced by an individual's culture and ethnicity. Different ethnic and cultural groups have varying norms related to the use of space. Nursing care involves close physical contact and communication, therefore, it is important to know cultural personal space preferences.

In addition to the preceding six phenomena identified, gender roles, family support, food and nutritional practices have also been identified as factors influencing health. These factors are influenced by culture and must be considered by the nurse if culturally competent care is to be rendered (Kozier, Erb, Blais & Wilkinson, 1995).

CULTURAL COMPETENCE AND CULTURALLY COMPETENT CARE DEFINED

The term culturally competent care is replacing culturally sensitive care because the latter term no longer accurately reflects the level of expertise needed by nurses who practice in our culturally diverse society (AAN, 1992). In order to become culturally competent, nurses must understand the concept, acquire the requisite knowledge and skills and then they must provide culturally competent care to clients of culturally diverse backgrounds. According to the American Academy of Nursing:

"Cultural competence is a complex integration of knowledge, attitudes and skills that enhances cross-cultural communications and appropriate/ effective interactions with others. It includes at least three perspectives:

(1) Knowledge of the effects of culture on others' beliefs and behavior, (2) Awareness of one's own cultural attributes and biases and their impact on others, and (3) Understanding of the impact of socio-political, environmental and economic context on the specific situation. It also includes an individual's ability to translate these perspectives into communication and interactions with other individuals and groups that integrate respect for cultural variation (Lenburg et al., 1995, p. 35). Cross-cultural nursing care is defined as care provided to individuals, families, or groups who are considered underserved as a result of race, culture, heritage, or sexual orientation. Culturally competent care is defined as care that takes into account issues related to diversity, marginalization, and vulnerability due to culture, race, gender, and sexual orientation (Meleis, Isenberg, Koerner, Lacy & Stern, 1995).

The definitions used here are from the monographs of the American Academy of Nursing. They have chosen to use the term cross-cultural in describing health care as opposed to transcultural because they consider cross-cultural to be more global, interdisciplinary and generic.

Dimensions of Culturally Competent Care

Five central dimensions of culturally competent care have been identified:

1. Awareness and sensitivity to cultural diversity.
2. Knowledge of cultural concepts/patterns.
3. Skills in the integration of cultural concepts into practice.
4. Focus on the interaction among the patient's ethnic/cultural, biological, psychological, sociological, spiritual, and economic systems rather than the function of the isolated elements.
5. Promotion of an environment context where values, customs, and beliefs of individual are respected (Warda, 1995).

Awareness involves recognition of issues that relate to cultural diversity. Sensitivity implies understanding the implications and meanings of the processes from the point of view of those directly affected. Cultural sensitivity involves learning new information so that various perspectives can be understood and appreciated (Pedersen, 1988 cited in Warda, 1995). Nurses must be aware of and sensitive to their own values, beliefs, and traditions. They must be aware of their own cultural biases and prejudices and respect both the differences and similarities among cultures. Awareness that there are commonalities among all cultural groups but that each group is different can do much to reduce the feelings of frustration for a nurse trying to provide care to clients of diverse cultural backgrounds (Busby, 1995). Awareness of one's thinking and behavior patterns can help accommodate those patterns to situations when differences arise as a result of cultural factors. For any one to work effectively with culturally/ethnically diverse groups they must begin with cultural awareness and sensitivity and accept the underlying premise that cultural differences exist and cultural uniqueness is a valid and integral part of each person (Warda, 1995). When the nurse is able to convey awareness and sensitivity to clients' unique health and illness beliefs and practices, good rapport is established. This promotes the delivery of safe and culturally competent care.

The second dimension, knowledge of cultural concepts and patterns, is essential to understanding cross-cultural health care issues. Because cultural differences can be critical in health care, nurses must be able to understand the cultural backgrounds of each client including his or her behaviors, beliefs, and expectations. Knowledge of patterned cultural characteristics and the symbolism and meaning attached to those characteristics broaden one's perspectives in caring for patients of diverse backgrounds (Warda, 1995). Learning about other cultures increases one's options by providing a wider perspective out of which decisions can be made. Enhancement of clients' health practices is contingent on the nurse's ability to use the individual's culturally based beliefs and values in the design of nursing interventions (Rojas, 1994). When nurses lack basic knowledge of culture, clients of diverse cultural backgrounds receive less than optimal nursing care (Kirkpatrick & Deloughery, 1995).

The third dimension is using skills in the integration of cultural concepts into practice. An essential part of practicing cultural competence is the learned and deliberate use of respectful behaviors and interactions. When interacting with culturally diverse groups it is essential to show respect for differences in values, beliefs, mores, and preferences of individuals, families, groups and communities (AAN, 1995). Clinical experience, cultural awareness, and bilingual ability have been identified as basic components of cross-cultural practice (Applewhite, Wong & Daly, 1991 cited in Warda, 1995).

The fourth dimension, the interaction of the patient's ethnic/cultural, biological, psychological, sociological, spiritual, and economic systems, must be considered in order to provide culturally competent care. The influence of socioeconomic status on health care is widely accepted. Socioeconomic status provides an indication of the person's style of living and the material resources upon which a person has to draw (Roy and Andrews, 1991). It is well documented that access to health care by individuals who are poor, minority, especially black and Hispanic, and/or uninsured is limited. In the United States health care disparities exist along racial lines. This problem is so severe that it is addressed by goals two and three of Healthy People 2000 (U.S. Department of Health and Human Services, 1990). People with low incomes, people who are members of some minority groups, and people with disabilities have been identified as those population groups that are at especially high risk and those that now experience above average incidence of death, disease, and disability. Healthy People 2000 acknowledges that even though these special population groups often need targeted preventive efforts, such efforts require understanding the needs of these groups. They further acknowledge that the special populations themselves are extremely heterogeneous and that variations within each group are extensive. Generalizations, which characterize population profiles by definitions, are dangerous because the exceptions are many.

The psychological system which addresses the mental and/or behavioral processes and characteristics of individuals and groups must also be addressed if nurses are to provide culturally competent care. The spiritual system of individuals and groups is often overlooked and/or neglected but must be considered. The nurse must be aware that ethnic differences in spiritual orientation among various groups exist and that the spiritual dimension is essential to overall good health (Andrews & Boyle, 1995, Edelman & Mandle, 1994).

Promoting an environment where values, customs and beliefs of individuals providing care are respected is the fifth dimension. This dimension is just as important to the provision of culturally competent care as awareness and sensitivity to cultural diversity and the understanding of cultural concepts and patterns of patients receiving care. Sociocultural assessments should be implemented to identify strengths and deficits in the system in which care is given so that if needed change can take place effectively (Warda, 1995).

The following strategies have been suggested for the implementation of culturally competent care:

1. Careful assessment of cultural background and individual factors which can help to identify patterns that may assist or interfere with a nursing intervention or treatment regimen.

2. Cross-cultural communication skills which enable problem solving processes that are acceptable and appropriate to the client.

3. Cultural context approach which assumes that patients are ethnically distinct based on their country of origin, historical point of entry, the degree of acculturation, and language proficiency (Warda, 1995).

An Afrocentric Approach for Providing Culturally Competent Care

Baldwin, Johnson, Cotanch & Williams (1996) have suggested an Afrocentric approach for assisting undergraduate and advanced practice nursing students to become culturally competent. The Afrocentric approach seeks in every situation the appropriate centrality of the African person. This approach, which is based on the theoretical constructs of the Afrocentric framework, can be applied to most African American populations. Afrocentrism is a theoretical approach used in many of the social sciences which focuses on the African heritage and the American experience of African Americans. Afrocentrism provides a frame of reference wherein phenomena are viewed through the lenses of the African experience (Asante, 1991, cited in Baldwin et al., 1996). The Afrocentric methodology provides an opportunity to study the world and its people utilizing an African world view.

The African world view has a holistic conception of the human condition and serves as a framework for the experiences of African Americans in this country. This view suggests that there is a resemblance between African ethos and the African American world view in terms of the focus on emotional vitality, interdependence, collective survival, oral tradition, perception of time, harmonious blending, and role of the elderly (White and Parham cited in Baldwin et al., 1996). Baldwin et al., developed a teaching module for undergraduate nursing students and advanced practice nursing students for teaching low-income African American women the importance of participation in breast and cervical cancer early detection and screening services. Based on their research findings and the work of Asante, Baldwin et al., developed a new model for organizing the content of the teaching module.

The model which uses an Afrocentric framework includes three components, 1) African world view, 2) Lived experience of African American women, and 3) Decision-making practices. The model offers a human science framework (phenomenological approach) and seeks to understand the behaviors of African American women, rather than focusing on predicting their behaviors. The teaching-learning process focuses on the strengths of African Americans including their resiliency, competencies and strong sense of survival in spite of social barriers. The instructional goals for the module include helping students develop respect for ethnically diverse populations and providing culturally congruent human caring. Content for the module includes such topics as developing cultural awareness, developing cultural knowledge and developing cultural skill. The authors believe that as students become culturally competent they develop respect for ethnically diverse populations and are able to provide culturally congruent care.

With the support of the Center for Disease Control (CDC) and the American Nurses Association, Baldwin et al., have published the teaching module as an Educational Program to provide a national curriculum guide aimed at teaching undergraduate and advanced practice nursing students useful approaches for counseling, and teaching low-income African American women about breast and cervical cancer screening practices. The model continues to be refined and tested in practice (Baldwin, 1995, personal communication).

The model was also tested in my research with elderly African American women. The purpose of the study was to determine the breast cancer knowledge of elderly African American women and their level of confidence when performing breast self-examination directed toward enhancing cancer knowledge and increasing utilization of breast cancer screening modalities. By demonstrating respect for the women, we were accepted and encountered little difficulty with the subjects sharing information. Additionally, we made every effort to understand the women's behaviors and did not try to predict what they would do. Rather than telling them what to do we asked them what they did and how we could help them. We were supportive of their behaviors and offered encouragement. Findings from the study showed that there were positive differences in cancer knowledge scores, in performance of monthly breast self-examination practices, and in self-efficacy (level of confidence) scores between pretest and posttest. The improvements were maintained one month following training. Subjects learned breast self-examination technique better and felt confident in their ability to initiate breast self-examination activity.

The subjects maintained self-efficacy at follow-up because they had confidence in their ability to perform breast self-examination correctly. In addition, subjects whose self-efficacy (level of confidence) scores were increased were more likely to have made an appointment for clinical breast examination and for mammogram.

Developing Cultural Competence

To become culturally competent requires an integration of knowledge, attitudes, and skills (Rooda, 1993). Nurses can take a number of actions or engage in a number of activities to develop this capacity. Hamilton (1996) suggests the following eleven ways to become culturally competent: 1) Gain an understanding of your own values and beliefs; 2) Recognize that your own culture conditioned your point of view; 3) Develop a perspective of cultural relativism; 4) Appreciate that cultural values are ingrained and therefore difficult to change; 5) Look at people as individuals, not as members of an amorphous group; 6) Seek information from others, including beliefs and practices about family roles, the meaning of health and illness, and healing practices; 7) Give safe, effective care to all clients regardless of their culture or diagnosis; 8) Be willing to modify health care delivery to accommodate the culture of your client; 9) Be aware of stereotyping; 10) Embrace other caregivers from other cultures; 11) Allow caring to guide you (p. 130).

A community-based curriculum in a culturally diverse environment requires that the faculty give high priority to cultural competence and culturally competent care. A variety of strategies can be used to help students develop cultural competence.

When the student body consists of African American students from all over the United States, students from several African countries, several Caribbean Islands, several Asian countries, and Muslim countries, and are diverse in both age and gender, the classroom can serve as a laboratory for helping students to acquire knowledge and skills in cultural competence. The curriculum is based on Sister Callista Roy's Adaptation Model and culture is viewed as a common influencing stimulus affecting behavior (Roy & Andrews, 1991).

The first step in assisting students to become culturally competent is to have them examine their own cultural values and beliefs concerning such areas as health practices, home remedies/folk medicine, customs, food practices, and other racial/ethnic groups. In the beginning of this activity, some students are reluctant to share their experiences. After what is called a warming up period and encouragement that it is a safe environment to share, students begin to share. As students become more comfortable, they open up and share more readily. Eventually all students are actively participating. This activity is a very revealing one. Personal biases, prejudices, stereotyping, and myths that students were not aware of are expressed. Students share beliefs and practices of "their parents and grandparents," which they eventually admit are some of their own beliefs and practices. This experience helps students to see the differences and the commonalities among the group. They learn that among the same cultural group there are many differences.

This activity raises awareness, helps students to understand their own behavior better, to be more sensitive to their classmates, especially those of a different racial/ethnic group, and to show respect for the values and beliefs of others. Students are taught that when behavior is taken out of its context and we try to explain it within our context, we create misinterpretation. For example, the following situation occurred during one of the classes. One student made a comment about the personal hygiene practice of "Africans." Her comment was supported by some of the other students. Every African student in the class was offended and felt that the student was making a generalization about something that was not true. Further discussion revealed that the student had no real basis for her statement. The student making the comment was not aware that she was demonstrating cultural insensitivity toward her classmates. The situation provided a learning opportunity for helping students to develop awareness and sensitivity.

Another step in developing cultural competence is knowledge of culture and relevant concepts. Culture as a concept provides the direction for students to understand their own behavior as well as the behavior of others. A strategy to facilitate students' learning includes a group activity in which students are assigned to research and present on a specific cultural group. Students self select one of several cultural groups which may include, but are not limited to, African American, Asian, Caribbean, Hispanic, Native African, or Native American cultures. Using specific objectives and guidelines students research the particular cultural group and present their findings to the class. There are specific assigned readings for all students but students are expected to include readings which they have identified. There is only one stipulation to this assignment, students cannot read to the class. They can be as creative and as innovative as they would like to be but must address specific objectives.

Students are particularly creative in this activity. Some groups have focused their presentations on the food practices of the cultural group and have included those foods in their presentations. Others have organized their presentation around the health practices and used role playing as the strategy for presentation. Following each presentation there is a question and answer period which provides an opportunity for the rest of the class to interact with the group and to clarify any inaccuracies. As a result of this experience students acquire knowledge and skills of the beliefs, values and practices of the various cultural groups and learn the differences and similarities of these groups as well.

The activities are implemented with beginning nursing students in their first nursing course. Expected outcomes are that students will show respect for values and beliefs of people of different cultural backgrounds and integrate knowledge of culture and cultural variations into their practice. In every nursing course the concept of culture as a common influencing stimulus affecting behavior is addressed and students continue to develop cultural competence as they move through the curriculum.

Conclusion

As the society becomes more diverse and health care focus moves from illness care to health promotion and prevention, nurses, along with other health care providers, will interact with individuals, families and groups from all over the world. To meet the health care needs of this diverse population the nurse must acquire the knowledge and skills to become culturally competent and provide culturally competent care.

REFERENCES

Alpers, R. R., & Zoucha, R. (1996). Comparison of cultural competence and cultural confidence of senior nursing students in a private southern university. *Journal of Cultural Diversity*, 3(1), 9–15.

American Academy of Nursing: Expert Panel Report. Culturally Competent Care (1992). *Nursing Outlook*, 40(6), 277–283.

Andrews, M., & Boyle, J. (1995). *Transcultural concept in nursing care*, (2nd. ed.). Philadelphia: J. B. Lippincott.

Baldonado, A. A. (1996). Transcending the barriers of cultural diversity in health care. *Journal of Cultural Diversity*, 5(1), 20–22.

Baldwin, D., Johnson, P., Cotanch, P. & Williams, J. (1996). An *Afrocentric approach to breast and cervical early detection and screening.* Washington: American Nurses Publishing.

Brink, P. (1990). Cultural diversity in nursing: How much can we tolerate? In J. E. McCloskey & H. H. Grace (Eds.) *Current Issues in Nursing.* Baltimore: Mosby.

Busby, A. (1995). Ethnocultural sensitivity and measurement of consumer satisfaction. *Journal of Nursing Care Quarterly, 9*(2), 16–25.

Compinha-Bacote, J., Yahle, T., & Langenkamp, M. (1996). The challenge of cultural diversity for nurse educators. *Journal of Continuing Education in Nursing, 27*(2), 59–64.

Clinton, J. F. (1996). Cultural diversity and health care in America: Knowledge fundamental to cultural competence in baccalaureate nursing students. *Journal of Cultural Diversity, 3*(1), 4–8.

Department of Commerce, Bureau of Census. Populations projections of the United States by age, sex, and Hispanic origins: 1990:2050. Washington, DC: Printing Office, 1992.

Edelman, C. L., & Mandle, C. L. (1994). *Health promotion throughout the lifespan* (3rd ed.). St. Louis: Mosby Year-Book.

Eliason, M., & Macy, N. (1992). A classroom activity to introduce cultural diversity. *Nurse Educator, 17*(3), 32–36.

Giger, J. N., & Davidhizar, R. (1990). Transcultural nursing assessment: A method for advancing nursing practice. *International Nursing Review, 37*(1), 199–202.

Giger, J. N., & Davidhizar, R. (1995). Transcultural nursing: Assessment and intervention (2nd ed.). St. Louis: Mosby.

Giger, J. N., Davidhizar, R. E., & Wieczorek, S. K. (1994). Transcultural nursing: Have we gone too far or not far enough? In O. L. Strickland & D. J. Fishman (Eds.). *Nursing Issues in the 1990's* (pp. 491–504). Albany, NY: Delmar Publishers.

Hamilton, P. M. (1996). *Realities of contemporary nursing* (2nd ed.). Menlo Park, CA: Addison-Wesley.

Healthy Mothers, Healthy Babies Coalition (1993, August). *Unity through diversity: Report on healthy mothers, healthy babies coalition communities of color leadership roundtable.* Washington, DC.

Kirkpatrick, S. M., & Deloughery, G. L. (1995). Cultural influences on nursing. In G. L. Deloughery (Ed.). *Issues and trends in nursing* (2nd ed., pp. 173–198). St. Louis: Mosby.

Kozier, B., Erb, G., Blais, K., & Wilkinson, J. M. (1995). *Fundamentals of nursing: Concepts, process, and practice* (3rd ed.). Redwood City, CA: Addison-Wesley.

Lenburg, G. B. (Ed.), Lipson, J. G., Demi, A. L., Blaney, D. R., Stern, P. N., Schultz, P. R., & Gage, L. (1995). Promoting cultural competence in and through education. *Monograph by the American Academy of Nursing.*

Leininger, M. (1991). Transcultural nursing: The study and practice. *Imprint 38,* 55–56.

Leininger, M. (1994). Transcultural nursing education: A worldwide imperative. *Nursing and Health Care*, 15(5), 254–257.

Meleis, A. I., Isenberg, M., Koerner, J. E., Lacey, B., & Stern, P. (1995). Diversity, marginalization and culturally competent care: Issues in knowledge development. *Monograph by the American Academy of Nursing.*

Rojas, D. (1994). Leadership in multicultural society: A case in role development. *Nursing and Health Care*, 15(5), 258–261.

Rooda, L. (1993). Knowledge and attitudes toward culturally different patients: Implications for nursing education. *Journal of Nursing Education*, 209–213.

Rosella, J. D., Regan-Kubinski, M. J., & Albrecht, S. A. (1994). The need for multicultural diversity among health professionals, *Nursing and Health Care*, 15(5), 242–246.

Roy, C., & Andrews, H. A. (1991). *The Roy adaptation model: The definitive statement.* Norwalk, CT: Appleton & Lange.

Specter, R. E. (1996). *Cultural diversity in health and illness* (4th ed.). Stamford, CT: Appleton & Lange.

Taylor, C., Lillis, C., & Lemone, P. 1993. *Fundamentals of nursing* (2nd. ed.). Philadelphia: Lippincott.

United States Department of Health and Human Services (1990). *Healthy people 2000: National health promotion and disease prevention objectives.* (Pub. No. PHS 91-50212). Washington: Government Printing Office.

Warda, M. R. (1995). Dimensions of culturally competent care. In J. F. Wang (Ed.). *Proceedings of the Second International and Interdisciplinary Health Research Symposium: Health care and culture* (pp. 173–178). Morgantown, WV: Department of Health Systems, West VA University, 173–178.

8

Teaching Issues in Health of Underserved and Diverse Populations—Challenges and Opportunities for Multicultural Nursing Education

Shirlee Drayton-Hargrove

As our society continues to become increasingly culturally diverse, there is a concomitant need for a workforce that reflects societal multiculturalism and nurses who can provide culturally-competent care. Our common vision for nursing in the 21st century embraces awareness and sensitivity to multiculturalism, knowledge of cultural patterns, skill in integrating cultural concepts into practice, and promoting an environment in which values, customs, beliefs, and culturally-based health traditions are respected (AAN Expert Panel Report, 1992; Jezewski, 1993; Malone; 1993; Outlaw, 1994; Warda, 1995).

Being culturally competent implies an awareness and sensitivity to race, gender, class divisions, shared history, values, celebrations, and ways-of-being for diverse populations. Being culturally competent denotes the ability to shift and view multiple perspectives of reality in interpersonal encounters. To prepare nurses for culturally-competent practice, programs must educate caregivers to effectively work with multicultural populations. Nursing curricula should be sensitive to racial, ethnic, and cultural diversity (AACN, 1993). There is a critical need for a shift in nursing curricula. Planned classroom inquiry must explore uncomfortable topics such as cross-cultural communication, ethical problem-solving, ethnocentricity, and institutional racism in the health-care delivery system.

Higher education must engage multiculturalism as a phenomenon to be seriously embraced. The concept of multiculturalism in higher education is in direct opposition to assimilation perspectives. According to Steele (1995), proponents of multicultural education challenge the assimilation position, opting for content more relevant to egalitarian ideas, inequity, discrimination, lack of access to, and unfair distribution of resources. Although there are core course requirements in many universities on racism, offerings in professional socialization can play a critical role in the preparation of nurses who are culturally aware and sensitive. Nurse educators with the courage to facilitate learning in these potentially uncomfortable areas must be supported by the entire faculty.

The objective of this chapter is to entreat an earnest dialogue on the strategies in education to facilitate student learning and to manage difficult domains. Its focus is on the development and pilot study evaluation of a nursing course designed to facilitate nursing knowledge in disease prevention and health promotion among medically underserved and diverse populations, and to teach skills as providers of culturally-competent care. Educational strategies and issues that present challenges and opportunities for nursing students and nurse educators will be discussed.

COURSE DEVELOPMENT: ISSUES IN HEALTH OF UNDERSERVED AND DIVERSE POPULATIONS

In 1994 a two-credit graduate course, "Issues in Health of Underserved Populations," was developed in a new curriculum for advanced practice nurses at Temple University. The University's mission is grounded in a strong social commitment to medically underserved and diverse populations. The course was designed for advanced practice nurses committed to work with low income and minority populations after completion of the graduate program.

The North Philadelphia area surrounding the University is populated predominantly by African Americans, Hispanic, and white ethnic groups. The course addressed the epidemiological health and disease issues, ethical problem-solving, racism and ethnocentricity in health care delivery, and cross-cultural communication in providing family-centered health promotion and disease prevention services. Course content varied since 1994, influenced by each teacher's differing philosophies and life experience related to these complex and often controversial issues. The following prototype, however, reflects the original 1994 course design whose over-arching course objectives were to:

1. Critique health problems and issues surrounding medically underserved populations in the United States.

2. Analyze the multiple cultural and societal factors that influence lifestyle, beliefs, and health care needs of ethnically diverse and medically underserved populations.

3. Design advanced practice intervention strategies that are effective in meeting the health care needs of multicultural and underserved urban populations.

4. Analyze ethical issues associated with the health care delivery system in the United States utilizing an ethical problem solving model.

5. Evaluate health-care delivery services for a selected underserved patient population.

Significant Social Influences on Course Development

People of color—African Americans, Hispanics, Asian Americans, and Native Americans are highly represented in the ranks of the medically underserved. The epidemiological facts reveal a major health crisis seen in the health status outcomes of minorities and low-income populations (US: DHSS, 1990). According to the Department of Health and Human Services Secretary's Task Force on Black and Minority Health in 1985, the health gap between white and African American populations is widening (US: DHHS, 1993, p. 3). All health status indicators demonstrate that members of ethnic minority groups fare more poorly than the general population (US: DHHS, 1993, p. 3).

Non-white males have the shortest life expectancy. Black males can expect to live 64.9 years, while their white counterparts can expect to live 72.3 years (US: DHHS, 1991, p. 11). Minority children under the age of one have death rates nearly double that of white infants. Maternal mortality rates for blacks remain high when compared to white populations. Blacks are 1.5 times more likely than all other groups to be uninsured (US: DHHS, 1991). Among the 37-plus million Americans who are uninsured, 23.9 percent are black and 32.9 percent are Hispanic (US: DHHS, 1993, p. 363). Minorities have less access to health care and less health care coverage when compared to whites (US: DHHS, 1991). To further complicate the problem, minorities are more likely to live in poverty.

Therefore, the course focused on cultural practices and implications for health promotion and prevention, high-risk populations, the examination of inequity, access to health care services, as well as, discriminatory practices, racism inherent in the health care delivery system, and the impact of culture on health behaviors. African American, Hispanic, Asian American, Native American , and low-income white groups were closely studied since these populations are disproportionately represented in the ranks of the nation's underserved. Major topical areas, educational strategies, and evaluation methods are reflected in Table 8.1.

Evaluation of Instructional Design and Social Significance

The science and the scholarship of teaching must be taken seriously by academicians who are committed to the development of socially responsible curricula in higher education. There are 4,200 federally designated medically underserved areas in the United States due to health professional shortages (Federal Register, 1994). Shortage areas include urban and rural geographic locations, selected population groups, and certain medical facilities. The sprawling north Philadelphia community encompassing Temple University has been designated a Health Medically Underserved Area and Professional Shortage Area. It has one of the lowest per capita incomes in the Commonwealth of Pennsylvania. This very large geographic area is 95 percent African American and Hispanic. It has a high communicable disease rate for HIV, tuberculosis, and hepatitis (A, B, and Viral), (Philadelphia Department of Health, 1990). Heart disease, malignant neoplasms, cerebral vascular accidents, influenza, pneumonia, diabetes, and homicide are among the most common causes of adult mortality among these residents (Philadelphia Department of Health, 1990).

As students prepare to work in areas such as urban Philadelphia, there must be exploration into the effects of instruction on student learning and student responsiveness to societal needs. For this reason during the fall semester of 1994, the course faculty performed a preliminary and post-course descriptive study to describe and explore the intentions, in-

Table 8.1
Course Structural Design

Content	Education Strategies	Evaluation	Objective Rationale
An overview of the health care system in the United States	Lecturette-critique of empirical data and clarification of terminology Discussion Group report on opinion exercise: The overarching issues are? Discussion of important points Small groups, then group reports Clarification of meanings Exercise: Student identification of perceived meaning-underserved, disadvantaged, under-representation, ethnic minority, race	Problem-solving-critical thinking paper	Objective #1, #5
Medically underserved populations: Issues and concerns of individuals, families, and the community	Lecture-epidemiological facts Student reaction forum and debate	Problem-solving-critical thinking paper	#1, #5
Application of theoretical models related to multicultural	Applications via lecturette group discussion	Problem-solving-critical thinking paper	#5

Table 8.1   (*continued*)

Content	Education Strategies	Evaluation	Objective Rationale
populations, including transcultural theories, self-help theories, family systems	Case study presentation by teacher and critique: examination of the role of advanced practice nurses		
Social factors and health services: Unintentional injury, housing, nutrition, education, infectious diseases	Student-assigned topics Student presentations of findings and reactions	Oral presentation	#1, #2, #3, #5
Stress and psychosocial issues and the underserved community	Case presentations and critique by students and teacher	Problem-solving-critical thinking paper Oral presentation	#1, #5
Ethnocentricity, racism and the health care system: The image of service professionals "Establishing meaningful dialogue"	Lecturette-research critique Case study Exercise: Dyads "Identify as Bias" followed by sharing of discussion and reaction Role play exercise: Planning a community-based health center-collaboration in the neighborhoods	Ethical analysis critical thinking paper	#3, #4, #5
Access to services, health promotion,	Values/health services Planning exercise: A boat load of new		#1, #4, #5

Table 8.1   (*continued*)

Content	Education Strategies	Evaluation	Objective Rationale
and disease prevention	people are arriving in our country		
Ethical concerns: Access, rationing, "haves deciding for the have-nots" Frameworks for ethical decision making	Lecturette-worthy vs. the unworthy Dilemma of who decides services Universal or a basic package Followed by student critique and reaction assignment Student application and critique of problem-solving framework-oral presentation on selected ethical dilemma reaction, critique		#4, #5
Cross-cultural collaboration	Lecturette on cultural aspects of selected populations Role play exercise: Planning a community-based health center-collaboration in the neighborhoods	Oral presentation Class participation	#2, #3, #5
Family friendly, culturally competent services	Student reaction to discussion points Obtaining cultural knowledge, awareness, and sensitivity	Problem-solving-critical thinking paper Oral presentation Class participation	#2, #3, #6

centives, and disincentives to work in underserved communities, as well as student perceptions of major problems facing underserved populations.

Forty-four graduate nursing students enrolled in "Issues in Health of the Underserved and Diverse Populations" were surveyed with consent. Graduate students were surveyed on their intentions to work in underserved areas, their perceptions of incentives and disincentives for such work, and their perceptions of major problems facing underserved populations. Upon completion of the course, an examination of students regarding their perceptions and plans to work with underserved populations was again performed.

Students were asked to participate in this study to obtain comparison data on employment intentions. The students were informed that the data would be used to examine factors related to their plans to work in underserved populations and for course evaluation purposes. On the first and last class session of the course, students who consented participated in completing a questionnaire (see Table 8.2).

Findings: The data was analyzed using descriptive statistics. Basic demographic data revealed that of the 44 students who initially enrolled in the class, 43 were female and one was male. Seventy percent of the respondents were white, 27 percent were black, 3 percent were Hispanic. Sixty-eight percent of the respondents were part-time students and 32 percent were full-time students, yet 98 percent were employed and only 2 percent were not employed. Students were asked to indicate the graduate track in which they were enrolled. Seventy-eight percent of the students were in the adult nurse practitioner track while 32 percent of the respondents were in the nurse clinical specialist track of Temple's Master of Science in Nursing program.

Students were asked to indicate their intention to work with underserved populations on the first night of class. Prior to the class 59 percent of the students intended to work with the underserved after graduation, 11 percent had no such intent, and 30 percent were undecided.

When the respondents were asked to identify the major problem facing underserved populations, 50 percent reported that access to quality care was the major problem, 16 percent reported a lack of health-related knowledge, and 9 percent identified poor compliance with prevention behaviors. Respondents reported that crime (5 percent), the identification of those who are underserved (5 percent), poverty (5 percent), malnutrition (5 percent), lack of insurance (5 percent) and mistrust of the health care delivery system (5 percent) were among the top problems. Illegal drugs were ranked as the top problem by only 2 percent of the respondents.

Table 8.2
Issues in Health of Underserved and Diverse Populations
Class Questionnaire

(Please circle descriptions that apply)

1. Race/Ethnicity:
      White (Non-Hispanic)
      Hispanic
      Asian
      African American
      Native American
2. Gender: a. Male   b. Female
3. Track: a. Clinical Nurse Specialist   b. Nurse Practitioner
4. Student Status: a. Matriculated   b. Non-Matriculated
                                a. Full-time   b. Part-time
5. What do you see as top problems in underserved communities?
      1st
      2nd
      3rd
      4th
      5th
6. What are the incentives for you to work in an underserved area?
7. What are the disincentives for you to work in an underserved area?
8. Do you plan to work in an underserved area? (please circle)
      a. Yes   b. No   If yes where?

Half of the respondents (50 percent) reported personal satisfaction as the major incentive to work with underserved populations. The need for health services was identified as the top incentive by 39 percent of the respondents. Five percent reported exposure to diversity. Education was reported by 2 percent and salary by 2 percent of the respondents. The disincentives to work with underserved populations included fears of risk to personal safety due to crime (48 percent), frustration with "system malfunction" (18 percent), poor salaries (11 percent), fear of not being accepted by the people (9 percent), poverty (2 percent) and driving long distances from their homes (2 percent). However, 9 percent of the respondents reported having no disincentives to work with underserved populations.

In contrast to the initial response on the first session of class at the last class, 33 of the original student respondents completed the second questionnaire. Several students had dropped out of the class for personal reasons and some students were absent the last night of class. Of the 33 participants on the second inquiry, 73 percent now expressed their intention to work in underserved populations, 18 percent were unsure, and 9 percent reported no intent to work with underserved populations. Incentives to work with underserved populations included personal satisfaction (45 percent), the need for quality care in underserved populations (30 percent), educational opportunity to learn (6%), good salary (6%). Twelve percent of the students did not respond to this item.

Disincentives were reported as crime (45 percent), poor salary (27 percent), and "frustration" (9 percent). Twelve percent of the respondents stated that they had no disincentives to work with underserved populations. Non-probability, purposive sampling and the sample size preclude the generalizability of results beyond the sample.

Although only 33 students responded on the last night of class to the questionnaire, proportionately more students expressed their intent to work with underserved populations and less students were unsure of their intent after completion of the course. For the 33 students responding to the second survey, the major incentive to work with underserved populations was the sense of personal satisfaction and the need for quality accessible health care in underserved communities. The major disincentive reported by this group of student respondents is the fear of personal injury due to crime, frustration, and poor salaries. The term "frustration" was documented but the source of this emotion was not clearly stated and warrants further investigation.

QUALITATIVE REFLECTIONS: IMPLICATIONS FOR THE 21st CENTURY

Challenges

The classroom is a microcosm of our society at-large. The same challenges faced by diverse populations everyday are often played out in the arena of the classroom. As evidenced in the survey, many students openly expressed professional commitment to helping others. However, even in a class comprised of nurses who profess caring, indices of insensitivity, expressions of moral and cultural superiority can surface. Students come into the academic environment with learned rules, preconceived notions, and varied experiences. The challenges to nursing faculty and students include: ethnocentricity, depreciation and rejection of the contributions of others, distrust, and complacency regarding the health dilemma of others.

During a values clarification exercise, students were told to pretend that they were a panel of experts. They were told that boatloads of people were coming into our country from another place on the globe. The immigrants were described as having poor health and limited financial resources. Student groups were to decide how to handle the new arrivals. As the exercise was in process, comments surfaced such as, "They must learn to fit into our society," "They will have to do things our way." This spontaneity provided opportunities for teachers to point out the dangers inherent in the inability or unwillingness to conceive of a diverse view or ways of being. During the exercise a student became upset and blurted out, "Why don't you just lecture and give us the information?" Such rejection may reveal the unconscious values of ethnocentricity.

Learned predisposition affects the manner in which individuals think, feel, and often how they behave toward persons, objects, and ideas (Steele, 1995). Many students may feel more comfortable as passive recipients of empirical data, health promotion, and disease prevention recommendations. However, if nurses are to become leaders in culturally competent care, then the educational process must engage students in often painful explorations. Individuals may need to immerse themselves in difficult explorations of supposed personal beliefs in their superiority, of which they may be unaware, and which may present barriers to cultural sensitivity (Warda, 1995). A lack of understanding and awareness may require examination of the meaning of culture and ethnicity (Outlaw, 1994). Therefore, course content may make students uncomfortable.

During the classroom experience some students may devalue or reject the contributions of others. One day when a guest was sharing an uncomfortable experience waiting for services in the health care system, a student questioned, "Are you saying that because you're black you had to wait?" Another individual commented that the discussion was uncomfortable. The student lamented, "People need to stop talking about racism and mistreatment. It's very uncomfortable." Students stated that they did not trust their classmates enough yet to share ideas. Other students refrained from class discussions. Distrust, complacency, resistance to self assessment and sharing, and meaningful dialogue are barriers to the development of awareness and sensitivity.

Educators must seize the opportunity to invite students to express their views and confront perspectives different from their own. Although the area of dialogue may be uncomfortable, the educator must be sensitive to achieve a balance of comfort. Malone (1993) questions, "Is nursing a profession that espouses a belief of cultural and racial sensitivity while behaving in a culturally and racially insensitive manner?"

Messages that certain people and ideas are unworthy may surface, as well as covert and overt hostility. Students were asked how many could speak multiple languages. One student responded with a question, "Why is so much emphasis placed on those groups? There are nice white poor communities too, you know. They need to learn to speak English." The student further noted that "there will always be poor people, we need to accept this fact." These are not strange or unusual ideas. Students come to the classroom with a set of preconceived notions. Again a challenge is presented. The educator needs to employ the nonthreatening and flexible use of questioning to help students probe the integration of proclaimed professional values in daily nursing practices.

Opportunities

Masters-prepared advanced practice nurses can play a critical role in the provision of accessible high quality primary care in underserved and multicultural communities (American Nurses Association, 1992). "Issues in Health of Underserved and Diverse Populations" provided an important opportunity for inquiry and discourse into sensitive areas in the educational process. Students and the faculty gained many personal insights. Students reported growth and expanded their knowledge.

Students' insights are clearly reflected in the following statements:

- "I realized the lengths people will go to maintain the status quo. This was evident in the energy exerted to resist meaningful classroom discussions."

- "Discussions were thought-provoking. It made me analyze my own attitudes toward racism, ethnocentricity, and the needs of minorities."

- "I became more aware of erroneous notions that I have utilized to make judgments about others. I learned a lot about feelings of others."

- "I believe I am more sensitive but I still have a journey."

- "I learned the value of listening and taking time to appreciate cultural influences. Most of all I learned to appreciate the art of caring."

Educator Learnings and Considerations for Nursing Education

The nursing profession has not excelled with achieving diversity within the profession nor in the development of widely agreed upon models for multicultural education (AAN, 1992; Brink, 1990). Awareness, sensitivity, and knowledge about diverse populations must be integrated throughout the educational socialization process of the professional nurse. Higher education has traditionally been an appropriate arena for critical discourse and multiculturalism must be engaged as a serious phenomenon within it. It must be incorporated not simply because accrediting organizations demand inclusion of multicultural concepts in curricula, but because we believe in its value. Nursing curricula must stimulate awareness and sensitivity through affective learning strategies such as values clarification exercises, case studies, role play, and critical, meaningful dialogue.

Nurse educators teaching courses with sensitive affective and cognitive implications require the support of the entire faculty. Student discomfort can easily be displaced into anger, and this anger may indicate that students are experiencing cognitive dissonance. Even though course content may make students "uncomfortable," the skillful educator needs to foster the notion of the classroom as a "safe place." The faculty must remain open-minded enough to engage in exploration with the student even when there is disagreement. It is too easy to allow students to remain passive recipients of didactic materials. Faculty should realize that students may find it easier to hear the facts without examining their attitudes or engaging in a critical dialogue on emotionally charged issues. The educator can stand at the podium and recite the epidemiological facts, and health prevention and promotion strategies; however, the meaningfulness of knowledge of facts without awareness and sensitivity is of questionable applicable value. To ignore these challenges is to deny students and faculty the opportunities for growth and change.

REFERENCES

AAN Expert Panel Report (1992). Culturally competent care. *Nursing Outlook*, 227–283.

American Association of Colleges of Nursing (1993). *Nursing Education Agenda for the 21st Century*. Washington, DC.

American Nurses Association (1992). Advanced practice nursing: A New age in health care. *Nurse Facts*. Washington, DC: ANA.

Brink, P. (1990). Cultural diversity in nursing: How much can we tolerate? In J. C. McCloskey & H. K. Grace (eds.), *Current issues in nursing* (pp. 521–527). St. Louis: Mosby.

Jezewski, M. A. (1993). Culture brokering as a model for advocacy. *Nursing and Health Care*, 14(2), 78–85.

Malone, B. L. (1993). Caring for culturally diverse racial groups: An administrative matter. *Nursing Administration Quarterly*, 17(2), 21–29.

Outlaw, F. H. (1994). A reformulation of meaning of culture and ethnicity for nurses delivering care. *Medical Surgical Nursing*, 3(2), 108–111.

Philadelphia Department of Public Health. 1990 Vital Statistics Report.

Steele, R. L. (1995). Diversity in Academia: Some Reflections. *The ABNF Journal*, 6(3) 84–86.

U.S. Department of Health and Human Services, *Healthy People 2000: National health promotion and disease prevention objectives*. (1990) Washington, DC: DHHS Publication No. (PHS) 91–50212). Washington, DC. U.S. Government Printing Office.

U.S. Department of Health and Human Services. *Towards equality of well-being: Strategies for improving minority health*, (1993). Washington, DC: DHHS Publication No. (ISBN-0-16-041714-1). Washington, DC. U.S. Government Printing Office.

U.S. Department of Health and Human Services, *Health status of minorities and low income groups*, (1991). Washington, DC. U.S. Government Printing Office.

U.S. Department of Health and Human Services, Federal Register. List of designated primary medical care health professionals; shortage areas: Notice. 59(14). January 21, 1994. Washington, DC. U.S. Government Printing Office.

Warda, M. R. (1995). Dimensions of culturally competent care. In Janet Wang (Ed.) *Proceedings of the Second International and interdisciplinary health research symposium: Health care and culture*, 1995, pp. 173–178, West Virginia University School of Nursing, Department of Health Systems: USA.

9

Nursing Education for the 21st Century— Preparing Culturally Diverse Minority Nurses

Jane M. Brennan

As *the 21st century* rapidly draws near, individuals in all walks of life are concerned with meeting the challenges which are sure to arise in the next millenium. The health care professions in particular recognize the demands created by changing demographics and new health care delivery approaches. Integrated health services and community partnerships are the delivery models of the 21st century. For nursing, the changes in the delivery of health care services have resulted in a return to the community as the major focus of primary health care.

"Nursing is a profession that historically has rendered unique and significant service to society" (Smith, 1995, p. 188). Changes in the demographic composition of American society have implications for how nursing can and will meet societal needs for health care. Minorities currently comprise approximately 25 percent of the United States population, but are expected to constitute one-third of the population by the year 2020 (Rosella, Regan-Kubinski & Albrecht, 1994; Ross, 1996). Nonwhite and Hispanic minorities represent approximately 10 percent of all nurses (Minnick, Roberts, Young, Marcantonio and Kleinpell, 1997). While this percentage is well lower than that of the overall minority population of the United States, it is less disproportionate than the percentage of minority health care providers in all professions (Campbell & Davis, 1996; Rosella, Regan-Kubinski & Albrecht, 1994). The disparity between numbers of minority clientele and available minority nurses impacts the availability of culturally sensitive nursing care providers, since studies show that nurses with minority backgrounds tend to work with people of color (Keklak, 1996; Minnick et al., 1997). Lack of cultural congruence between health care providers and clients can impact access to and compliance with therapeutic regimens, resulting in unfavorable consequences for the client and frustration for the care provider (Crawford & Olinger, 1988; Leininger, 1994; Minnick et al., 1997; Russell & Jewell, 1992). As the focus of health care returns to community based and home care settings, patients will expect sensitivity to their unique cultural values (Gibson, 1996).

Issues related to cultural diversity may be viewed from two perspectives: preparing nurses to care for clients with culturally diverse backgrounds, and preparing culturally diverse nurses to meet society's health care needs. This chapter will focus on the preparation of culturally diverse or minority nurses for practice in the 21st century in the United States. The culture of nursing education is described, and cognitive and noncognitive variables are discussed. Minority nursing students' stories of selected experiences in nursing education help to illustrate some of the themes described in the nursing literature, and suggestions intended to enhance faculty development in the area of cultural awareness are included.

THE CULTURE OF NURSING EDUCATION

Most definitions of culture include the concepts of values, beliefs, norms and practices that are shared and which guide thinking and acting in patterned ways (Giger & Davidhizar, 1995; Leininger, 1978). The culture of nursing education, like most of higher education in America, is largely Eurocentric, reflecting the dominant culture achieved by assimilation (Davis, 1995; Pacquiao, 1996). Within the Eurocentric tradition, linear learning, deductive logic, hierarchical organization, competitive ethics and authoritarian ideology are the norm (Harris, 1993). According to Fitzsimons and Kelley (1996), "A nursing education curriculum is really an introduction to, and some level of mastery of, the culture of the profession" (p. 8). The culture of the nursing profession is acquired through a process of professional socialization. Does the goal of professional socialization translate to an implicit goal of homogeneity through assimilation? Would not a goal of biculturalism in which students learn to affirm their own individuality while respecting the cultural differences in others be a more suitable goal for nursing education? (Pacquiao, 1996).

Yoder (1996) studied how nurse educators teach diverse ethnic students. Five patterns of faculty response emerged from the informants' descriptions of their experiences in nursing education. Three of the patterns and the bulk of the behaviors described reflected a strong Eurocentric tradition with little consideration for differences in ethnic cognitive and learning styles and communicative patterns.

Many faculty assume that all students' needs are similar and that the same teaching approach is suitable for all students, thus ignoring cultural differences. Other faculty expect students to conform to the mainstream culture, but help students acquire the skills needed to assimilate the mainstream expectations. Some faculty are perceived as unwilling to tolerate cultural differences at all (Yoder, 1996). Crow (1993) challenges faculty to question the biases and assumptions underlying both the culture of nursing education and the culture of nursing practice.

Recruitment and Retention Issues

Documents such as the *Essentials of College and University Education for Professional Nursing* (AACN, 1986) and the *Criteria and Guidelines for the Evaluation of Baccalaureate and Higher Degree Programs in Nursing* (NLN Accrediting Commission, 1996) contain language which speaks to cultural, ethnic and racial diversity. The issues of recruitment and retention have been addressed periodically in the nursing literature for the last 30 years (Dowell, 1996; Fitzsimons & Kelley, 1996; Heydman, 1991; Saucier, 1994). Heydman (1991) noted a lack of studies related to the recruitment and retention of minority students and evaluation of program outcomes. Heydman (1991) concluded that the existing nursing literature offered little direction for nurse educators pertaining to the issue of retention of minority nursing students.

Saucier (1994) observed that a need for nursing to increase both recruitment and retention efforts for underrepresented groups continues to exist, despite the fact that nursing actually has better minority representation than other disciplines. After reviewing the nursing literature on intervention strategies for retention of nursing students, Saucier (1994) concluded that while information on a variety of retention strategies is available, not enough is known about the financial and organizational factors which influence retention of students. Although the numbers of minority students enrolled in nursing education programs have increased slightly, the number of ethnic minority nursing graduates in all educational programs has declined in recent years (Fitzsimons & Kelley, 1996). Without an increase in the pool of baccalaureate prepared minority nurses, there will continue to be a dearth of minority nurses prepared at the graduate level for leadership roles.

Performance Predictors

Minority students generally perform less well on standardized tests which measure componential intelligence than do their white counterparts (Korngruth, Frisch, Shovein & Williams, 1994). Garcia and Pearson (1994) conclude that poverty and English proficiency are the major factors in explaining the performance discrepancies between African American, Latino, Native American, Anglo and English as second language students. In research focused on retention and attrition of students, Sedlacek (1987) and his associates identified eight noncognitive variables related to academic success of all students, especially minority and nontraditional students. These noncognitive dimensions include self-confidence, realistic self-appraisal of academic abilities, community service, culturally related ways of learning, long range goals, an ability to understand racism, leadership, and strong support persons (Boyer & Sedlacek, 1988; Korngruth et al., 1994). Self-confidence and realistic self appraisal were important to academic success across all semesters for both black and white students (Tracey & Sedlacek, 1985). Korngruth and associates (1994) used Sedlacek's tool to investigate factors related to attrition of nursing students. The researchers found that the variable of understanding racism was most predictive of academic success among minority nursing students.

The word racism can trigger many heated emotional responses when discussed, whether in academia or in general conversations. Racism refers to prejudicial and oppressive behaviors aimed at particular groups based on physical or cultural attributes (Steele, 1995). The history of racism in the United States evolved from a need for social control in the early colonies. The term *white* disregarded European cultural differences and implied racial unity and superiority based on ancestry and physical characteristics (Bowser, Auletta & Jones, 1993).

Racism may exist on personal or institutional levels or both. Institutional racism is legitimized through policies, procedures, and normative patterns, such as those found in academia. Many minority authors speak to the existence of racism in academia in general (Bowser, Auletta & Jones, 1993; Steele, 1995). Racism may be overt or covert. The latter is often subtle, insidious and masked by the rhetoric of ideology. Covert racism impacts political and social affiliations, intellectual perspectives, and mentoring opportunities (Steele, 1995). Gonzalez (1993) noted that "fear, anxiety and deep seated feelings" frequently arise in faculty discussions about the admission and education of diverse [minority] students (Gonzalez, 1993, p. 5). A commonly expressed fear is that changes in the normative patterns of the university will lower the quality of the education. It is interesting to note that this argument has been advanced about every suggested curricular change in universities for close to 100 years (Gonzalez, 1993).

Both faculty and higher education institutions must assume the responsibility of developing responsive curricula which incorporate the diversity of the students' culture, and learning styles, while maintaining the expected standards (Gibson, 1996). Unless racism is acknowledged and challenged by institutional leadership in academia, minority faculty will be neither recruited nor retained, thus diminishing the potential for mentoring and modeling of minority students by minority faculty (Steele, 1995).

Vaughn (1997) observed that many black professional nurses and nursing faculty believe that racism exists in nursing today, evidenced by stratification of enrollment in various nursing education programs and lack of efforts to recruit and maintain minority faculty role models. The number of minority students in baccalaureate nursing programs is far less than in associate degree and diploma programs (Fitzsimons & Kelley, 1996).

Differences in learning and cognitive styles are part of cultural diversity (Sims & Baldwin, 1995). Educational research suggests that ethnicity does play an important role in individual learning and that accommodation of various learning style preferences and strengths has not been addressed through teaching strategies and methods geared to a diversity of styles (Huber & Pewewardy, 1990 as cited in Carter, R. T. & Goodwin, A. L., 1994). Both teachers and students come to a teaching-learning interaction with a biopsychological history that includes cognition, problem solving ability, interpersonal and communication skills, and cultural and family values and traditions (Rew, 1996).

The concept of primary and secondary cultural differences among minority groups (Ogbu, 1992) is useful in understanding differences in learning among and between various groups. Voluntary minorities are those groups of individuals who have recently come to the United States seeking economic and educational opportunities and/or political freedom (Ogbu, 1992). Some examples of voluntary minorities who have relocated to the eastern United States include recent immigrants from Asia, West Africa, and the Caribbean Islands. For these minority groups, the primary cultural differences experienced include world views, language, and teaching and learning styles. International students would be classified as voluntary minorities, since their presence in American educational institutions reflects a choice of pursuit of opportunities not available in their native countries.

Involuntary minorities, according to Ogbu (1992), are those ethnic groups whose presence in the United States originated from slavery, colonization, or conquest. Included in this classification of ethnic minorities are Black Americans, Native Americans, early Mexican Americans, and some Puerto Ricans. Whereas voluntary minorities have chosen to leave their homes and families in pursuit of a particular goal or goals, involuntary minorities experienced oppression. Voluntary minorities compare themselves with peers in their native country while the frame of reference for involuntary minorities is comparison with white Americans (Ogbu, 1992). Involuntary minorities tend to develop secondary cultural differences which are based on opposition to the majority values. These secondary differences negatively affect learning to a greater degree than do primary differences because academic success and loss of ethnic identity are not separated (Ogbu, 1992).

An additional barrier to success in higher education experienced by many minority students is that of poverty. The discrepancies in standardized test scores between minority and majority populations is strongly related to poverty and language facility (Garcia & Pearson, 1994). The *culture of poverty* has long been accepted as an explanation for the production of educationally disadvantaged students in urban schools. Lack of financial support for minority nursing students continues to create additional barriers to increasing both recruitment and retention of minority students.

Student Voices

The following stories of minority students illustrate how noncognitive factors, especially understanding of racism, realistic self-appraisal, positive self concept, long range goals, and cultural ways of learning impact on the minority students' educational experiences. Hearing the voices of nursing students provides nursing educators with an opportunity to increase their awareness of the diverse cultural needs of students. The stories of Black American and "English as Second Language" students portray vividly how noncognitive variables and primary and secondary cultural differences influence academic achievement and learning experiences.

Diane

Diane is a twenty-two year old who graduated from a private high school in Connecticut and attended a baccalaureate nursing program in a university in another state. Although the university had a number of culturally diverse students, the majority population of both students and teachers was white. Throughout her first three years at the university, Diane had felt fully integrated into the culture of the school. She had many friends among both races and both genders. Academically, Diane had performed well and she felt socially comfortable in the setting. Diane's confrontation with racism occurred as part of a clinical rotation in her senior year.

Diane was assigned to a clinical rotation at a suburban hospital where the patient population and vast majority of nursing staff were white, while the housekeeping and cafeteria workers were black. At the end of the clinical rotation, Diane confided to the clinical instructor how difficult the experience had been for her. Not only were there no role models of black nurses for her to emulate, but she felt ostracized in the cafeteria when she joked with and hugged a white male classmate. Diane was able to recognize the existing racism in the setting and discuss it with the instructor without becoming hostile or angry. Diane's positive sense of self-esteem and realistic self-appraisal enabled her to acknowledge and deal with the racism which she encountered in the clinical setting.

William

William is a twenty-one year old black male. Unlike Diane, William came to the predominantly white university from an inner city public school background. By choosing to attend college and majoring in nursing (a predominantly female profession), William has gone against the prevailing culture of many young black males from low socioeconomic backgrounds. William struggled with the basic science courses during the first two years of the program, but was able to progress by repeating courses. William demonstrated leadership qualities as a resident assistant, and the ability to make friends with fellow students. He also was actively involved in the university community. These noncognitive factors are related to predicting academic success. As William began his clinical courses, his academic performance slowly deteriorated. William identified personal problems related to family support as a major concern at this time. He was encouraged to use the counseling services as well as the academic support services available at the university, and reported doing so. As the semester continued, William's academic performance continued to decline, and he withdrew from two courses. In spite of this reduction in course load, William failed the third course. Although he was advised to continue school on a part-time basis rather than a full-time basis to shore up his academic foundation, William insisted upon returning as a full-time student the following semester. This decision seemed based upon an unrealistic self appraisal of his academic skills and an emphasis on short term goals (staying in school full time) rather than on long term goals (successfully completing the program). The noncognitive factors of decreased family support, unrealistic self-appraisal and focus on short term goals reduce the likelihood of William's academic success.

Eugene

Eugene transferred to the university program after taking a few courses at a community college. Eugene is a nontraditional student, married with two children. Eugene admits that his interest in academics is a newly acquired one. In the first two years of the nursing curriculum, Eugene encountered several academic difficulties. During the course of his junior year, Eugene began missing classes, though never clinical, and missed turning in several written assignments for grades. As a result, he failed a nursing course and had to repeat it, thus slowing down his progression in the curriculum. When discussing the semester with his advisor after the fact, Eugene described a number of personal problems which he had encountered during the course of the semester. He had not shared these problems with the faculty in the course at the time, because he felt they were his problems and he had to solve them. Eugene's financial problems were so severe that at times he had to make choices between buying books and feeding his family. Eugene explained that sometimes he lacked the carfare (approximately $4.00 each day) and could not attend class or extra study sessions. In spite of these obstacles, Eugene continues to maintain a positive self-image, believing that he can succeed. Although Eugene feels supported by his family members in regard to his academic goals, he feels as if he is letting family members down when his academic progress is impeded. Racism is a factor in Eugene's case insofar as he carries the baggage of being financially and educationally disadvantaged.

Lisa

Lisa is a nontraditional black student who transferred into the university from a community college. Just prior to entering the university program, Lisa was involved in a serious automobile accident and had to delay starting school by one year. Lisa lives at home with her elderly parents for whom she feels responsible. She commuted to school and clinical via public transportation, a trip which could take up to two hours, one way. As a senior nursing student, Lisa's confidence in herself as a student was shaken when she failed a nursing course and had to repeat it. As a result, her academic progression was somewhat different from most of her classmates. Lisa took the expected heavy credit clinical course for second semester senior year with her classmates while also repeating the failed course.

Lisa was the only black student in the clinical group at a predominantly white hospital. She had not worked in the nursing field outside of school and seemed intimidated by her classmates familiarity with clinically related knowledge and skills. During the course of the rotation, Lisa complained several times to the clinical instructor that the other students in the group ignored her and discriminated against her. She expressed her feelings of isolation and anger. The faculty member confronted the group members with the concern, and heard the other students describe how their efforts to be friendly and inclusive had been rebuffed. At that point, the other students in the clinical group decided to ignore Lisa. In turn, Lisa interpreted this behavior as racist.

Lisa also expressed concern at the insensitivity of the white students about what financial hardship is. After hearing Lisa discuss how difficult it was to commute by public transportation, a classmate commented that Lisa ought to get a car. This remark offended Lisa, because she would like to have a car but could not afford one at this time. Lisa's interpretations of events seem to fit with Ogbu's (1992) description of ways of thinking among involuntary minority members.

For Lisa, a relative lack of experience and her diminished academic self confidence were two factors which acted as barriers to academic success. Lisa also tended to interpret all her interactions with her classmates as being the result of racism. The instructor worked with Lisa on increasing her self-esteem by providing clinical learning opportunities for Lisa and offering positive feedback. In spite of these problems, Lisa successfully completed the nursing curriculum.

Suzie

Suzie is a perky young Korean American student. She arrived in the United States when she was three years old. Although Suzie is Asian in appearance, she speaks flawless English. Suzie described an experience of racism during her first year of college. She was the only minority student in a predominantly white rural college. Shortly after her arrival, several students assumed she could speak no English because she looked Asian, and would talk about her as if she were not even present.

Suzie was raised with traditional Korean values. Her family values education very highly. Her parents work long hours in a small grocery store to enable her to attend school. Suzie notes a difference between many American students' attitudes and her own: "American students tend to party and yet make it through school. I was raised with the traditional Korean values—STUDY, STUDY, STUDY. Asian parents came to the United States so that their children could get an education. Children pay back their parents by doing well in school."

Although Suzie's verbal English skills are excellent, she thinks bilingually and has had difficulty with some of the science courses. Suzie sees the role of teacher as pivotal for the student who experiences language related problems. "The most important thing for students is that you must feel comfortable with the teachers, especially when your language skills are poor. Teachers need to be understanding and offer extra help."

Suzie has described problems associated with primary cultural differences: world views, values and language difficulties. The noncognitive factors which increase Suzie's probability of academic success include the ability to focus on long range goals, strong family support, and a cultural norm that highly values education and studying.

Li

Li graduated from high school in Vietnam and then came to the United States at age 18 with her parents. Although she had studied English in her native country, Li has found it challenging to read and understand the English textbooks used in her classes. "In Vietnam, teachers lectured in a very detailed fashion, and the textbook was seldom used." Li thinks in two languages, English and Vietnamese. "I take notes in English in the classroom, but if I cannot think of how to write an English word, I will use the Vietnamese word. It takes me more time to read the text and to take a test because of thinking in two languages. In Vietnam, tests were mostly short essay." Li finds it difficult to try to pick out answers in multiple choice tests. When teachers announce "only five minutes more," Li panics and tries to answer the questions quickly. As a result, she does not take the time to think through the answers. Li has experienced academic difficulties as a result of poor test taking skills. On the positive side, Li has strong family support and a cultural ethic which values studying hard to master a subject. Li is able to offer suggestions about strategies which may help students such as herself.

Li notices a great difference between students in Vietnam and in the United States. Education is highly valued and parents expect to pay the cost. In Vietnam, therefore, students focus on school and do not work to support themselves. Li observed that American students do not allow sufficient time to study.

Li offered several suggestions to assist students like herself. Pairing strong students with weak ones would be helpful, because it is easier to ask a peer than to ask a teacher. Li is afraid the teachers may think she is stupid. Another suggestion that Li offered was having teachers schedule brief review sessions—just five or ten minutes at a time. "If a teacher shows interest in the student, the student will work harder so that they do not waste the teacher's time. If a teacher spends time with the student and the student does not study, the student feels guilty."

Anh

Anh came to the United States with her family when she was eleven years old, after spending three years in a refugee camp. When she started in American schools, she spoke no English and no one at the school spoke Vietnamese. "It was very hard at first—no one was there to help you. At home, no one in my family spoke English, and at school, no one spoke Vietnamese." Even in the English as a Second Language (ESL) classes, Anh found that the ESL students represented a variety of minorities, and no other Vietnamese students were in the class. Anh describes her goal of assimilation into the new culture by saying, "I had to go with the flow and depend upon the American school system." Anh is still self conscious about her English and prefers to ask questions of the teacher privately after class. Anh survived the isolation and loneliness of language differences and has long range goals for education. Her experience in secondary school taught her that she can succeed and has helped develop self confidence in her academic capabilities.

Jeanmarie

Jeanmarie is a 20-year-old student who came to the United States at the age of 12. Although Jeanmarie had studied English in Haiti (along with Greek, Latin, and Spanish), she did not *know* English. Her native tongue is both French and Creole. Jeanmarie "attended ESL classes and every school related activity I could find to help me learn English." Language differences have created some academic difficulties for Jeanmarie. "In nursing classes we are taught in English; if I don't understand something the professor said, I will try to think of it in my native language. I do not like to ask questions in class because many people cannot understand me. I would rather talk privately to the teachers in their offices."

Hands on learning in the clinical area is especially helpful. "When a teacher talks about something in class, you have to try to imagine what it is like. In class we learned that a patient in shock is 'cold and clammy.' Once I saw that in a patient, I really understood what it meant. Videos are also very helpful in understanding what the book is saying."

Jeanmarie likes caring for clients from other cultures. "Here I am the one with the different background. I try to accommodate them, to put myself in their place, and treat them the way I would want to be treated."

Jeanmarie's experiences reflect primary cultural differences. She has tried to adapt her cultural ways of learning to her present situation. Language differences create difficulties for her. Jeanmarie demonstrates a high level of cultural sensitivity to her clients because of her own personal experiences.

Gisele

Gisele also came to the United States from Haiti as a teenager. "It was really hard to go to high school because I did not speak English, only

French and Creole. School is still hard for me because I think and feel in three different languages. Nursing is still another language. Sometimes when you speak with an accent, people think you cannot understand English. Just because you speak with an accent does not mean you are stupid."

"I have to work twice as hard as American students because of the language differences. I always prepare for class and try to understand what the teacher will be talking about. Some professors don't allow enough time for students who think in several languages. You can tell from the expression on their faces. The teachers say they want you to ask questions and then make you feel stupid when you go to their office and they say, 'This is the fifth time you are here.'"

Gisele was very anxious before her first clinical rotation. "I had lots of thoughts on my mind. If I have to spend twice as long in the classroom, what will it be like in the clinical setting?" For Gisele, her saving grace was her clinical instructor. "My clinical instructor built my confidence. I never got frustrated because she was there for me. A good clinical instructor is really important for foreigners."

Gisele's cultural background made it especially difficult when she failed a course. "My parents have very high expectations. It used to be 'don't come home.' Living in the United States, people learn to think differently. Now my mother encourages me."

When asked what suggestions she would make to nurse educators, Gisele responded, "I would like for nursing instructors to appreciate who I am as an individual. I don't want more time; I don't need more time. If I go to a professor's office with a question, I would like to feel respected because I want to better understand the material."

The Haitian students shared some similar primary cultural differences with the Asian students. The Haitian students also have a deep sense of respect for teachers and education, and are shocked by the disrespect which they observe in the American student population. Education and educated persons are highly valued. Only a few individuals in Haiti, Korea and Vietnam have the opportunity to go to college, so these students feel privileged to have the opportunity to go to school.

Implications for Faculty Development

Tanner (1996) identified the need for faculty development in the area of cultural diversity as the major issue of curriculum reform for the 1990s.

One of the qualities ascribed to successful teachers of nursing consists of creating an environment conducive to learning through conveying a deep respect for students. Another attribute of the successful teacher is the ability to utilize a variety of teaching methods according to class character-istics (Anderson, 1997). Cultural awareness by faculty involves the recog-nition of individual differences among ethnic minority groups.

A variety of suggestions to assist faculty in the development of cultural awareness in their teaching can be found in the literature (Gonzalez, 1993; Huff, 1993; Lou 1993; Rew, 1996; Roberts, 1993; Vaughn, 1997; Yoder, 1996). Among the strategies suggested are the following:

- Get reacquainted with yourself and your beliefs and values (Out-law, 1994; Roberts, 1993; Vaughn, 1997).
- Get to know the students "a whole lot better" (Roberts, 1993).
- Learn to listen (Vaughn, 1997).
- Accept students' cultural backgrounds and encourage sharing of personal insights in class discussions (Gonzalez, 1993; Rew, 1996).
- Practice behaviors which denote respect, such as calling students by name (Gonzalez, 1993).
- Do not blame the students for failure to learn (Lou, 1993).
- Reject the traditional model of college, teaching that the student must conform to the norms of the professor (Lou, 1993).
- Don't pretend (even to yourself) that you can enter the world of the minority student (Huff, 1993).
- Incorporate new scholarship about minorities into your teaching (Lou, 1993).
- Provide landmarks and warning signs to guide students safely through the "landscape of learning" (Rew, 1996).
- Eliminate stereotyping (Vaughn, 1997).
- Provide role models (Nelson, 1996; Steele, 1995; Vaughn, 1997; Yoder, 1996).
- Be a mentor (Gonzalez, 1993; Huff, 1993).
- Confront racism directly (Gonzalez, 1993; Steele, 1995; Vaughn, 1997).

Benediction

This chapter has explored the issue of educating culturally diverse minority students for the 21st century. What is known from research about assessments, interventions and evaluation of outcomes has been reviewed. Theoretical frameworks from the discipline of education suggest ways of thinking about the culture of education in America. Personal stories of nursing students are provided to help faculty "get to know" what the students experience. Finally, practical tips are offered to assist nursing faculty to become even more successful teachers. May you go forth blessed with new insights and strategies as you educate nurses for the next millennium.

REFERENCES

American Association of Colleges of Nursing. (1986). *Essentials of college and university education for professional nursing: Final report.* Washington, DC: Author.

Anderson, C. A. (1997). Nursing faculty. In McCloskey, J. C. & Grace, H. K. *Current issues in nursing,* (pp. 34–40). St. Louis: Mosby.

Bowser, B. P., Auletta, G. S., & Jones, T. (1993). *Confronting diversity issues on campus.* Newbury Park, CA: Sage.

Boyer, S. P., & Sedlacek, W. E. (1988). Noncognitive predictors of academic success for international students: A longitudinal study. *Journal of College Student Development, 29,* 218–223.

Campbell, A. R., & Davis, S. M. (1996). Faculty commitment: Retaining minority nursing students in majority institutions. *Journal of Nursing Education, 35* (7), 298–303.

Carter, R. T., & Goodwin, A. L. (1994). Racial identity and education. *Review of Research in Education, 20,* 291–336.

Crawford, L., & Olinger, B. (1988). Recruitment and retention of nursing students from diverse cultural backgrounds. *Journal of Nursing Education, 27*(8), 379–381.

Crow, K. (1993). Multiculturalism and pluralistic thought in nursing education: Native American world views and the academic world view. *Journal of Nursing Education, 32*(5), 198–204.

Davis, S. P. (1995). A challenge to develop a new paradigm shift in nursing education. *Journal of Cultural Diversity, 2*(4), 124–130.

Dowell, M. A. (1996). Issues in recruitment and retention of minority students. *Journal of Nursing Education, 35*(7), 293–297.

Fitzsimons, V. M., & Kelley, M. L. (1996). *The culture of learning.* New York: NLN Press.

Garcia, G. E., & Pearson, P. D. (1994). Assessment and diversity. *Review of Research in Education, 20,* 337–391.

Gibson, D. M. (1996). The humanistic edge. In Fitzsimons, V. M. & Kelley, M. L. *The culture of learning.* New York: NLN Press (pp. 17–21).

Giger, J. N., & Davidhizar, R. E. (1995). *Transcultural nursing: Assessment and intervention.* St. Louis: Mosby.

Gonzalez, J. C. (1993). Once you accept, then you can teach. In Roberts, H., Gonzalez, J. C., Harris, O. D., Huff, D. J., John, A. M., Lou, R., & Scott, O. L. (1993). *Teaching from a multicultural perspective,* (pp. 1–16). Thousand Oaks, CA: Sage.

Harris, O. D. (1993). Equity in classroom assessment. In Roberts, H., Gonzalez, C., Harris, D., Huff, D. J., Johns, A. M., Lou, R. & Scott, O. L. *Teaching from a multicultural perspective,* (pp. 77–90). Newbury Park: Sage.

Heydman, A. (1991). Retention/attrition of nursing students: Emphasis on disadvantaged and minority students. In Baj, P. J., & Clayton, G. M. *Review of Research in Nursing Education, Vol. IV,* (pp. 1–29). New York: NLN Press.

Huff, D. J. (1993). On becoming a mensch or mentor. In Roberts, H., Gonzalez, C., Harris, D., Huff, D. J., Johns, A. M., Lou, R. & Scott, O. L. *Teaching from a multicultural perspective,* (pp. 91–96). Newbury Park: Sage.

Keklak, M. M. (1966). The nursing academic support center: High visibility for an Hispanic nurse mentor. In Fitzsimons, V. M. & Kelley, M. L. *The culture of learning,* (pp. 39–48). New York: NLN Press.

Kornguth, M., Frisch, N., Shovein, J., & Williams, R. (1994). Noncognitive factors that put students at academic risk in nursing programs. *Nurse Educator,* 19(5), 24–27.

Leininger, M. M. (1978). *Transcultural nursing: Theories, concepts and practices.* New York: Wiley.

Locke, D. C. (1992). *Increasing multicultural understanding: A comprehensive model.* Newbury Park, CA: Sage.

Minnick, A., Roberts, M. J., Young, Y. B., Marcantonio, R., & Kleinpell, R. M. (1997). Ethnic diversity and staff employment in hospitals. *Nursing Outlook,* 45(1), 35–40.

National League for Nursing Accrediting Commission. (1996). *Criteria and guidelines for the evaluation of baccalaureate and higher degree programs.* New York: NLN.

Nelson, L. R. (1996). Mentoring African American students: One Path to Success, in Fitzsimons, V. M. & Kelley, M. L., *The culture of learning,* (pp. 91–94). New York: NLN Press.

Ogbu, J. G. (1992). Understanding cultural diversity and learning. *Educational Researcher,* 22(8), 5–14.

Outlaw, F. H. (1994). A reformulation of the meaning of culture and ethnicity for nurses delivering care. *MEDSURG Nursing,* 3,(2), 108–111.

Pacquiao, D. F. (1996). Educating faculty in the concept of educational biculturalism: A comparative study of sociocultural influences on nursing students' experiences in school. In Fitzsimons, V. M. & Kelley, M. L. *The culture of learning,* (pp. 129–162). New York: NLN Press.

Rew, L. (1996). Affirming cultural diversity: a pathways model for nursing faculty. *Journal of Nursing Education,* 35(7), 310–314.

Rosella, J. D., Regan-Kubinski, M. J. & Albrecht, S. A. (1994). The need for multicultural diversity among health professionals. *Nursing & Health Care*, 15(5), 242–246.

Ross, L. L. (1996). Minorities in the mainstream. *Minorities: Pathways to the Health Professions*. Philadelphia: Allegheny University of the Health Sciences (brochure).

Russell, K., & Jewell, N. (1992). Cultural impact of health care access: Challenges for improving the health of African Americans. *Journal of Community Health Nursing*, 9(3), 161–169.

Saucier, B. L. (1994). Retention of nursing students: Intervention strategies. In L. R. Allen (Ed.). *Review of research in nursing education, Vol. VI* (pp. 107–126). New York: NLN Press.

Sedlacek, W. E. (1987). Should higher education students be admitted differentially by race and sex? The evidence. *Journal of the National Association of College Admissions Counselors*, 22, 22–24.

Sims, G. P., & Baldwin, D. (1995). Race, class and gender considerations in nursing education. *N&HC: Perspectives on Community*, 16(6), 316–321.

Smith, G. R. (1995). Lessons learned: Challenges for the future. *N&HC: Perspectives on Community*, 16(4), 188–191.

Steele, R. L. (1995). Diversity in academia: Some reflections. *The ABNF Journal*, 6(3), 84–86.

Tanner, C. A. (1996). Cultural diversity in nursing education. (Editorial). *Journal of Nursing Education*, 35(7), 292–293.

Tracey, T. J., & Sedlacek, W. E. (1985). The relationship of noncognitive variables to academic success: A longitudinal comparison by race. *Journal of College Student Personnel*, 26, 405–410.

Vaughn, J. (1997). Is there really racism in nursing? *Journal of Nursing Education*, 36(3), 135–139.

Yoder, M. K. (1996). Instructional responses to ethnically diverse students. *Journal of Nursing Education*, 35(7), 315–321.

Part V

New Phenomena and
New Partnerships

At *the turn of* the 20th century, infectious diseases were a leading cause of illness and death. Nursing's work was shaped to respond to the care of those affected. Long life was a rare occurrence for so many. Since that time, advances in medical science have lowered the mortality rate of infectious diseases, while chronic and degenerative disorders have increased in prevalence. There is a striking increase in the number of older Americans. By the year 2025, nearly one in five Americans will be over 65 bringing to the care scene new challenges and opportunities for nursing leadership.

Many of the chronic disorders experienced by both the young and old are diagnosed earlier and treated more aggressively. Amidst these new realities nursing's work continues to change in response to what presents itself.

The observations of Given, Given and DeVoss remind us that as nurses are educated for the future, providing nursing services for those with chronic health problems, new competencies, including astute assessment and referral skills will be required.

The models of family care that are becoming known to nurses in the community are a new departure for most nurses who have provided care in hospitals. Responding to people in a different setting while considering family care systems is an exciting new challenge as meaningful partnerships are forged.

Tartasky predicts that the services provided by nurse practitioners will be in great demand as the chronically ill population continues to increase and be seen in a variety of settings beyond the hospital. The opportunity for nursing leadership in the prevention and the development of patient self-management skills is one example of a whole new frontier for nursing action in the provision of relevant care, the education of students, and research initiatives.

10

The Education of Nurses for the Future— Caring for Those with Chronic Health Care Problems

Barbara A. Given, Charles W. Given, and Danielle N. DeVoss

Nursing practice includes restorative, supportive, and promotive health care activities. Despite changes in sociodemographics and in the health care system, these areas provide foci for practice which will extend into the 21st century. Restorative practices will be targeted to modify the impact of illness or disease on the large number of individuals who are aging and who are living with chronic illness. Supportive practices will seek to modify environments to enhance personal and public health by prevention, early detection, and the reduction of morbidity from chronic diseases. Promotive care practices will be directed toward fostering personal and family growth and development and to help persons and families achieve self-defined health goals.

The scope of nursing practice will be dynamic and will continue to evolve as the health care system changes. Changes in nursing knowledge and research and the expansion of professional responsibilities will depend upon how political environments promote or inhibit such changes and how needs for services are defined. Nurses must assume leadership roles to be active participants in health care system transformation. The scope of nursing practice must be flexible and responsive to societal needs, responding to evidence-based approaches to care as well as to expanding and shifting professional collaboration (ANA Policy Statement, 1995). It is impossible to know precisely what the future will bring, but nurses must be educated and prepared to meet the changes and future demands of the health care delivery system. We may not know how the system of care will evolve, but we do know what some of the health care needs of society will be, and thus must prepare nurses to meet those needs.

In this chapter, then, we will focus on basic baccalaureate nursing practice for the next century, given the rapid changes in the health care system and the concomitant projected demographic and social changes in society. The growing population of elderly persons with chronic disease provides a context for much of the discussion.

What roles will the nurse assume and what skills will be required of the nurse of the 21st century? As we near the coming century, nurses will continue to be a central component in the health care system and will be expected to provide cost-effective quality services to influence patient and family outcomes. Nonetheless, *restructuring* or *reengineering* needs become apparent now, so that we can prepare graduates of nursing programs to meet the expectations and needs of our changing society. Nurses must be open to altering and evolving practices which will improve patient, family, and community care while recognizing and appreciating the constraints facing the system.

HEALTH CARE SYSTEM TRENDS

Most nurses being educated today will practice within large, integrated health care systems where care will be delivered across diffuse networks, with vertical and horizontal consolidation taking place even now at extraordinary rates. Attention will be especially redirected toward risk factors affecting substantial community segments. Most communities will find their care delivered by two or three major health systems, with payment mechanisms capitated and based on competition. Most individuals will have their health care services paid for by employment-based or by government-subsidized insurance. There will continue to be a pervasive concern for maintaining costs through mechanisms to control and limit expenditures (O'Neil, 1993). More and more care will be home and community care, external to the acute care system. Nurses of the future will need to be prepared to work in this environment and to match patient needs with health care specialties offering efficient services leading to effective health care outcomes.

DEMOGRAPHIC, SOCIAL, AND ECONOMIC TRENDS

Barzansky, Friedman, and Arnold et al. (1993) and Mundinger (1994) anticipate that within the next decade the largest percentage of health care clients will be of Hispanic, African American, and Asian descent. Cultural diversity will be the norm in many, if not all, communities. Differences between socioeconomic levels are expected to become more pronounced, the gap between rich and poor will widen, and more families will slide below the poverty level. More patients will be over 65 years of age, reside in urban areas, and have chronic diseases (cardiovascular, pulmonary, cancer, and depression, as well as AIDS or tuberculosis) or will be survivors of those diseases or other new diseases or syndromes that evolve.

The number of adults requiring long-term and supportive care has increased in large part because of the success of medical research and care. Individuals are now surviving with conditions that 20 years ago were fatal. In the United States, it is estimated that over 11.3 million adults depend on others for some degree of care due to chronic disabilities and that at least 10 percent of the U.S. population requires long-term care (Center for Vulnerable Populations, 1992; Komisar et al., 1996). Of those with chronic disabilities in need of care, 12.6 percent are age 50 to 59, and 43.6 percent are age 60 or older. The prevalence of disability increases with age and the elderly population is rapidly growing, with those over 85 years of age the fastest growing segment. Those Americans over the age of 85 are expected to reach a population of 4.6 million in the year 2000 and 8 million in the year 2030 (U.S. Bureau of the Census, 1992). Baby boomers will begin to turn age 85 after 2030, resulting in a dramatic impact on the demand for both formal and informal long-term care services.

The prevalence of limitations in daily activities increases to 56.8 percent among the oldest-old and is higher among women and African Americans than among men and Caucasians (Aday, 1993). The oldest-old are likely to have multiple health problems that result in physical and mental frailty and consequent dependency on long-term care services and family members for assistance. Individuals aged 85 and older are four to five times more likely to be disabled and to require assistance with personal care activities than those aged 65 to 74. Those over 85 are most often women living alone on inadequate incomes (Leutz, Capitman, MacAdam, & Abrahams, 1992). The life expectancy of persons with developmental disabilities is also dramatically increasing, resulting in a growing mentally-impaired geriatric population who experience an earlier onset of health-related problems such as respiratory disease, hearing loss, and dementia.

The exponential growth of the elderly population, especially that of the oldest-old and the multiple chronic illnesses and dependencies they face, will profoundly increase family and community responsibilities for care and add to the complexity of the coordination of care. Continued formal care restrictions and cost containment will, in the future, alter the availability of family caregivers to provide care to chronically ill family members. Enhanced and specialized care management systems will be required to work with a diverse population and manage complex acute and chronic problems to keep individuals out of the hospital, and, if admitted, to minimize the time they spend there. Most of the responsibility for restorative and rehabilitative care will be shouldered by families outside of the acute care setting. A component of care management is the advocacy of patient and family rights and support as they adopt new roles. The role of advocate is suitable for nurses and will, in fact, be required of nurses in the future.

The demand on long-term care facilities will increase as individuals and families find that they can no longer continue to provide care on a daily basis for long periods of time. In long-term care facilities, nurses will have a major role in the organization and management of care for the growing population of the chronically ill and/or dependent elderly, many of whom are women.

The least healthy and most disabled elderly tend to be older, poorer, single, minority, and female. Elderly persons of color experience greater degrees of functional and chronic impairment than whites but utilize fewer long-term care services (Leutz, et al., 1992). Thus, families are called on to provide more care. Many factors have affected family structures and the resources available for the community care of relatives: geographic mobility; escalating divorce rates; single parent families; greater public acceptance of single, cohabiting, and homosexual lifestyles; blended families with competing loyalties and responsibilities; larger numbers of women in the labor force; and growth in poverty. Today, families are smaller than they have been at any time in history primarily because of a decrease in the birth rate. The declining fertility rate and the increase in childless marriages will affect how the nurse of the future works with families. Ever-increasing numbers of individuals will outlive their families and their care resources. Who will these childless elders turn to for assistance with care in the future?

For many families, the lack of adequate income often leads to poor or substandard housing, poor nutrition and diet, and minimal or no health care. For many persons, minimal health care may result in delayed diagnoses and more severe conditions. Many of the stresses families of the future will face derive, directly or indirectly, from the lack of economic resources and will impact the health and general well-being of the family. Personal and family inadequacy may limit a family's ability to provide care for the chronically ill.

The shifting composition of the U.S. workforce—a growing number of women, single-parent, and dual-earner households—has led to a concern for how family care responsibilities, traditionally the onus of the family alone, will be carried out given the entry of family carers into the workplace. There has not yet been a widespread adoption of work-family benefits or programs to support the employed family caregiver.

The combined effects of demographic, social, and economic changes will continue to put pressure on families and make it less likely that they will be able to provide long-term care alternative arrangements, and assistance when needed. Families may find themselves sandwiched between increasing pressures for family care and an escalating demand for cost effectiveness in the health care system. Public policy, normative attitudes, and health care delivery changes advocating the cost-effectiveness of care have increased. As a result, families feel constrained both by the time required to care and economic pressures from both within and outside of the family. The expectation that families should provide the majority of chronic illness care to relatives will no longer be realistic; thus, the formal system will have to provide mechanisms for care. Nurses will be in the center of this dilemma and will be expected to assume a role of organizing care to meet the needs of the patients and family members functioning in new types of health care settings and interdisciplinary team arrangements.

Nurses of the future will need to care for persons in this changing sociodemographic environment and be comfortable with cultural diversity and families with complex special care needs (especially those of elderly clients who are chronically ill). Within a community-based practice, a working knowledge of cultural diversity will be an important foundation. Particular attention to personal health habits, stressors, and health risks will be necessary for health promotion and disease prevention within the family and the community.

THE PROVISION OF CHRONIC AND LONG-TERM CARE

Long-term care and chronic care in the United States is fragmented, inadequately financed, and biased toward skilled care needs and institutionalization (Estes, Swan, & Associates, 1994). Little support is available for families to meet the custodial and supportive care needs that would keep the elderly independent longer and add to the quality of life of the patient and the caregiver. As changes in health care and cost containment continue, increased pressure will be placed on family members who are available and capable to become the primary carers and to furnish millions of hours of informal, *unpaid* care. A critical component of the preparation of nurses of the future will be training and supporting nurses to work with families to enhance their capacity to care.

Variables Affecting the Provision of Care

Community-based care of the future will include determining how factors such as age, gender, employment, financial status, developmental status, marital status, living arrangements, and usual role obligations alter and influence the care situation. Age and gender characteristics directly influence family's availability, capability, and willingness to assist the patient with care. Chronically ill spouse caregivers provide care for patients who are sometimes no less diminished in self-care and mobility and yet do this with less assistance than nonspouses. As a consequence of the longevity of women's lives, elderly females generally are cared for by adult children, while older males generally are cared for by their spouses.

Given the chronic nature of many diseases and their impact on the large aging population, much focus will need to be on keeping individuals independent. Age not only affects how families respond to an *on time* diagnosis or heart problems in an older family member, but may influence the availability of support and the amount of effort invested in assisting the patient to recover. Family caregivers will be aided most by having mobile patients who are able to perform or assist in their own self-care activities. Patient gender may influence the usual household tasks and which tasks will be relinquished or realigned. Reassignment of the usual roles of patients due to the effects of the disease and treatment must be assessed so that patients and families can be linked to the community services and support needed.

In addition to the demographic trends of fewer children, impaired mobility, and blended family structures, adult children are caught between their work roles (professional and career-related) and life roles (family care-related). Parent care will be a major variable in the care provided in the next century, as competing roles—work, social, and family—add to the complexity of the care situation. These role demands will become a major societal issue. Middle-aged (intergenerational) caregivers are more likely to suffer role conflicts because of the multiple competing role demands placed on them. Income and overall financial status influence the resources families can bring to care. In the future, those who are underserved will suffer more than the *haves* as they will find fewer and restricted resources to assist them with care.

Employment retention does not necessarily result in reduced assistance to dependent elderly or chronically ill relatives. Women's employment will not necessarily pose a problem to the health care system, but rather, will create a problem for the women, as they will be required to perform a *double duty* which leads to increased burden and stress due to the multiple roles they perform. Stressors become compounded if the working female caregiver also has children of her own to care for and is the sole or primary source of support for those children. Health promotion activities for the employed caregiver will be needed and will become a part of the nursing care regimen.

The availability of care is also influenced by the employment status and living arrangements of patients and family members. Because some family members do not have the physical or emotional capacity to care, the capability of care providers must be assessed by the nurse in order to acquire needed support. Patients with no close relatives or those with poor prior relationships and intensive demands of care are at risk for institutionalization. Employed caregivers provide less care than nonemployed caregivers while caregivers who live in different households from their patients tend to provide only slightly less care overall.

Individuals who live alone are also at very high risk for institutionalization when they become dependent and have care demands. In addition, following current population trends, we will see aging children in their 60s and 70s caring for patients in their 80s and 90s. The availability and types of alternative living and care arrangements will grow as the chronically ill and dependent population grows. Identification and coordination of resources will be a major focus for the nurse when caring for individuals with chronic illness who live alone without an established or available care support system to enable them to remain as independent as possible.

Care Situations and Strategies

Care for the acute and chronically ill elderly includes a wide range of care activities and care that is provided during the day, at night, and on weekends, as well as *on demand.* Care includes custodial or maintenance help or services, yet is more than meeting physical needs. Care requirements that family members fulfill depend on the patient's physical, functional, and psychological capacity. *Caring for* encompasses both the performance and/or supervision of concrete care tasks along with monitoring emotional status and providing emotional support.

Family involvement in care tasks depends on patient functional disability in daily self-care activities and can include such tasks as bathing, dressing, eating, laundry, or transportation—custodial and predictable tasks which may not be difficult for family members to manage. Symptom management and control, however, may become major foci for both the patient and family as they struggle to manage the symptoms of disease and side effects of ongoing treatment for many of the chronic illnesses. These activities require much observation, supervision, and judgment— often beyond the knowledge, skill, and capacity of the family member. Because of the extent of problems, nurses will have to work in partnership with families to meet information needs and to model the care strategies that will result in families helping their family members to achieve maximum outcomes. Nurses will need to outline for families how their efforts will contribute to those outcomes.

Family involvement (assistance) in care management ranges from direct care to complex monitoring and decision-making to emotional comfort. Providing support and encouragement, and dealing with the patient's emotional status and psychological distress require caregiver attention and energy. This care taxes the caregivers, who often have their own unmet emotional needs. Caregivers may have few skills to manage effectively in this highly-charged emotional environment. Each form of care involvement demands different knowledge, skills, organizational capacities, role demands, and psychological strength from family members. With the chronicity and continued family responsibility, this family care demand may extend over a number of years. The health care system—which currently concerns itself with the patient and his or her medical and health care problems—will, in the future, need to address this hidden health care system, i.e., the family, and to recognize their influence on clinical outcomes. Nurses will need to be prepared to play a lead role in protecting the emotional integrity of families and ensuring that their psychosocial needs are addressed.

The survival rates for those with chronic illnesses will continue to climb and the aging population will continue to grow. Symptom experience will become a profound variable in the care of these individuals. Whether symptoms are the consequence of the disease or treatment, nursing-sensitive outcomes will focus more and more on symptom management and upon alleviation or reduction of symptoms to manageable levels. Symptom management activity will be directed toward improving and preserving functional outcomes. Family burden is seriously influenced by physical functioning, especially in social and personal care activities.

Family members already provide 80 percent of the in-home care to the elderly with chronic illnesses, even when formal services are used selectively (Leutz, et al., 1992; U.S. Special Committee on Aging, 1992). The need for in-home care provision is projected to dramatically increase, but families may not be prepared to care. Assessing the health status of family members and family needs will be critical skills for the nurse of the future. When adult children become involved in care, they may not live with the care-recipient. Planning and coordinating care will become a major task of the nurse. Care requirements dictate *who* cares and *what assistance* they receive. The nurse of tomorrow will need to be skilled to project and plan for needed care, assess the capacity of patient and family caregiver to ensure that needed care occurs, and to match unmet needs with the available health care systems and complement these resources with personal, family, and community resources. Coordination of a broad range of services will become a more complex task. Care coordination must occur in the context of the best possible patient and family outcomes.

Of the 5.5 million elderly with disabilities in 1990, about 1.5 million lived in nursing or residential care homes, with women comprising 75 percent of nursing home residents. This is, however, only a small proportion of the patients with chronic disabilities, but this number will markedly increase in the next two decades and family members will be required to provide care. In the coming years, more community and home-based support services will need to be made available and affordable to families. There are few paid home care resources, however, readily available to families. Family caregivers comprise the cornerstone of the provision of community-based long-term care (Estes et al., 1994). Without family care (seldom accounted for by the formal care system), the number of persons served by publicly supported long-term care services, particularly institutional care, would increase dramatically. Health education programs need to consider this as a factor influencing patient care.

Assistance to families may depend on roles within the family. Nonworking daughters and elderly spouses, especially females, often get the least formal and/or informal assistance. Initial assessment should include determining the patient's previous relationship with the caregiver and the existing network of secondary caregivers so that the health care provider is aware of all available supportive resources. It will be important that nurses acquire the skills to assess patient and caregiver needs and then determine the available and appropriate resources for family members (Zarit, Pearlin, & Schaie, 1993). Nurses will have to be aware of the existing resources in the community, and to creatively combine and coordinate these resources to best benefit the patient and family. Much more of the care of the future for all age groups will be self-provided and family-driven.

The nurse of the future will need to deal with the articulation of family care within the formal system. They will be expected to enhance the capacity of the family to care. Assessment will focus on unmet needs of patient and caregiver. In most instances, the health care professional will be dealing with a primary caregiver, typically a female (mother, daughter, wife, granddaughter, grandmother).

The provision of direct care imposes restrictions on family role responsibilities. Social activities influence the manner in which the family member views care. Changes and restrictions in work roles and career opportunities, coupled with economic costs such as loss of patient and family income and added out-of-pocket expenses are additional burdens that must be considered as essential to a broad health care assessment. Socioeconomic differences influence access to care as well as outcomes of care; socioeconomic status may allow families to purchase assistance and to spend a smaller percentage of their income on care costs, both formal and informal. The nurse will have an important role in functioning in multiple alternative settings in which traditional and new, alternative forms of long-term care will be provided.

Systems of Care

Current health and medical services are procedural, medical, and high-tech, oriented toward the short-term care of persons with acute illness rather than toward a continuum of care for chronically ill persons. The need for medical interventions will climb as mortality decreases. This, accompanied by a significant increase in loss of physical functioning, will allow for a growing disabled patient population. The medicalization of care, combined with capitated forms of reimbursement under managed care systems, have resulted in increased expectations that families can and will perform high-tech tasks previously administered by professionals in institutional settings. To compensate for this transfer, community and support service systems should be set up to assist families with skilled care procedures and techniques. Systems of care which reimburse for failing heart transplants and high tech procedures, but not for personal care or homemaker services essential to supporting chronically ill patients and their families in the community, compromise the legitimacy of family care. New systems of care will be needed to resolve this conflict and to meet the needs of family members.

The long-term care system of the future will, by necessity, need to offer a continuum of care: from simple, acute care to follow-up and recovery, rehabilitation and health maintenance and community-care services that could support both the dependent person or chronically ill patients and their families (Estes et al., 1994; Leutz et al., 1992). The transition to institutional and long-term care will also need to be a continuous and smooth process for patient and family.

In the future, family caregivers will require assistance to provide care in the home. Meeting the needs of growing, culturally diverse populations with chronic disabilities requires new professionals, new roles and new strategies for health care. Nursing should take a leadership role in meeting the needs of a transforming patient population and family care system. The nurse of the future will be most effective when practicing in partnership with the family and patient and providing appropriate access to the correct health professional as needs dictate.

A model of family care supported by nurses must consider the overall context of care for the individual and assess prior role relationships between the patient and caregiver. Family members assume care responsibilities as a part of expectations of commitment to the family, but many lack the capacity and capability to provide the needed care. Although multiple members may be involved in providing components of care, usually one person (typically a woman) is primarily responsible for direct care and coordination of care. Daughters are clearly the most frequent adult children caregivers.

Care expectations and opportunities are different for each family and influenced by multiple variables. For daughters and daughters-in-law, family caregiving is an *off time* phenomenon (out of the usual life cycle order) and is not a normative expectation in younger families. Care challenges are even more burdensome at this time since not only are these challenges unexpected, but the support needed to meet the challenges may not be available or offered to these families. When a male spouse falls ill and the wife becomes the sole wage earner *and* the family care provider, her ability to provide total care and fulfill her multiple roles is greatly diminished.

Time spent by the family members planning and providing care is time not spent in other family, social, or work-related activities and must be considered a social cost of care. The stresses and conflicts caused by the care requirements may be particularly problematic at certain stages of family or individual development, as well as certain career stages. Shortened lengths of hospital stays and shifts toward outpatients in the home will continue.

In the future, the nurse must be aware of these sociodemographic and developmental differences and discrepancies among clients. The nurse will need to determine the capability, availability, and capacity of families to care, as well as help patients' families reduce barriers and mobilize resources to allow continued employment and spousal care. Nurses will need to identify resources or appropriate assistive personnel to enable this to happen. The resources required to care will need to be matched at a patient-by-patient and family-by-family need level. Only through this prioritization can resource use be maximized and patient and family care needs be met.

Given the transfer of acute and chronic care to family members, the health and well being of the family unit is a crucial component of patient care and an important part of nursing assessment. Change in patients' conditions due to alleviation of problems, remission, or exacerbation of the disease processes necessitates an associate change in family care responsibilities. This can result in negative reactions, stress, and strain of the family care provider, especially as care becomes more comprehensive and exists over a long period of time, thus jeopardizing both care and clinical outcomes. Patients' dependencies on others to perform tasks of daily living, to aid in symptom management, and to help with mobility impact family members' daily schedules and, subsequently, may impact caregiver depression (Given, Given, Helms, Stommel, & DeVoss, in press). The patient's own psychological reaction to illness appears to influence the burden felt by the family caregiver, and, at times, family distress equals or exceeds that of the patient. Thus, a family care approach is an integral part of the planning of future care.

Family caregivers have been and will continue to be the primary source of assistance to those with functional disabilities who live in the community. A small percent of people with disabilities receive paid home care services. This is rapidly increasing, but containment is being placed on this care as well. Paid community-based services, such as adult day care, home-delivered meals, or transportation assistance, are important to families and will become more important. At any given time, seven out of eight disabled elders in the community rely on informal care and whatever formal care they can find and pay for themselves (Leutz et al., 1992). Mixing and matching formal and informal care will become an increasingly occurring family care activity in the future. This will necessitate communication in multiple settings among various branches and levels of the health care system.

The complex needs of the aging and chronically ill serve to illustrate the knowledge and skills that will be required of the nurse of the future. The next section provides further discussion of those requirements.

ROLES OF THE NURSE OF THE FUTURE

The Pew Health Professions Commission (O'Neil, 1993) identified seven areas of competency essential for all future health care practitioners. These include: 1) caring for the community's health, 2) providing contemporary/state-of-the-art clinical care, 3) functioning in emerging systems—new health care settings in which health care practitioners function in interdisciplinary teams with expanded accountability, 4) providing cost effective and technologically appropriate care, 5) supporting prevention and promoting healthy lifestyles, 6) empowering patients and families in decision-making processes, and 7) managing information and continuing education. These skills will be necessary in order to adequately deal with a demographically changing, chronically ill, and aging patient population in a rapidly transforming and chaotic health care industry.

Cost containment will certainly remain a primary concern in the future and will require nurses to focus on prevention, health promotion (among the total population as well as the elderly), and the maintenance of function and independence for those who are chronically ill and aging. At the same time, state-of-the-art care will be a requirement in most settings and a demand of many patients and families. The Pew areas of competence will be used to summarize the role of the nurse in addressing these issues or needs in the decades ahead.

Caring for the Community's Health

The days of lengthy hospital stays that incorporate recovery beyond physiologic stability are gone; the new focus of health care will be community care and health promotion. Nurses will practice within some type of population-based, capitated model of care that will seek to meet the changing needs of various communities. Training and socialization must occur so nurses can fit into future practice contexts.

The chronically ill will require assistance to stay in their homes. Nurses can contract directly with patients or with Medicare and insurance programs to provide a determined number of visits to assess the patient and the family member providing care, to check on medication administration, to observe the care environment, and to choreograph the use of social service, physical therapists, or nutritionists. Using the phone and electronic services technology will enhance the capacity of the nurse to stay in touch with individuals requiring assistance with their chronic health problems.

Clients with difficult and complex problems will be increasingly cared for in community and ambulatory settings through nurse case managers. Managed care systems already track high-risk clients in and out of the health care system to ensure efficient use of services that promote health, prevent illness, or monitor recovery and rehabilitation. A concern for the overall health of the community will be a priority.

Formal sources of supportive patient care in the community—in which the nurse of the future will play a larger part—include ambulatory care and general care provided through community-based agencies. The coordination of community care across settings and through the various transitions will be an important task for nurses. A case management role with specified outcomes and measures to achieve them will be important to ensure patient quality-of-life.

Nurses will likely be called upon to establish independent clinics in rural and urban underserved areas, with the added potential Medicare and Medicaid reimbursement. Poor nutrition, poor hygiene, poor self-care, and alcohol abuse are prevalent in these underserved populations and will complicate the management of care. Nurses can do a great deal to improve self-care capacity through health promotion, and dissemination of knowledge and skills that will enhance the quality of life for such populations. There will be a variety of new ways for nurses to function within the community, including new settings, role articulations, and coordination of care activities.

Formal agencies *do not* substitute for the care that family members provide, but they can provide a community-based platform of support that enables families to continue to care. This support will become more important in the future. Patients and families are often unaware of the existence of supportive agencies or are uncertain about how to find or gain access to them. Families may be reluctant to acknowledge that they need help, guidance, and teaching to enable them to accept needed services; and nurses often need to legitimize eligibility criteria and services to the family. Family attitudes related to use of services include: concern for opinions of others (fear of losing *face*), confidence in the service system, preference for informal care, belief in caregiver independence, and acceptance of government services (King, Collins, & Liken, 1995). Nurses will need to address and examine each of these factors. Socially adept family caregivers are able to identify and secure agency services more easily than those who have few social skills. It will be important to advocate for those with few social skills and assist them to gain skills. As change agents, the nurse of the future will require knowledge of community resources and entitlements and will ensure that supportive and appropriate community systems and services for needed care are available and utilized.

State-of-the-Art Clinical Care

Nursing professionals need to be able to define, market, provide, and, most importantly, document their role in delivering the quality services to health care consumers that, in new ways, link the processes with the outcomes of care. In the future, nurses will need to link their process of care with desired and expected outcomes. This will require that they engage in an evidence-based approach to care, one that links patients' medical and social characteristics with nursing interventions to produce the desired outcomes. Nurses functioning without state-of-the-art knowledge will not be familiar with the appropriate intervention most likely to produce a positive outcome for patient and family.

It is likely that for patients presenting complex multi-system chronic illnesses, nurses may have to specialize in order to focus on patient organ systems. This may become necessary as the number and complexity of drug regimens increase and as the intricacy of care for patients increases. For example, cancer treatments are becoming more complex and aggressive. Nurses will need to understand how a particular regimen may impact a patient, what the normal expected effects are, how long such effects may last, and when these effects are abnormal either in severity or duration. With the emphasis on ambulatory and home care, the nurse will be responsible for the early detection of problems, will implement appropriate therapy, and monitor and evaluate progress. The goal of these activities will be toward forestalling a hospital admission or other costly yet avoidable care.

In the future, managed care organizations will take responsibility for chronic illness across the disease trajectory. Nurses will be required to have the skills to anticipate needs and tailor the disease management approaches to the changing needs of the patients and family members, and determine when deviations occur. These skills will secure a necessary and important role for nurses in the health care delivery system.

New Health Care Settings and Expanded Accountability

Nurses will be working in and across sophisticated technology-based systems of care. The nurse of the future will work with the well and the chronically ill in settings across the continuum—from technologically sophisticated surgical centers to patient homes, clinics, day care centers, geriatric living communities, meal delivery sites, and foster care environments. There will be a variety of new living and health care opportunities in the community, such as day care centers—not just for the mentally impaired (e.g., the Alzheimer's population), but also for others who need care and supervision for a limited period of time each day. A variety of services geared toward assisting family members to continue to provide care, such as foster day care living arrangements, will become prevalent. These will be important community-based settings for nursing care and will link patients and families with medical specialties.

Professional nurses with higher degrees will function as managers of care, specialists in clinical areas, and case managers (Fagin & Lynaugh, 1992; Mundinger, 1994; Peterson, 1989; Safriet, 1992; Sullivan, Lee, & Warnick, 1987). Regardless of setting, nurses will assume more responsibility and accountability, be self-reliant, and familiarize themselves with current knowledge and expertise. Health care administrators demand clinical and systems outcome data for decision-making. Payers are demanding accountability while current health care systems are stressing cost-effective quality health care. Report cards and performance indicators for individual practitioners are the norm. Nurses will need to be attentive and understand how they contribute to the outcomes and develop nurse-sensitive indicators of these outcomes so that the relevance of the care they provide is noted.

Management tools (disease and demand management) will be needed to help guide patients through the continuum of care; health care professionals are currently calling these *care paths* and *clinical guidelines*. These tools must become more research and outcome-based and include the nursing component. Nurses require guidelines based on nursing in order to practice and should be involved in the development and utilization of these clinical guidelines.

Accountability and evaluation will become increasingly important in the future. Once plans are developed for the patient and family member, the nurse will use expected outcome criteria to evaluate the effectiveness of that plan. Follow-up monitoring of expected outcomes will become an important activity for the nurse, and accountability for patient satisfaction, efficient use of resources, and ethical behavior will be expanded.

Both process and outcome assessment evaluations will be important. Addressing accountability remains a difficult task, but must take place. Process and outcome variables must be defined, recognizing that many outcomes involve a number of other health care professionals. Development of nurse-sensitive indicators for functional status, mental health status, satisfaction with care, cost of care, and burden of care is critical to future accountability and credibility.

Functioning in Interdisciplinary Teams

Much more interdependence and broader service relationships will emerge as care is provided in a number of settings across the care continuum (New Roles, 1996), and interdependence will continue to be vital among parts of the system. Teams are managing health problems and nurses need to learn how better to work together—not in a hierarchical fashion, but as a collaborative team whose combination of skills meet a range of needs for patients and families. It will be vital to relate, communicate, interact, and contribute to a team-based approach to service delivery. Nurses must learn and demand the role of interdependence and collaboration, but be ever mindful of their own unique contributions.

Interdisciplinary functioning will be necessary to deal with both the complex needs of the patient, as well as the new interactions required by the changing health care system. There will be continued interdependence with the integrated systems. Nurses and physicians will, of necessity, require increasing interdisciplinary clinical training opportunities (Donaldson et al., 1996).

Providing Cost-Effective and Technologically Appropriate Care

Because the financial costs of care borne by the family may approach the cost of long-term institutionalization, support of the family caregiver may become a consumer demand and an important component of health care. In the future, nurses will need to carefully determine how best to support family care and mobilize resources to enhance care as a way to contain health system costs, as well as influence patient outcomes.

The nurse will need to have working skills in applying sometimes conflicting ethical precepts related to bringing about patient benefit, avoiding harm, enhancing patient autonomy, and increasing the well-being of a diverse group of patients and their family members. The vertically integrated systems will continue to focus on decreased costs, therefore mechanisms of gatekeeping, controlled referrals, and strict adherence to practice guidelines will predominate (Greenlick, 1995). Future nurses will need to develop creative clinical judgment and reasoning skills that can be applied in a variety of settings.

As nurses increasingly rely on informatics-driven resources to gain state-of-the-art knowledge, they will be influenced by scientific evidence, research-based practice guidelines, and benchmarks, among other factors. Both qualitative and quantitative data will be the cornerstone of work and activity. Patients and nurses will have access to information through electronic interaction and communication with expert systems to discuss therapies and treatment, and information databases will be used to compare care processes and outcomes of nursing practice (Zarit et al., 1993).

Families do not have readily available services or systems to address symptom management, equipment operation, criteria for patient assessment and monitoring, emotional or informational needs, and skill development. Trial and error constitutes how they learn to care. Services often are not available to patients and families during supportive and continuing care periods—when they need them the most. Along with mobilizing and coordinating resources, nurses will be important sources of information. With electronic linkages, nurses are enabled to retrieve and disseminate information in an inexpensive and almost instantaneous way. At present, no one agency or organization helps patients and families to meet the varying information needs that may arise during and/or following an episode of illness. Nurses will be able, however, to connect with the various organizations operating on-line and initiate the process of coordinating care.

In the coming years, the health care system will integrate more and more technology into the provision of care. Patients and families who do not function well in a high-tech realm and/or who are marginalized and restricted from access to high-tech care will continue to be disadvantaged. Delivering the medical plan of care via technological devices will be the norm. New applications of information technology relating to health and functional profiles of patients will be available to health care professionals. Complete patient records will readily be available to all providers no matter what setting. Protocols will determine how each individual is to receive medical and supportive services based on personalized profiles. The nurse of tomorrow will need to know how to integrate information systems *and* how to integrate and acclimate patients and families to these technological communication and information systems.

New technologies are making health care portable and non-institutional. These systems will be used to administer medications, retrieve laboratory results, document patient progress reports, measure patient status (such as blood pressure, heart rate, and glucose) from afar, and to permit patient interaction with the health care systems.

Supporting Prevention and Promoting Healthy Lifestyles

Nursing interventions of the future will focus on prevention and new and interesting ways to promote health and well-being. Although not the focus of this chapter, secondary prevention for those with chronic illness is and will continue to be a concern. New methods of motivating and stimulating individuals with chronic health problems to engage in preventive practices; to prepare themselves for behavioral, emotional, and physical changes due to an illness; and to adopt health behaviors to prevent relapse or continued deterioration of the chronic problem will be required. Given the prevalence of chronic illness in an aging population, major efforts will need to be on secondary prevention and ways to maintain independence. The success of the system will be measured by how cost-effectively consumer mental, social, and physical function is maintained. Nurses will be engaged in health promotion and disease prevention in community settings and other settings such as geriatric meal sites, elderly residential areas, and senior centers. Strategies for health promotion and self-care will become a major part of the patient outcomes on which nurses will be evaluated.

To capture a patient or family members' readiness to learn provides the best environment for teaching preventive strategies. Culturally sensitive interactions facilitate a sense of partnership required in the new era. Inventing, adopting, and implementing strategies to maximize a patient's or family member's participation in their own care will be a health care priority. Teaching and counseling, as well as strategies to assist the elderly and those with chronic illness to stay independent, will remain essential ingredients of health promotion and disease prevention. Additionally, partnership will allow for the blending of two important health care goals: preventing both acute and chronic disease and promoting health behaviors while allowing patients and families active decision-making and roles in their personal health care.

Reimbursement and entitlement programs often determine which services can be provided; thus, services offered do not always match patients' and families' actual needs. Services today are available when tied to an acute care episode. In the future, the most cost-effective mechanism for the care of the chronically ill will be a careful matching of services to needs. In the next decade, nurses will assume a major role in family preparedness to identify and acquire knowledge and skills needed for care. Nurses of the future will need to be active in more thorough assessment of the needs of both patient and caregiver, and ensuring that services are provided based on these actual needs.

Patient and Family Involvement in Care and Decision-Making

In the future, family members must interact, coordinate, and negotiate with the health care system across the continuum of care to obtain information, services, and equipment. The knowledge base of the family caregiver will include the ability to recognize and manage treatment effects and symptoms, to engage in personal and intimate care tasks, and to supervise and monitor overall patient health status. Nurses can have an active role in advocating for patients and empowering family members to make decisions about care.

Nurses will likewise need to assist the family to anticipate the needs that will arise during the disease course, given the illness, stage, age, and other patient and family factors. Encouraging and supporting the patient and family caregiver in decision-making will be an important component of family care. When assisting a family to plan for the future, the nurse will need to be informed about the illness trajectory, and sophisticated state-of-the-art treatment, as well as risk factors involved.

Nurses of the future will be case managers and need to ensure continuity of care as well as work in partnership with the family to mobilize resources. As changes in status and location of care occur, patients and families will face difficult decisions and nurses will be responsible to aid them in making critical care decisions. Nurses will note both patient and caregiver responses to changing health care problems, will welcome patients into the decision-making process, and will be responsible for assisting patients to gain access to the appropriate type and level of care as transitions occur. They will possess the knowledge and skills to assist family members so that they will accept and utilize the needed resources and do so without feelings of guilt and role conflict.

Managing Information and Continuing Education

Clinical epidemiology and the behavioral sciences will be beneficial to providing information and fostering the ability to build effective skills, such as information organization, methods of responding and communicating with culturally diverse patient populations, understanding verbal and nonverbal communication, and engaging the patient's and family's participation in the therapeutic plan. Theories of behavior change will help nurse clinicians to involve individual patients and family members in their own care, improve compliance with therapeutic regimens, understand causes and utilize effective interventions to reduce substance abuse and prevent relapses, and integrate the family in dealing with illness and health. A nurse's knowledge will include statistics, epidemiology, decision-analysis, cost-effectiveness analysis, economics, ethics, computer sciences, and health care organization and evaluative sciences.

The next generation of nurses will need to be independent, flexible, decision-makers skilled in computer usage, education and information provision, and systems approach tactics. Nurses will require the ability to communicate effectively, be self-aware, have an understanding of the effect of the self on others, be able to solve problems, and be able to reflect on life experiences. Continued learning will be the norm. Future education will be dynamic and continuous (Leners, 1996).

Summary

It is clear from discussion of the Pew Health Professions Commission competency areas, that the roles of the professional nurse in the future will be broad and require a high level of clinical and social competency and accountability. Continued professional growth and development will be required. Skills as a team member will be essential as more collaborative learning and health care coordination takes place in the community among health care professionals. The idea of community will continue to transform, including both virtual and actual populations.

The emphasis on cost-effectiveness will not diminish, but will instead continue with competitive managed care. The ability to operate in cost-effective, clinically-relevant evidence-based practice will be required. Marketplace forces and public policy forces will continue to bring change to the health care system; thus, the nurses of the future must stay attuned to the forces heralding change and be flexible to continue to evolve with and shape their practice. Nurses of the future must be positioned to make themselves clinically competent, cost-effective, contributing, and caring providers within a collaborative model. The changing sociodemographics and transforming family structures will require new and specialized skills of both the nurse and the family. Professional nurses will be in a favorable position to play a critical and vital role in the health care system of the future.

REFERENCES

Aday, L. (1993). At risk in America: The health and health care needs of vulnerable populations in the U.S. San Francisco: Jossey Bass.

American Nurses Association. (1995). *Nursing's social policy statement*. Washington, DC: American Nurses Publishing.

Barzansky, B., Friedman, C., Arnold, L., et al. (1993). A view of medical practice in 2020 and its implications for medical school admissions. *Academic Medicine*, 68, 31–6.

Center for Vulnerable Populations, (1992). *Familiar faces: The status of America's vulnerable populations—A chartbook*. Portland, ME: Center for Health Policy Development.

Donaldson, M. S., Yordy, K. D., Lohr, K. N., & Vanselow, N. A., (eds.) (1996). *Primary care: America's health in a new era* (pre-publication copy), National Academy Press, 4–4.

Estes, C. L., & Swan, J. H. (1994). Privatization, system membership, and access to home health care for the elderly. *Milbank Quarterly*, 72(2), 277–98.

Fagin, C., & Lynaugh, J. (1992). Reaping the rewards of radical change: A new agenda for nursing education. *Nursing Outlook*, 40, 213–20.

Given, B. A., Given, C. W., Helms, E., Stommel, M., & DeVoss, D. N. (1997). Determinants of family caregiver reaction to care and depression: New and recurrent cancer. *Cancer Practice*, 5(1), 17–24.

Greenlick, M. R. (1995). Educating physicians for the twenty-first century. *Academic Medicine*, 70(3), 179–185.

King, S., Collins, C., & Liken, M. (1995). Values and the use of community services. *Qualitative Health Research*, 5(3), 332–347.

Komisar, H., Lambrew, J., & Feder, J. (1966). *Long-term care for the elderly, a chart book*. New York: The Commonwealth Fund.

Leners, D., Beardslee, N. Q., & Peters, D. (1996). 21st century nursing and implications for nursing school admissions. *Nursing Outlook*, 44(3), 137–140.

Leutz, W. N., Capitman, J. A., MacAdam, M., & Abrahams, R. (1992). *Care for frail elders: Developing community solutions*. Westport, CT: Auburn House.

Mundinger, M. (1994). Health care reform: Will nursing respond? *Nursing and Health Care*, 15, 28–38.

New roles, new responsibilities for health: Responding to imperatives for change. (1996). Irving, TX: VHA, Inc.

O'Neil, E. (1993). *Health professions education in the future: Schools in service to the nation*. San Francisco: Pew Health Professionals Commission.

Peterson, S. (1989). Designing continuing education programming based upon futurist literature. *Journal of Continuing Education in the Health Professions*, 9, 87–93.

Safriet, B. (1992). Health care dollars and regulatory sense: The role of advanced practice nursing. *Yale Journal of Regulation*, 9, 417–88.

Sullivan, T. J., Lee, J. L., & Warnick, M. L. (1987). Nursing 2020: A study of nursing's future. *Nursing Outlook*, 35, 233–5.

United States Bureau of Census. (1992). *Households, families, and children: A 30-year perspective*. Washington, DC: Government Printing Office.

United States Special Committee on Aging. (1992). *Aging America: Trends and projections, 1990–1991.* Washington, DC: U. S. Department of Health and Human Services.

Zarit, S., Pearlin, L., & Schaie, K. (1993). *Caregiving systems: Informal and formal helpers.* Hillsdale, NJ: Erlbaum.

11

Understanding the Trajectory of Chronic Illness Using Asthma as a Prototype

Donna Tartasky

As the 21st century approaches, the number of individuals with chronic illness will increase due to several factors. First, there has been an unprecedented growth in the elderly population. Second, changes in the way diseases are being treated have transformed many acute illnesses into chronic illnesses. For example, heart disease, cancer and AIDS, once considered acute illnesses have moved to a chronic illness trajectory. Moreover, people with other diseases such as sickle cell anemia and cystic fibrosis are now being more successfully treated and have had their lives extended. As a result of these trends, the demand for care related to chronic illness is growing. In 1987, 22 million people had an activity limitation caused by a chronic condition. By 1993, this number had increased to 27 million. By 2020, it is projected that 134 million people will have chronic conditions, and 39 million will have a major activity limitation.

Data on the incidence and prevalence of chronic illness is aggregated through surveys on chronic conditions, a term that includes both chronic diseases and impairments. A recent analysis of the National Medical Expenditure Survey provides estimates of the prevalence and direct costs associated with chronic conditions (Hoffman, Rice & Sung, 1996). Approximately 90 million persons have chronic conditions that are associated with medical care use or disability days. Rates of chronic conditions are highest in the elderly. However, one in four children younger than 18 years have a chronic condition.

Costs related to chronic illness include direct and indirect expenditures. Direct costs include: hospitalization, physician and other professional visits, emergency department visits, home health care visits, dental visits, prescription medication and medical equipment and supplies. Indirect costs include estimates of morbidity (days lost from school or work) and mortality (loss of work productivity based on income and usual life expectancy). While only 46 percent of the noninstitutionalized population reported chronic conditions, they accounted for 76 percent of the direct medical costs in this country in 1987. Similarly, projections of expenditures for people of all ages with chronic conditions show they disproportionately use health care services. Recent estimates of the number of persons with chronic conditions in 1995 were almost 100 million. The importance of this number is underscored by several facts. First, the majority of people with chronic conditions live normal lives but are faced with recurrent exacerbations, higher health care costs, the risk of long-term disability and more days lost from school and work. Second, persons with chronic conditions are at greater risk for being underinsured. Costs associated with chronic conditions have been noted to be three times higher compared to people without such illnesses. Persons with chronic conditions are less attractive to insurance companies, particularly managed care companies and often must supplement their coverage. Third, since over 100 million Americans have chronic conditions, almost every family is affected. Next, because our elderly population is growing, the cost of health care related to chronic conditions and long-term care will rise. Last, and most importantly, the health care needs of people with chronic illness are complex. The need for comprehensive care that includes prevention, availability of technology and services is limited by a system that focuses on offering benefits for acute services.

Most discussion of costs has focused on chronic conditions, a term that includes both chronic diseases and impairments. However, the term illness is often used to describe the same phenomena. Some discussion of these terms is important in order to understand the meaning of chronic illness.

TERMINOLOGY

Dimond & Jones (1983) noted the term *disease* denotes a state of non-health; whereas *illness* denotes phenomena that are apparent to the ill person only. Disease, however, is considered to be a cause of illness. Oftentimes an ill person may have a disease and be unaware of it. Illness refers to the subjective perception of a symptom and imputing meaning about that symptom. Individuals with chronic illness fall along a broad spectrum of symptomatology that ranges from asymptomatic to symptomatic. Symptoms are important in that they influence the way in which people define their situation and seek help (Dimond & Jones, 1983). While each chronic illness has its own pathophysiology, symptomatology and treatment, commonalities across illnesses exist.

Characteristics of Chronic Illnesses

In general, chronic illnesses are long-term, characterized by exacerbations and remissions and have the potential to be life-threatening. In spite of this, however, most people with chronic illnesses manage to lead productive lives. In fact, working-age adults 18 to 64 years of age account for 60 percent of all noninstitutionalized people with chronic conditions (Hoffman et al., 1996). This is in part due to the episodic nature of such illnesses, as well as recent innovations in treatment and in particular pharmacological therapy. Yet, many issues confront the individual with chronic illness. Of primary consideration is the fact that over one-quarter of young adults, half of middle-aged adults and 69 percent of the elderly have more than one chronic condition or comorbidity (Hoffman et al., 1996).

As a result, for many the sequelae of chronic illnesses include: activity limitations, social isolation and being underinsured. Escalating out of pocket costs for the chronically ill are a relatively new phenomenon related to rising co-payments and managed care. As a result, many individuals who have health insurance cannot afford to comply with their treatment regimens or even utilize preventive care.

Problems with medication adherence and treatment compliance are another issue for the chronically ill. This is in part due to the fact that the individual with chronic illnesses may delay seeking care and sometimes does not respond to worsening symptoms. In addition, chronic illnesses are characterized by exacerbations and remissions. Persons who are asymptomatic may forget and or not think they need to take their prescribed medications. Asthma is one chronic illness that has recently been the focus of attention in the popular press and medical literature. As such, it typifies some of the issues affecting the chronically ill. An overview of asthma followed by a discussion of a conceptual model of symptom management will be used to understand some of the complexities of chronic illness.

Overview of Asthma

During the past decade the incidence of asthma has steadily increased as has the frequency and severity of illness (National Institutes of Health, 1995a). Most of this increase has occurred since 1990. Currently, asthma-related morbidity and mortality account for approximately one percent or six billion dollars in health care costs annually (Weiss, Gergen & Hodgson, 1992). Inpatient costs, medications, emergency room use and physicians' services account for most of these expenditures. In fact, of all visits to office-based physicians and hospital outpatient departments, asthma was the sixth most frequent morbidity-related principal diagnosis and the eleventh most reported principal diagnosis in emergency departments (Burt & Knapp, 1996). Emergency room usage has been noted to be higher for children under 15 years of age and in African Americans. In a study of asthma in New York City, hospitalization rates and emergency room usage for blacks and Hispanics were 3 to 5.5 times that of whites and were highly correlated with poverty (Carr, Zeitel & Weiss, 1992).

   Increases in asthma prevalence, morbidity and mortality despite the availability of effective treatment led to the formation of The National Asthma Education Program (now known as The National Asthma Education and Prevention Program-NAEPP) by the National Heart, Lung and Blood Institute of the National Institutes of Health (NIH). The goal of the NAEPP is to decrease asthma morbidity and mortality and increase the quality of life of persons with asthma. Publication of the *Expert Panel Report: Guidelines for the Diagnosis and Management of Asthma* (NIH, 1992), has led to an increased emphasis on asthma education and self-management. Another publication, *Nurses: Partners in Asthma Care*, has provided nurses with asthma information specific to their role as health care educators (NIH, 1995b). More recently, new guidelines referred to as the Expert Panel Report II (EPR-II) were released that expand on the 1992 report. Despite widespread dissemination of these documents, asthma remains an illness that is undertreated particularly in minority communities.

Pathophysiology

Asthma is a lung disease that is characterized by: 1) airway obstruction that is reversible (although not completely in all patients); 2) airway inflammation; and 3) increased airway responsiveness to a variety of stimuli (NIH, 1992). Wheezing, dyspnea, cough and the sensation of tightness in the chest are due to airflow obstruction. People with asthma are considered to have an increase in airway responsiveness to a variety of stimuli which leads to an inflammatory response. Airway inflammation produces: acute bronchoconstriction, swelling of the airway wall, chronic mucus plug formation and airway obstruction (NIH, 1995a).

Exacerbations of asthma are characterized by mucousal swelling, excess secretions and increased airway responsiveness, which are part of the inflammatory response. Even when symptoms are absent, there is some airway inflammation and airway hyperresponsiveness. When asthma is severe and death results there is extensive infiltration of the airways with eosinophil mast cells, and mononuclear cells with involvement of both the large and small airways. The extent of airflow obstruction can be determined through pulmonary function evaluation which provides an objective measurement of airflow such as forced expiratory volume in one second (FEV_1) and peak expiratory flow rate (PEFR). Measurement of FEV_1 and its accompanying forced vital capacity (FVC) are done during a forced expiratory maneuver using a spirometer. Although measurement of pulmonary function using peak expiratory flow (PEF) is an important technique, it does not reflect the status of small airways in the lung as it is totally effort dependent (NIH, 1992).

Risk Factors Involved in the Development of Asthma

Several risk factors for asthma have been discussed in the literature. A frequently asked question is whether or not asthma is genetic. Asthma is associated with atopy which is defined as "the propensity, usually genetic, for developing IgE-mediated responses to common environmental allergens" (NIH, 1995a). Studies have shown that atopic diseases tend to occur in families and that IgE is partly under genetic control. Others have noted that there is a higher prevalence of asthma in racial/ethnic subgroups. While differences in the prevalence of asthma have been noted in black versus white children, this has been attributed to socioeconomic and environmental factors. Childhood asthma is more prevalent in boys than girls, however, this disappears after the age of ten when airways mature. Other causal factors related to asthma are environmental and inhaled allergens such as cigarette smoke, pollens, dust mites, cockroaches and animal related agents. These causative agents lead to sensitization in the atopic individual which in turn leads to allergic inflammation and the development of asthma.

Diagnosing Asthma

The diagnosis of asthma is based on medical history, physical examination and objective measures of pulmonary function (Janson-Bjerklie, 1993). In order to assess symptomatology, medical history should be careful and comprehensive. Most clinicians would agree that the major symptoms of asthma are wheezing, dyspnea, chest tightness, sputum production, nighttime awakenings and cough (Sullivan et al., 1996). Chronic cough is often indicative of asthma and may be the presenting symptom in children or adults with asthma. The diagnosis of asthma may be difficult but practitioners can easily do a spirometry to determine airflow obstruction. Some individuals and children in particular, have completely normal airway function measurements on spirometry (Tinkelman, 1996). In order to make a diagnosis of asthma, airway responsiveness testing is done (histamine or methacholine provocation challenge). During this test, forced vital capacity or FEV_1 is measured before and after the administration of methacholine or histamine.

Overall, pulmonary function testing is important for the diagnosis and management of asthma. In the initial assessment of complaints, it can aid in differential diagnosis and can be used to monitor the efficacy of therapy and also offer an objective means of following a patient's asthma over time. Peak flow meters are used in the home to determine peak expiratory flow rate (PEFR). PEFR may be assessed by a number of hand-held devices specifically designed for this function. When the peak flow meter is used appropriately, it is an important tool that can be used to understand day-to-day variation of expiratory flow and as an indicator for medication and emergency action. Once asthma is diagnosed, effective therapy must begin.

Asthma Therapy

Appropriate therapy is dependent on assessing the severity of asthma. Classifying patients according to symptoms is important in determining treatment. The EPR-II Guidelines for the Diagnosis and Treatment of Asthma classify asthma into four categories based on clinical features before treatment (NIH, 1997). These include: mild intermittent, mild persistent, moderate persistent and severe persistent asthma. Individuals with symptoms that occur less than twice a week, nighttime symptoms that occur less than twice a month, brief exacerbations, an FEV_1 or a PEF equal to or more than 80 percent of predicted value and PEF variability of less than 20 percent, and are asymptomatic and have a normal PEF between exacerbations are characterized as having mild intermittent asthma. These individuals do not need daily medication and use short-acting bronchodilator or inhaled beta$_2$-agonists for quick relief of symptoms. The management of mild persistent, moderate persistent and severe persistent asthma is more complex.

Patients with mild persistent asthma need medication every day to achieve and maintain control of their asthma. These are individuals with symptoms occurring more than twice a week but less than once per day, nighttime symptoms more than twice per month, exacerbations which may affect activity, FEV_1 or PEF equal or more than 80 percent of predicted and PEF variability in the 20–30 percent range. Individuals with mild persistent asthma need to use an anti-inflammatory medication daily for long-term control and an inhaled beta$_2$-agonist for quick relief of symptoms. Moderate persistent asthma is characterized by daily symptoms, daily use of inhaled short-acting beta$_2$-agonist, nighttime symptoms more than once a week, exacerbations which affect activity and exacerbations which occur more than two times per week and may last for days. In these individuals, peak flow variability is more than 30 percent and FEV_1 or PEF is more than 60 percent but less than 80 percent of predicted value. Once treated, these patients need an anti-inflammatory agent; or inhaled corticosteroid or an inhaled corticosteroid and a long-acting bronchodilator for long-term control. Patients with severe persistent asthma have continual symptoms, frequent exacerbations, limited physical activity, frequent nighttime symptoms, PEF variability more than 30 percent, and FEV_1 or PEF equal or less than 60 percent of predicted value. Such individuals need a long acting bronchodilator and inhaled corticosteroid daily and long-term corticosteroid oral therapy. Although medical management differs based on the severity of asthma, the goal of therapy is to stabilize individuals and use a step wise approach to therapy. This means that treatment should be reviewed every one to six months to increase or decrease treatment when appropriate, based on these guidelines.

Asthma can be managed through education, control of factors contributing to severity, assessment and monitoring of pulmonary function and pharmacological therapy. Several types of interventions specific to these areas are discussed separately and present their own specific challenges.

Patient education is a continual process. Most importantly, in order to be effective the provider and client must form a partnership and agree on goals. Those outlined by the NAEPP guidelines include: maintain (near) normal pulmonary function rates, maintain normal activity levels, including exercise, prevent chronic and troublesome symptoms and recurrent exacerbations of asthma and avoid adverse effects from asthma medication (NIH, 1992). In order to achieve these goals clients need to understand that self-management skills and adherence to treatment are the keys to reducing episodes, emergency room visits, hospitalizations and work or school absences. Patient education is most important in order to control symptoms. The "Five Rs of Teaching" provide a framework for viewing effective asthma management. They are: reach agreement on goals, rehearse asthma management skills, repeat messages, reinforce appropriate behavior and review (Taggart & Rachelefsky, 1996). For the clinician, these are time-consuming tasks which may yield more favorable outcomes in high risk or more costly patients (Sullivan et al., 1996). Most importantly, the need to educate patients to develop a partnership in asthma management which includes the health care professional, the patient and the patient's family should be emphasized (NIH, 1995a). The EPR-II recommends that all asthmatics monitor symptoms to recognize early signs of deterioration. In addition, the EPR-II emphasizes the importance of patient-provider communication, patient satisfaction and the importance of quality of life and functional status.

Factors contributing to asthma severity include: irritants or allergens, viral respiratory infections, rhinitis, sinusitis and gastroesophageal reflux. Control of some of these factors is difficult, particularly for clients of lower socioeconomic status. Many of the steps that can be taken to combat indoor allergens require expenditures for items that are not covered by most insurers or Medicaid. Some of these include: hand-held peak flow meters, spacers, home air filters, removal of carpeting, air-conditioning and the use of mattress covers to prevent the build up of dust mites. For adults, exposure to other allergens such as cigarette smoke are more easily controlled. Children, however, may have significant exposure to adults who smoke. Indeed, parental cigarette smoking has been associated with increased asthma related morbidity (Weitzman, 1990).

Gastroesophageal reflux (GER) is associated with a variety of pulmonary disorders including asthma. Estimates of the incidence of GER in asthmatics range from 34–89 percent (Sontag et al., 1987). In a recent study of adult minority asthmatics, 83 percent of participants noted symptoms indicative of GER (Tartasky, 1997). The exact nature of the relationship between GER and asthma is unclear but has been attributed to a few factors. Both beta$_2$-agonists and theophylline contribute to lower esophageal sphincter pressure which may facilitate backflow of gastric contents. Next, GER may trigger asthma by causing microaspiration into the tracheobronchial tree. In addition, cough and greater inspiratory effort that accompany asthma increase abdominal pressure and force secretions past the lower esophageal sphincter (Field, Underwood, Brant & Cowie, 1996). Most importantly, antireflux therapy has been noted to improve asthma symptoms and improve pulmonary function in 73 percent of patients (Harding et al., 1996). Given the incidence of GER in asthmatics, clinicians need to assess their patients for symptoms.

Assessment of pulmonary function is essential for measuring airway hyperresponsiveness and response to therapy. Spirometry is recommended at the time of initial assessment and should be done periodically in selected individuals who use PEFR to monitor their asthma. Home peak flow monitoring is an important and useful tool in overall asthma management and requires teaching of the technique, reviewing and interpreting of a written log which the patient maintains at home, and writing of an action plan for care based on peak flow values. Baseline peak flow readings taken when the patient is stable, and the individual's personal best or predicted value are used to help determine when variability is significant and to establish an action plan. The personal best can best be estimated after a two to three week period in which the patients record their PEF two to four times a day. The recorded PEF should be the best of three blows. Once stabilized, the peak flow monitoring can be done daily in the morning. If the reading is less than 80 percent of the personal best, more frequent monitoring may be needed.

Pharmacological therapy is key to effective asthma management. The EPR-II recognizes inappropriate therapy as a major contributor to asthma morbidity and mortality. The goals of asthma therapy are: to prevent chronic and troublesome symptoms, maintain pulmonary function, maintain activity levels, prevent recurrent exacerbations, provide optimal pharmacotherapy and minimize medication side effects and to achieve patient satisfaction (NIH, 1997).

The two main types of medication for treatment of asthma are long-term control medications (anti-inflammatory agents) used to achieve and maintain control of persistent asthma and quick-relief medications (bronchodilators), used to treat symptoms and exacerbations. Most often, these medications are administered through multiple dose inhalers (MDIs). The EPR-II emphasizes the importance of anti-inflammatory agents in achieving long-term control. Bronchodilator medications include $beta_2$-agonists, theophylline and anticholinergics. These medications relax bronchial smooth muscle and dilate the airways. Patients need to be taught to properly use their $beta_2$-agonist inhaler. This includes taking a deep inhalation following administration, holding one's breath ten seconds and waiting five minutes between inhalations.

Inhaled corticosteroids are safe and effective and can be the primary therapy for many patients with asthma. If using an inhaled bronchodilator and an inhaled anti-inflammatory agent, the bronchodilator medication should be used first. When using an inhaled corticosteroid, patients should also take a deep inhalation and hold their breath for ten seconds, and wait one minute between inhalations. Following use of the corticosteroid inhaler, patients need to rinse their mouths with water to prevent oral candidiasis. Combination therapy, consisting of both types of medication, is recommended for persons with moderate to severe asthma and has been found to produce positive clinical outcomes (Sullivan et al., 1996). Despite evidence that these medications can effectively control asthma, many clients do not adhere to their prescribed regimen. A recent study of children's use of medications which employed electronic monitoring, revealed more than 90 percent of patients exaggerated their use of inhaled steroids (Milgrom et al., 1996). It was not determined in this study if exaggeration of inhaler use was intentional or accidental. Others have studied problems associated with medication compliance and noted patients sometimes do not receive adequate instruction in taking inhaled asthma medications (Creer & Levstek, 1996). Since asthma can be episodic as can medication use, repeated instruction is necessary as are periodic checks of inhaler use. Often the use of an assistive device such as a spacer, which is used in conjunction with an inhaler, is necessary.

While patient education, environmental control, objective management of pulmonary function and pharmacologic therapy have been discussed separately, they are closely intertwined and constitute interventions that affect asthma management. Other interventions such as immunotherapy (desensitization), acupuncture and other nontraditional approaches have been used to treat asthma. Some have noted that asthma is exacerbated by stress and psychotherapy may be beneficial, however, effectiveness of this intervention is not known. Asthmatics like other chronically ill individuals, often do not react quickly to symptomatology and need to be assessed by clinicians. A symptom management model used to understand how patients respond to symptomatology is important in understanding chronic illnesses such as asthma (see Figure 11.1).

Model for Symptom Management

Much has been written about the ways in which symptoms are perceived and acted (or not acted) upon by different people (Mechanic, 1972). Given the subjective nature of symptoms, they are generally regarded by most people as a call to action or the reason why people seek care. A conceptual model of symptom management has been used to describe the symptom experience, symptom management strategies and symptom outcomes (Larson et al., 1994).

Using this model, the symptom experience involves the interaction between the patient's perception of a symptom, meaning of a symptom and response to a symptom. Perception of symptoms is based on a host of factors including person, environment and health/illness variables. Demographic variables such as age, gender, and ethnicity as well as psychological traits such as motivation and environmental factors such as one's home all influence perception of symptoms. Imputing meaning about a symptom is a difficult task for the person with a chronic illness such as asthma. If asthmatic individuals are asymptomatic, they may not respond to their illness using appropriate self-management techniques. For example, some asthmatics need to utilize their inhalers, even when asymptomatic. Using medication when asymptomatic may be illogical for some people. For other asthmatics, availability of medications and environmental factors such as cigarette smoking may play a role in responding to symptomatology.

Evaluation of symptoms reflects a complex set of variables that interact and influence behavior. These include: intensity, location, temporal nature, frequency, and the associated pattern of disability. Asthma is characterized by a host of symptoms such as coughing, wheezing, and dyspnea. In a study of asthmatics, patients' evaluations of the intensity and danger

Figure 11.1
Conceptual Model of Symptom Management

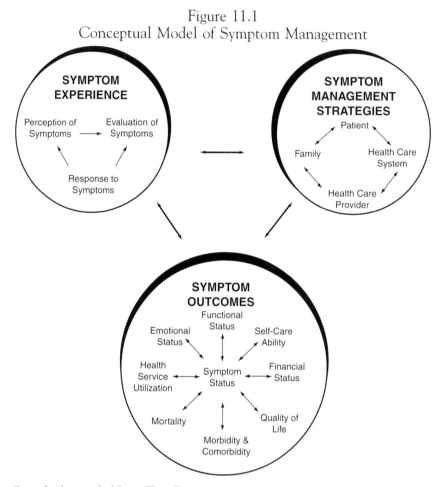

associated with their dyspnea were the most important predictors of seeking medical care (Janson-Bjerklie, Ferketich, Benner & Becker, 1992).

Symptom-management strategies are used to avoid or delay negative outcomes associated with illness. Management begins with assessment of symptoms by the patient and is followed by identification of the intervention, implementation of the intervention and evaluation of the intervention. Symptom management may require changes in strategies over time, and requires a patient-family-clinician partnership. An example of symptom management is use of the peak flow meter and inhalers by the asthmatic patient. Peak flow meters can be used by the asthmatic patient daily. If the asthmatic patient is symptomatic, the peak flow meter reading can be used to obtain an objective measure of pulmonary function. The PEFR can then be used to adjust inhaler usage.

In this model, symptom outcomes are characterized as ten multidimensional indicators including: self-care ability, financial status, morbidity, and comorbidity, mortality, quality of life, health service utilization, emotional status and functional status. Symptom status is at the core of this model and the other indicators are related. This is because symptom status may affect functional or emotional status, self-care ability, health care utilization, financial status, or quality of life and may result in increased morbidity and mortality. In the asthmatic patient one symptom, dyspnea, can affect other dimensions such as self-care ability and quality of life. Symptom outcomes are complex and interrelated and need to be part of teaching self-management skills to asthmatics. Psychosocial factors are an important variable in symptom outcomes in asthma and other chronic illnesses and are described separately.

Psychosocial Factors in Asthma

At one time asthma was considered a psychosomatic disease. In the last few decades, asthma has been acknowledged as a disease related to bronchial hyperreactivity. Successful management of a chronic illness such as asthma requires that the patient obtain regular medical care, comply with a therapeutic regimen and make lifestyle changes. While these tasks are not difficult for most people, they can be problematic for inner city populations who live in old housing, lack transportation, insurance and other resources.

Other patients with chronic illness manifest psychological dysfunction that interferes with appropriate health behaviors. In addition, strong emotional responses such as anxiety and anger can exacerbate symptoms specific to a chronic illness. In a study which examined the effect of emotion on bronchoconstriction, 40 percent of participants were found to have a decrease in pulmonary function after exposure to an emotional trigger (Isenberg, Lehrer & Hochron, 1992). Social support can also be a key factor in asthma management, especially when friends, family, and co-workers can assist with avoidance of asthma triggers (Gaioni, Fisher & Strunk, 1996).

Psychosocial factors can take on even more importance in chronic illness as the individual often experiences symptom exacerbation, failure of therapy and physical deterioration, and must cope with a variety of illness related stressors. Several concepts related to coping have been widely explored in the literature. These include: attribution theory, locus of control, helplessness and hardiness. Although some of these factors are closely intertwined, researchers have demonstrated that greater feelings of control have a positive impact on psychological well-being and physical health (Rodin, Bohm & Wack, 1982; Felton, Revenson & Henrichsen, 1984). Since inner-city minorities have less control over their environment and health, this finding may provide some explanation as to why their asthma related morbidity and mortality exceeds that of white populations.

Conclusion

During the next few decades, there will be a rapid increase in the number of people with chronic illness. As this population grows, nurses will increasingly help manage the chronically ill. In order to do so, nurses will continue to move from acute care sites into community based care which will include alternative delivery models and settings. Each of these settings will provide unique practice opportunities for the nurse clinician or practitioner, nurse educator or nurse researcher. Asthma is one of many chronic illnesses that nurses can target in their practice area.

Presently, nurse practitioners are managing the health care needs of many chronically ill people in consultation with physicians. As the chronically ill population expands, needs for these services will likewise increase and nurse practitioners will increasingly see patients in nurse managed centers, managed care environments, assisted living facilities, home care and ambulatory care settings, parish and life care settings. Indeed, management of chronic illnesses such as asthma will increasingly be done by nurse practitioners, particularly in managed care environments.

Nurse educators will also be working with their students to care for the chronically ill. Because the health care needs of the chronically ill are complex, and the health care system is cutting services, nursing students will be providing more comprehensive services in alternative environments. One of the most difficult tasks will be providing services to chronically ill patients whose insurance and resources are limited. Nursing students under the supervision of faculty, can provide services that are otherwise not reimbursable and make a valuable contribution to patient care. This is particularly true in the area of patient education. Much of the asthma related morbidity and mortality could be prevented through instruction and development of patient self-management skills.

Nurse researchers will continue to target the chronically ill by testing intervention strategies that improve health outcomes. Studies that explore the physiological, environmental and psychosocial variables that affect the chronically ill are necessary to decrease related morbidity and mortality. Asthma is one chronic illness that has not been explored in depth in the nursing literature. Developing and testing interventions in different populations of asthmatics, is a challenge for nurse researchers.

REFERENCES

Burt, C. W., & Knapp, D. E. (1996). Ambulatory care visits for asthma: United States, 1993–94. *Advance Data, 277*, 1–15.

Creer, T. L., & Levstech, D. (1996). Medication compliance and asthma: Overlooking the trees because of the forest. *Journal of Asthma, 33*, 203–211.

Dimond, M., & Jones, S. (1983). *Chronic illness across the life span.* Norwalk: Appleton-Century-Crofts.

Felton, B. J., Revenson, T. A., & Hinrichsen, G. A. (1984). Stress and coping in the explanation of psychological adjustment among chronically ill adults. *Social Sciences, 18*, 889–898.

Field, S. K., Underwood, M., Brant, R., & Cowie, R. L. (1996). Prevalence of gastroesophageal reflux symptoms in asthma. *Chest, 109*, 316–322.

Gaioni, S. J., Fisher, E. B., & Strunk, R. C. (1996). Identification and management of psychosocial factors. In C. W. Bierman, D. S. Pearlman, C. G. Shapiro, and W. W. Busse (Eds.), *Allergy, asthma, and immunology from infancy to adulthood* (pp. 256–267). Philadelphia: W. B. Saunders.

Harding, S. M., Richter, J. E., Guzzo, M. R., Schan, C. A., Alexander, R. W., & Bradley, L. A. (1996). Asthma and gastroesophageal reflux: Acid suppressive therapy improves asthma outcome. *The American Journal of Medicine, 100*, 395–405.

Hoffman, C., Rice, D., & Sung, H. (1996). Persons with chronic conditions. *JAMA, 276*, 1473–1479.

Isenberg, S. A., Lehrer, P. M., & Hochron, S. (1992). The effects of suggestion and emotional arousal on pulmonary function in asthma: A review and a hypothesis regarding vagal mediation. *Psychosomatic Medicine, 54*, 192–216.

Janson-Bjerklie, S. (1993). Assessment and management of adults with asthma: Guidelines for nurse practitioners. *Nurse Practitioner Forum, 4*, 23–29.

Janson-Bjerklie, S., Ferketich, S., Benner, P., & Becker, S. (1992). Clinical markers of asthma severity and risk: Importance of subjective as well as objective factors. *Heart and Lung, 21*, 265–272.

Larson, P. J., Carrieri, V., Dodd, M. J., Faucett, J. S., Froelicher, E. S., Gortner, S. R., Halliburton, P., Janson-Bjerklie, S., Lee, K., Miaskowski, C., Savedra,

M., Stotts, N. A., Taylor, D., & Underwood, P. (1994). A model for symptom management. *Nursing Research, 26*, 272–276.

Mechanic, D. (1972). Social psychological factors affecting the presentation of bodily complaints. *New England Journal of Medicine, 286*, 1132–1139.

Milgrom, H., Bender, B., Ackerson, L., Bowry, P., Smith, B., & Rand, C. (1996). Noncompliance and treatment failure in children with asthma. *Journal of Allergy and Clinical Immunology, 98*, 1051–1057.

National Institutes of Health (1992). *Teach your patients about asthma: A clinician's guide* (NIH Publication No. 92-2737). Washington, DC: U.S. Government Printing Office.

National Institutes of Health (1995a). *Global initiatives for asthma* (NIH Publication No. 95-3659). Washington, DC: U.S. Government Printing Office.

National Institutes of Health (1995b). *Nurses: Partners in asthma care* (NIH Publication No. 95-3308). Washington, DC: U.S. Government Printing Office.

National Institutes of Health (1997). *Highlights of the Expert Panel Report II: Guidelines for the Diagnosis and Treatment of Asthma* (Draft) Washington, DC: U.S. Government Printing Office.

Rodin, J., Bohm, L. C., & Wack, J. T. (1982). Control, coping and aging: Models for research and intervention. *Applied Social Psychology Annual, 3*, 153–180.

Sontag, S., O'Connell, S., Greenlee, H., Schnell, T., Chintam, R., Nemchausky, B., Chejfec, G., Van Drunen, M., & Wanner, J. (1987). Is gastroesophageal reflux a factor in some asthmatics? *American Journal of Gastroenterology, 82*, 119–126.

Sullivan, S., Elishauser, A., Bust, A. S., Luce, B. R., Eisenberg, J., & Weiss, K. B. (1996). National asthma education and prevention program working group report on the cost effectiveness of asthma care. *American Journal of Respiratory Critical Care Medicine, 154*, S84–S95.

Taggart, V. S., & Rachelefsky, G. S. (1996). Patient education: Creating a partnership for effective asthma care. In C. W. Bierman, D. S. Pearlman, C. G. Shapiro, and W. W. Busse (Eds.), *Allergy, asthma, and immunology from infancy to adulthood* (pp. 268–281). Philadelphia: W. B. Saunders.

Tartasky, D. S. (1997). Community based assessment of adult minority asthmatics. Unpublished manuscript, Southern Illinois University at Edwardsville.

Tinkleman, D. G. (1996). Evaluation of the patient with chronic respiratory symptoms. In C. W. Bierman, D. S. Pearlman, C. G. Shapiro, and W. W. Busse (Eds.), *Allergy, asthma, and immunology from infancy to adulthood* (pp. 135–143). Philadelphia: W. B. Saunders.

Weiss, K. B., Gergen, P. J., & Thompson, T. A. (1992). An economic evaluation of asthma in the United States. *The New England Journal of Medicine, 326*, 862–866.

Weitzman, M., Gortmaker, S., Walker, D. K., & Sobol, A. (1990). Maternal smoking and childhood asthma. *Pediatrics, 85*, 505–511.

Part VI

Maximizing Modalities for
State-of-the Art Practice

Many of today's commonly accepted nursing practices were not known at the beginning of the 20th century. Some have been kept, some others have been modified, while still others have been discarded as ineffective based on scientific evidence.

Similarly, some modes of communication, which are well known and used by so many of us in our work, had not even been discovered. In some instances, the discoveries of bench scientists held promise but had yet to be marketed for mass consumption. Distance learning technology is a striking example of a useful, new and widely accessible mode of communication which connects people and ideas across large areas. The efficiencies which are possible, along with the availability and positive outcomes attributed to its use, bode well for its wider use in the education of the 21st century nurse.

Dr. Beason's discussion of the potential distance learning holds for the ongoing education of the nursing workforce and the model that she describes provide a good case for greater use of this technology. Evaluative research focused on further assessment of the true value of distance learning technology to users and purchasers is needed. In addition, ways of enhancing its usefulness as an educational tool should be ongoing.

Dr. Cournoyer reminds us that the profession's research for the future is dependent on the significant involvement of baccalaureate nurses for they represent the pool from which further investigators come. She challenges us to attend to research career development. As we enter the 21st century unlimited opportunities remain for conducting practice based research and of using that which is known as nurses practice.

12

Distance Learning—Education to Prepare Nurses for Practice in the 21st Century

Charlotte F. Beason

From rural elementary schools in Kentucky, corporate training sites and executive board rooms, to the universities of the countries of the European Union and the lone individual who settles in front of a computer screen at eleven p.m. when children are finally asleep, distance learning is improving access to education for growing numbers of individuals. Distance learning is not a new technology. Correspondence courses, training films and television broadcast curricula have been available for several decades. What is leading to the growth in this educational approach, however, is the application of rapidly developing information technology to the concepts and principles that have traditionally made distance learning an attractive option. *US News and World Report* (1995) estimated that approximately four million Americans were involved in on-line academic education endeavors, only one form of distance learning. At the time of the report, some 75 universities and colleges offered on-line degree programs. Information technology will continue to expand at an exponential rate. In the 21st century, use of this education modality will

The views expressed in this paper are those of the author and are not meant to represent the policies of the federal government or the Department of Veterans Affairs.

increase; and, as technology evolves, distance learning will move from current types of activities that mimic present classroom applications to new and innovative methods that use all types of media, artificial intelligence, desktop applications, and information management technology yet to be invented.

For the purpose of this chapter, the author defines distance learning as an educational approach in which students and faculty are physically distant. From this rudimentary definition, the methods by which the education process takes place are many and varied. In the most basic approaches, interaction is minimal, students complete correspondence courses or view previously recorded classroom videos which may be accompanied by written assignments. As additional technology is incorporated into the delivery mode, interaction becomes more complex, progressing from one-way and two-way audioconferencing to more sophisticated applications in which faculty provide real-time presentations through interactive audio and video linkages. Distance learning utilizing state of the art technologies can employ two-way interactive videoconferencing and make extensive use of computer capabilities such as utilizing the Internet to distribute syllabi and teaching materials. Today, students may access interactive chat rooms on the Internet for discussion with instructors or other class participants. They may complete group assignments using software designed to link individuals over wide geographic distances, e-mail assignments to instructors and complete tests on the Internet.

Rapid changes in health care leading into the 21st century will make distance learning a creative alternative for registered nurses and others who find that they must augment existing skills or develop totally new skills to remain competitive in the health care job market. In addition, health care organizations will increasingly purchase, support and/or produce distance learning as a method to strategically plan and implement education and training activities to achieve the workforce skill mix needed to meet the projected needs of the organization.

This chapter discusses the potential distance learning holds as a teaching strategy to meet the ongoing education and training needs of a nursing workforce in the 21st century health care arena. Issues surrounding the implementation of distance learning strategies are considered not only from the perspective of educators and students but also from the viewpoint of corporate consumers—health care organizations that may purchase distance learning services as a strategy for meeting workforce skill requirements. Finally, one health care organization's beginning effort to implement a distance learning strategy and the lessons learned through the process are described.

21st CENTURY HEALTH CARE

There is little doubt that the practice of nursing reached a significant turning point with the advent of health care reform activities in the early 90s. In response to a public mandate to control health care spending, offer services to greater numbers of individuals, and provide cost effective and efficient health care, the health care industry began far reaching restructuring activities that continue to this date.

In these years immediately prior to the 21st century, professional nursing is witness to rapidly changing economic and social forces that are catalysts for wide scale reorganization and reduction of the nursing workforce. Newly implemented models of care delivery focus on primary and preventive care provided through ambulatory treatment. As a result of this shift in focus, inpatient hospital beds are being cut across the nation and fewer numbers of nurses are required to provide bedside nursing care. At the same time, new models of care delivery are creating a widespread demand for certain advanced practice nurses, especially nurse practitioners. While there is likely to be no immediate shortage of nurses, many of the nurses in the workforce are not skilled to provide the types of care which are needed in evolving health care organizations (Aiken & Salmon, 1994).

As a corollary to the numerous changes taking place in the health care system, many nurses, for the first time in their careers, are faced with the prospect that they may not have lifelong employment at the work site of their choice. Nurses now see that future employment will be linked to knowledge and expertise that can be applied to a restructured and dynamic health care environment. As a result, many nurses now view life-long learning as vital to maintaining employment in an ever changing health care environment. Perceptive nurses realize that the way to cope with organizational change is to identify new opportunities and develop those skills that are necessary to take advantage of those opportunities.

Further, a need for additional education and training for nurses will arise from a demand for creativity and innovation in the nursing workforce. Even as nursing functions are being realigned, nurses in all roles are being tasked to identify and implement highly innovative clinical and managerial practices. This need for innovative nursing practices will be accelerated by forces both internal and external to the profession. In the years approaching the 21st century, nurses will be challenged to prove that, as caregivers, they add value to health care goals. In response, nurses will implement effective practices to assure the quality, cost efficiency and accessibility of care. Innovative nursing practice will need to be a hallmark of 21st century health care. Just as corporate America has learned that an innovative workforce moves the organization toward attaining and exceeding corporate goals; health care executives will expect an innovative workforce to meet and exceed their corporate goals. While there are numerous forces which influence an organization's ability to support an innovative workforce, certainly one of the strongest is the training and education of employees to promote creativity and risk taking behaviors.

Finally, 21st century health care will be marked by strong corporate support of employee learning. Through corporate benchmarking, health care executives have found that successful organizations value employee learning. The nation's leading companies identify learning needs, budget regularly for employee education and training, and routinely align education with corporate goals (Meister, 1994). These companies act on the principle that education and training strengthens the employee and strengthens the likelihood that strategic goals and activities will be met. In short, successful organizations invest in employees so that they are able to deliver the right service, to the right customer, at the right time and in the right place. As health care executives restructure organizations they will create learning environments that enhance employee performance and understanding.

DISTANCE LEARNING AS AN EDUCATIONAL APPROACH

Distance learning, which originated as printed correspondence courses in the 1930s (Lytle, Lytle, & Youmans, 1995), is today as varied in approach as the forms of information technology used to convey it. There are distance learning formats that can accommodate as many types of technology as the user may possess; and whether high tech or low tech, each approach can be beneficial when matched appropriately to the topic being presented.

The viability of distance learning as an educational approach for the 21st century was considerably strengthened with the passage of the Telecommunications Act of 1996. This law required carriers to provide telecommunication services at reasonable rates to any rural public or nonprofit health care provider. It further directed that access to advanced telecommunications and information services be enhanced for "all public and nonprofit elementary and secondary school classrooms, health care providers and libraries" (P.L. 104-104, 1996).

With this legislative support, affordable distance learning services will increasingly be within reach of a significantly larger audience with widely divergent needs. Affordable distance learning will be sought to support groups as divergent as kindergarten students in urban classrooms and rural nurse practitioners scattered over several states. Videoconferencing and other types of computer mediated communication will be available to enhance diagnosis, treatment, and care planning as well as the education of health care providers. In support of patient education, distance learning strategies will be used to educate patients, their families and non traditional caregivers in a variety of settings.

In the 21st century, distance learning will be commonly accepted as a cost effective method to provide education and training to single employees at individual sites or to several hundred individuals at multiple sites. The traditional classroom will be irrevocably changed as distance learning modifies teacher and student activities in the nation's classrooms at all levels. Virtual classrooms will become common and the likelihood of numerous virtual universities that have neither campuses nor geographical locations will be a part of our imminent future.

The current explosion in information technology brings with it responsibilities for the design and use of distance learning. Individuals and organizations take pride in acquiring and using the latest computer hardware or software, yet designing an education program for the purpose of using a type of technology simply because it is available without considering learner needs can have ruinous effects on the educational experience. A principle most educators learned very early in their careers is that delivery methods should fit the content and objectives of the topic being taught. This principle, however, can be casually or even deliberately abandoned in the enthusiasm of implementing a distance learning program. Information technology will be successful only as long as it is appropriately matched to the audience and the topics being presented. Each new technology that is incorporated into distance learning methods changes the dynamic of the learning experience and impacts faculty teaching techniques, curriculum design and student expectations.

DISTANCE LEARNING TECHNOLOGY

Satellite Transmissions

Until recently, distance learning was hampered by limited or no interactivity. Satellites have been used to visually transmit courses live from one site to others while communication has generally been provided through audioconferencing (one-way video, two-way audio). This enables participants to see and communicate with the instructor, however, they are unable to see or communicate with each other. Instructors teaching from a studio environment are hampered in this process because they receive no visual cues from students to indicate understanding, confusion, the need to ask questions or any of the countless other nonverbal responses to which instructors in traditional classrooms become accustomed (Shomaker, 1993). Modifications to this process include the installation of responsive key pads which, when activated by a student, alert the instructor that one or more students has a question or does not understand a concept. The instructor can then repeat and clarify details.

Computer Mediated Communication

In computer mediated communication (CMC) students and instructor are linked to a computer network which enables them to communicate from any location at the same time (synchronously) or at different times (asynchronously). Since participation requires only an existing telephone line and a modem, CMC offers easy access as students share information or work together in groups to complete assigned projects. Using this medium, instructors can also administer tests and provide remedial instruction (Phelps, Wells, Ashworth & Hahn, 1991). This approach is used in work environments as a cost effective method of providing continuing education, and executive training. As an added advantage, CMC offers administrators the option of having workers from several locations engage in problem solving with the flexibility of jointly designing, implementing and monitoring projects.

Videoconferencing

Another approach to distance learning is videoconferencing, considered by many to be the most reasonable delivery format for interactive training. Videoconferencing offers flexible, high quality delivery and is easily adapted to varying educational formats. To date, these systems remain costly although those costs are declining. Distance learning using videoconferencing technology requires the use of high speed transmission lines or private telephone networks. Research and development of equipment in this area is intensive; desktop videoconferencing over personal computers, full motion technology, and other improvements can be expected (GAO, 1995; Satterlund, 1993).

In an optimal videoconferencing environment, the instructor presents from a modified classroom or studio equipped with one or more cameras, microphones, fax machine, computer and monitor for viewing students (often built into a custom made teaching desk). Students gather in classrooms that are equipped with monitors that display the teacher or teacher projected images. In the classroom, students also have access to a fax machine, computers and voice activated microphones. The teacher can control the camera to switch from one site to another allowing students to view central or other distant classrooms. In the process of the class, students will talk with the instructor or with students at other locations; at the same time, students may access the Internet and download specific materials sent by the instructor, scan written documents onto the computer or fax documents to other classrooms and the instructor.

Internet

The Internet offers a dynamic and effective method of distance learning in which learners can interact across the country or around the globe. In the privacy of their own homes, students can enroll in classes, communicate with instructors and other students and complete courses. The Internet cannot as yet mimic interactive multimedia, however, it is increasingly being used in business as a tool for performance support. A major advantage to Internet education is that products can be developed and posted for use very quickly (Wulf, 1996). There are drawbacks to distance learning via the Internet. Copyright laws and regulations are unclear as to the ownership of materials placed on the Internet. Potential users continue to find accessing and downloading information a difficult and arduous process; and, in addition, Internet transmissions are slower than with other forms of computer based training (Gurvey, 1997). These barriers will be overcome, however, and use of the Internet for distance learning will grow. While the Internet cannot as yet accommodate real-time video and audio, such transmissions will likely be available in the future.

Benefits

The benefits of distance learning are many and varied. Distance learning is viewed as cost effective, providing wider access to academic and continuing education and maximizing access to qualified instructors (Billings & Bachmeir, 1994). There are little if any differences between the outcomes of distance learning students when compared with traditional students (Keck, 1992; McClelland & Daly, 1991; Barry & Runyan, 1995). In a review of distance learning and its effectiveness, the Office of Technology Assessment (OTA) found that "In most instances, distance learning appears to be as effective as on-site, face-to-face instruction in the classroom" (OTA, 1989). This educational format extends academic education to individuals within their home or work site at times when they are able and willing to learn. Distance learning provides opportunities for students to hear and interact with nationally known experts who may never come to a geographic site near them and it extends educational opportunities into rural and underserved areas. Within traditional academic settings a college or university offering unique areas of concentration can extend its courses to students at other colleges and universities. The distance learning process provides opportunities for collaboration and the formation of a variety of consortia among academic, business and health care organizations.

In the corporate environment, convenience and cost savings are the more obvious reasons for employing distance learning strategies. Corporate sponsors have found that distance learning provides a savings in travel funds that is coupled with the convenience of custom designed courses offered at the work site. Business schools are meeting the need for executive education via distance learning replacing standard residential courses with satellite classrooms (*Business Week*, 1995).

A survey of Fortune 1000 companies found that on the average about one quarter of all employees have access to the Internet. More than 70 percent of these companies cluster some computers into special learning centers to support employee education (*Training*, 1996). Organizations as varied as the Federal government and Ford Motors have implemented distance learning activities with success. Most conclude that distance learning participants achieved course objectives as effectively as did students in traditional classroom training. The Federal Aviation Administration (FAA), the General Accounting Office (GAO) and the Department of Veterans Affairs (VA) have moved to distance learning technologies, successfully making training available to increasingly large audiences within the confines of budget constraints (GAO, 1995).

Future Applications

One commonality among successful Baldridge award winning organizations is an emphasis on learning for all ranks of the organization. In the 21st century, distance learning will be commonly utilized by corporate America. Distance learning will not only extend the college and university classroom into corporate settings, it will also enable executives, researchers and other experts to teach and interact with distant academically based students, providing valuable linkages to the preparation of students wishing to assume roles in business and industry. Business leaders will collaborate with collegiate and secondary schools to prepare employees to assume greater or more complex responsibilities. Distance learning will also enable employees to acquire academic degrees or complete courses which support broader job responsibilities and meet corporate human resource development needs.

The process by which distance learning is delivered will lead future academic educators and purchasers to examine traditional pricing methods. Organizations that have equipped reception sites for employees enrolled in distance learning programs will be unlikely to support per capita tuition costs because they will recognize that costs do not mount significantly as additional numbers of students are enrolled in classes. Additionally, in corporate settings, distance learning will eliminate or greatly reduce the need for off-site travel and enable education and training officers to use limited resources more effectively. Corporate leaders will be unlikely to sacrifice the potential cost savings from implementing distance learning programs on a per capita pricing plan, rather, they will seek to contract all inclusive fees for employee education and training. Astute managers will negotiate distance learning contracts to insure meeting organizational learning objectives. At the same time, they will install technology which can be used not only for distance learning but also to support meetings, teleconferencing, just in time training and myriad other needs within the organization.

The distance learning sites of the 21st century will bear little resemblance to the learning sites now commonly in use. Equipping collegiate and corporate classrooms for distance learning will be the norm. Computers, fax machines, interactive video equipment and technology yet to be developed will be common on the desktop and in the classroom. Individual workstations will be equipped for interactive educational activities giving students and employees the ability to view and interact with instructors— asking individual questions and responding when called upon by faculty. While large organizations may outfit and maintain their own transmission sites others will form consortia to jointly support satellite uplinks, videoconferencing networks, telephone networks and high speed transmission lines.

In the next decade, it will be common for organizations and academic institutions to include distance learning capability in their plans and contracts for telecommunication services. While the number of organizations and schools that build their own production studios will increase, the need for elaborate production facilities will be greatly impacted by continued refinement and sophistication of the technology and a movement on the part of providers to form consortia in which they pool resources for production purposes.

Increased use of distance learning will also foster collaboration. A survey of the Internet already lists a number of collaborative education programs. It will be common for academic providers to pool their resources in cost saving approaches to provide distance learning. Education and training providers may jointly equip and utilize production facilities, share the purchase of blocks of satellite transmission times or join consortia that purchase videoconferencing transmission lines to provide wider availability of transmission options at cost effective and competitive rates.

With wider access to affordable telecommunication and information services, the market for distance learning education will grow and the number of providers will increase. Health care service organizations will require a broad array of high quality services in varying formats and levels of sophistication and complexity. Both academic and proprietary educators will recognize that nursing and health care education is a profitable niche for developing and marketing products. As a result, distance learning will become a highly competitive buyers' market. While increased access and competition will surely benefit consumers, all must be aware that as the numbers of high quality programs increase, the number of providers with lesser qualifications offering poor quality programs will also increase. Now and into the future, both nurse consumers and health care organizations should investigate the abilities of distance learning providers and the quality of the programs they offer.

MAKING A CASE FOR DISTANCE LEARNING IN NURSING EDUCATION

Distance learning programs can provide much of the education and training nurses must have in order to develop new skills for successful practice in the 21st century. As an educational process that benefits populations requiring flexibility and efficiency in both time and costs, distance learning will uniquely accommodate the lifestyle and work schedules of many nurses who will seek formal learning opportunities.

Of those men and women entering nursing in the future, a growing number will be entering their second or even third careers. These 21st century students will be closely linked to communities and they will have social and economic responsibilities that, in effect, bind them to both geographic areas and work commitments. Nurses enrolled in earlier nursing distance learning programs were found to be older than their counterparts in traditional programs, worked longer hours, had more children and commuted farther to the education site (McClelland & Daly, 1991). To a group such as this, the possibility of completing all or a portion of course work required for a generic degree, advanced degree or certificate in nursing through a distance learning curriculum will be highly attractive.

Health care organizations can also benefit from the distance learning process. Organizations can contract with a college or university to provide site specific education or to provide general academic education for a segment of the workforce. Depending on the technology utilized, students can gather in classrooms, access programs from their worksite or individual students may complete all course work in the privacy of their homes. Courses are offered at a time convenient to students and the work environment.

The need for degree completion, skill acquisition and certificate nursing education will proliferate in the future. With the shift in restructured health care environments to emphasis on primary and ambulatory care provided in clinic, community and other settings, nurses seeking to remain competitive in the health care marketplace will need the community assessment, problem solving and clinical management skills that are taught at the baccalaureate level. The U.S. Department of Health and Human Services, Division of Nursing (DHHS), reports that 34 percent of all registered nurses listed the diploma as their highest level of education while 28 percent reported an associate degree as the highest degree attained (DHHS, 1994). Combined, these groups represent a significant number of nurses who will need additional education or training and can be expected to seek out educational programs to acquire the knowledge and skills for primary care, community and ambulatory practice. Additionally, some of the essential skills necessary to the restructured care environment such as case management, interdisciplinary approaches to patient care and financial management have not been part of most traditional baccalaureate programs. Therefore, it can be expected that many nurses prepared at the baccalaureate level and above will require continuing and academic education to prepare for future health care roles.

The move to ambulatory and primary care practice has greatly increased the demand for primary care providers, particularly for nurse practitioners. In 1994, the Pew Health Professions Commission set a goal of doubling the number of nurse practitioner graduates by the year 2000 (Pew, 1994). Since that time, the number of nurse practitioner education programs has increased modestly, however, the demand for accessible, quality nurse practitioner education continues to grow and the capacity of programs to produce nurse practitioners does not appear to be keeping pace. Distance learning nurse practitioner education is an approach that can yield positive results in meeting this need. The most effective and expedient approach to increase numbers is to educate clinical nurse specialists (CNS) in the skills needed to become certified nurse practitioners. This approach effectively redirects an existing resource—clinical nurse specialists— when jobs in specialty areas may have been eliminated or relocated and affords new job opportunities for the CNS group that might otherwise be faced with unemployment.

Growing emphasis on primary and preventive care, has led to increased needs for primary care providers in the health care work force. The numbers of nurse practitioners and certain advanced practice nurses must be increased if national health care goals are to be reached (Pew, 1994). At the same time, the number of bedside nurses and clinical nurse specialists is being reduced within many restructured organizations. These nurses will provide a ready and growing audience for advanced practice education.

Distance learning also provides opportunities for health care employers to strategically plan for meeting the need for additional nurses with critical job skills such as physical assessment or case management. Employers can target training dollars toward meeting organizational objectives. Educating existing employees to new skills required in the organization saves the costly outlay of funds for employee recruitment and orientation. By supporting distance learning opportunities, the health care employer is positioned to provide an employee benefit that also meets the organization's need for employees with a different skill mix. It additionally can move the organization toward becoming an employer of choice—a valuable designation in a competitive health care market place that now has too few primary care providers. Finally, by educating existing workers to new role requirements, employers invest in individuals whose value to the organization is already known. At the same time, employees have access to job enhancements and are able to retain employment as health care networks are restructured.

In the competitive world of health care delivery, implementation of a distance learning curriculum provides the opportunity for collaborative efforts among health care networks and academic institutions. Several health care organizations may band together to purchase distance education, sharing the up front investment costs in hardware and software that support the educational effort. In taking this approach, organizations define common needs among the workforce and purchase services that will be of benefit to all. In the future, such distance learning consortia will be commonplace enabling remote health care sites to be active participants in continuing and academic education.

As with any educational approach, distance learning will not meet the needs of all nurse learners. The need for self direction, relative isolation of the student and lack of a traditional face to face education approach may prove uncomfortable and distracting to some. In addition, distance learners must be active listeners and they must make the effort to interact with the instructor whatever the medium used. The distance learner must have a degree of comfort to query instructors and enter discussions in order to obtain the greatest benefit from instruction. In the absence of such interactions, the learner may not fully grasp course content and may become dissatisfied with the teaching process.

Nurses who take part in a distance learning modality will likely be highly motivated students. Forces in the health care workplace have demonstrated the need to acquire new skills and new abilities. The significant restructuring taking place within the workplace has resulted in a *teachable moment* for many. Future job viability and employability is viewed as hinging on the acquisition of new skills. On the other hand, this same group of motivated learners will likely experience a number of difficulties as they engage in the education activity. Experienced and successful clinicians entering a new realm of practice will likely have to *unlearn* certain habits, skills and practices in order to adapt to new roles and practice patterns in newer health care organizational settings. The relative isolation of distance learning students makes it more difficult for instructors to pattern or guide a student toward new roles.

Today's motivated nurse learners may have all the skills which ensure a successful education experience but lack one essential ingredient—they are prevented by geography, time constraints, family commitments or other circumstances from traveling to a traditional classroom setting to take part in the educational offering in a traditional manner. Even when costs are not a consideration for adult learners, circumstances may prevent participation in traditional classroom instruction.

Nurses preferring education and training offered at non traditional times and in convenient locations find distance learning a viable alternative to campus-based programs. Organizations, faced with a need for increased numbers of primary care and ambulatory care providers, can sponsor distance learning programs for their employees to develop the right skills mix for ambulatory and primary care patterns. There are indeed many advantages to distance learning education or training.

CONSIDERATIONS IN MOVING TO A DISTANCE LEARNING CURRICULUM IN NURSING

Moving to a distance learning format can not be viewed as simply taking the classroom to the air waves. A number of issues should be considered in planning for the implementation of a distance learning curriculum. Implementing a distance learning program requires careful consideration by the teaching institution, the student and/or the health care organization contracting for the distance education service. Employing distance learning strategies should be considered whenever large numbers of individuals over geographically dispersed areas have similar learning needs. Distance learning is indicated when local resources are not sufficient to meet the learning needs evidenced in the community; when expertise is centered in one area and those learners who need to avail themselves of the expertise are in another area; and when commuting is not feasible due to excessive distances.

Technical assistance will be required in order to effectively plan and carry out each step of the implementation process from planning, through transmission, to evaluation. Successful distance learning providers will have well skilled production experts, instructional designers and learning resource managers as part of the planning team and as permanent staff.

Once the commitment has been made to move to a distance learning format a number of issues should be considered. Equipping either a studio or classroom for distance learning applications requires strategic acquisition rather than the random purchase of equipment. Absent or poor planning can result in incompatible equipment or a configuration of equipment that yields poor audio and/or visual results. Television production specialists and instructional design technicians should be consulted throughout this process. Since technology changes rapidly, planners must decide if they will purchase or lease necessary equipment. While purchasing equipment can be viewed as a long term investment in building a telecommunications department, leasing offers the flexibility of upgrading equipment as technology changes. Organizations should be careful to purchase or lease equipment that meets projected needs rather than to be swayed by persuasive technology which will not be utilized effectively in the type of approach being implemented. Equipment too sophisticated for the task at hand can be as problematic as equipment which is not adequate for the production being transmitted. Upon review, some organizations may find the initial outlay of funds required to purchase or lease equipment and modify or construct classroom facilities prohibitive. This does not preclude participation in distance learning production, rather, it points to a need for fostering creative collaborative relationships that will support production and transmission activities.

Clearly the type of course to be taught will influence the technology required in the distance learning approach. Theory courses may not require the detailed real-time transmissions that a physical assessment course may require. Lessons learned from a decade of business teletraining should be put to use as distance learning is planned. One such lesson is that poor picture and sound quality can interfere with, if not ruin, a distance learning presentation. Poor sound and visual quality will rapidly produce dissatisfied learners and course dropouts. While a number of students learn quite adequately using only two-way audio transmissions, those transmissions or recordings must be of the highest caliber. Any production that is geared toward sight and sound should be the highest

quality the equipment and technological linkages will provide. In addition, planning must be extensive before activities begin. Starting the
process with inadequate tools, inadequate preparation and inadequately
equipped classrooms will doom the process to failure.

Faculty Preparation

Faculty teaching strategies and skills are challenged in a distance learning
format. It is not only the students who will acquire new skills. Even when
teaching a class taught numerous times before, care must be taken to
format the content for distance learning transmission. Faculty must think
visually, planning carefully how each aspect of the narrative lesson plan
can be illustrated. The appropriateness of handouts, graphics, pictures
and films should be evaluated in light of how they will be transmitted
to the student. It cannot be overemphasized that such planning takes
time; it may take as long as a month to receive the copyright release
required to broadcast a single illustration during the course of the class.
Given that technological difficulties can arise without warning, some
materials may need to be mailed to students prior to the class both to
prepare for coming classes and to augment any equipment failures that
may occur (Fulmer, Hazzard, Jones, & Keene, 1992).

Similarly, faculty must give careful consideration to verbal interactions
with class participants and the teaching techniques that will be used.
While most courses can be taught through a distance learning format,
each type of course requires special consideration and requires unique
adaptations. Lectures should be animated and interactive, incorporating
principles of adult education. Games and group exercises can and should
be utilized. Rather than using flip charts, students can document activities
completed by groups or teams and fax these to all sites for immediate
discussion and feedback (Shomacher, 1993; Crowley, Russell, & Martin, 1995).

There are also certain technical skills that faculty should master. Even
though technicians are often available during presentations, faculty should
acquire rudimentary skills in operating a personal camera, cueing the use
of films and graphics, and paying attention to monitors which indicate
whether students have questions or are unable to understand the point
just raised. Some new skills are quite simple, e.g., faculty must know
how to use a microphone, recognize where they can move and learn to
incorporate movement into their teaching strategies.

Student Expectations

Nurses like other adult learners of the day are far more familiar with technology of all types and are sophisticated in the use of basic information technology such as fax machines, modems, and e-mail. With increased use of computers in clinical care settings, as well as expanded access and use of the Internet, most nurses are familiar with data entry and the concept of interacting with other individuals at distant locations. These abilities can foster student comfort with distance learning. However, there are probably still ample numbers who continue to *break out in a cold sweat* at the prospect of touching a computer keyboard. These nurses will expect and require careful orientation to the process and activities of distance learning.

The distance learning approach may not be acceptable to all learners. Some students may require and prefer to commute to the structure of the traditional classroom, feeling that they will learn more easily when they are physically present with the instructor. Others may need the contact and exchange with other students and the opportunity to question and exchange views within the classroom. Still others may be ill at ease using electronic equipment or simply prefer to be in the same room with the instructor as demonstrations are presented.

The distance learning experience places more responsibility on students to be self-directed than does traditional classroom education. While little research has been conducted to identify characteristics of successful distance learning students, study has shown that the most successful distance learning students are self-directed and highly motivated to complete the course of study (OTA, 1989).

Coordination

Education and training providers, sponsoring health care organizations and individual students should agree to clearly defined responsibilities before entering any distance learning agreement. It is the responsibility of the academic site to maintain quality of the total presentation to provide guidance and consultation to both site coordinators and remote faculty.

It is likely that the remote site will be asked to provide a site coordinator whose responsibilities may include assuring that equipment is available and in working order, acting as a resource to students or even supervising return demonstrations. In all cases the duties and expectations of this individual should be clearly spelled out. Remote sites may also be asked to provide library resources, Internet access or other similar support. There should be a clear understanding of the type of records to be kept by the provider and the responsibility for record keeping at the remote site. Questions should be asked regarding any restrictions or requirements of accrediting agencies with which the host site must comply.

The integrity of testing materials must be maintained and students should have access to faculty as outlined in course materials. The education provider should answer questions such as how many sites can participate and how many participants can be at each distant site. Further, a clear understanding among the academic site, the classroom site and learning expectations for each group must be well delineated. For instance, will a computer be required of each student? Should the reception site videotape and store lectures? Will each classroom be required to have faxing capabilities, monitors, televisions, Internet access, and video recorders? When agreement is reached and all equipment is in place, it will be both valuable and prudent to conduct a preliminary test of the transmission and use of all equipment prior to initiating classes.

CHALLENGES TO SUCCESSFUL IMPLEMENTATION

The implementation of a distance learning curriculum presents a number of challenges. Having identified that the implementation of nurse practitioner distance learning programs would be beneficial in meeting existing workforce needs, it must be pointed out that the implementation of such a curriculum presents two significant challenges. The first is conveying clinical concepts and providing for a clinical teaching component. The second is providing for the socialization of distance learning students to their role as either nurse practitioners or baccalaureate prepared nurses.

Implementing Clinical Courses

Clinical courses offer the greatest challenge to a distance learning modality. Even with the requisite system of two-way interactive media in place, faculty are challenged to demonstrate clinical assessment and care skills in manners which are clearly viewed and clearly understood. Interacting with the class verbally may not provide satisfactory feedback to determine if the student can demonstrate the skill. As a result careful planning for follow-up and return demonstrations of clinical skills are required (Crowley, et al., 1995). With this approach also comes the need to ensure the quality of clinical faculty as well as to ensure that clinical practica are carried out in a manner consistent with the curriculum and course requirements. Further clinical supervision must be ensured to oversee skill acquisition that is consistent with practice standards. How the educational institution and faculty train distant clinical faculty preceptors and bring about the clinical competence of students remains a nearly uncharted journey. There is little in nursing literature to assist faculty in planning for teaching clinical courses through a distance learning format.

Approaches to ensuring quality of the clinical portion of the education process are varied. Clearly, clinical faculty who are geographically distant from the educational institution require orientation and a level of oversight. Training films for clinical faculty/preceptors may be developed; preceptors may be visited on site by regular faculty to observe some portion of clinical supervision. However, if the geographical distance between students and the education faculty is great and there are multiple off campus teaching sites, both the logistics and costs of such endeavors can be prohibitive. Clinical preceptors may be required to come into the campus teaching site for periodic review, discussion and counseling if necessary. Again, there may be prohibitive aspects to this practice. One solution in part may be to use the same distance learning technologies, such as videoteleconferences or satellite conferences. Interactive sessions using videoconferencing can be scheduled periodically with clinical preceptors to provide oversight for the clinical component.

Socialization

An issue receiving increasing prominence in distance learning literature is that of how students become socialized to their professional roles if they are educated through a distance learning format in the absence of role models such as faculty and others in the academic environment. In some course work this may pose little or no problem, however, for RN-BSN and expanded role students the inability of students to communicate freely with peers and to learn from the experiences of others eliminates an important part of the teaching process. In addition, students derive both benefit and confidence from a verbal exchange and validation with the instructor and peers.

While the socialization process is obviously hindered, studies of nurses and other professional groups have shown that professional socialization does take place with distance learning students (Cragg, 1991). This occurs through the faculty making special efforts to incorporate interactive strategies and socialization activities into courses (Penney, Gibbons, & Bushy, 1996). The professional socialization process can also be fostered by the site coordinator through formation of discussion groups, and the process of matching students with practitioner mentors and offering feedback to students (Crowley, et al., 1995). Students involved in computer mediated conferences have been found to form cohesive and friendly groups through the computer which allows for sharing experiences and providing feedback (Cragg, 1994).

Development and Marketing

The development of high quality distance learning programs is costly in both human and fiscal resources, requiring careful planning and investigation of methods and technology research followed by equipment purchase and curriculum development. Increasingly, numbers of academic institutions are looking toward health care organizations as partners in agreements to subsidize the development of distance learning curricula and course delivery with the assumption that the particular academic institution will meet the distance learning needs for the service setting. Such arrangements do have relative merit; organizations are able to obtain customized education and training while colleges and universities receive the preliminary support which enables the establishment of divisions or departments of distance learning.

There are cautions, however, to the preceding practice. In the future, health care networks will change missions and practice patterns in rapid response to consumer needs and to accommodate advances in patient care. Health care organizations will modify their strategic plans and corporate goals and objectives will change. In such a dynamic environment, the traditional time consuming college and university approach to course development and the modification and preparation of classes will not be adequately responsive to needs in the health care service sector. On the other hand, health care organizations will recognize that because of their diversity, one education provider can meet certain of their education and training needs while unable to meet other needs. In the future, it will be common for an organization to contract separately with a number of education providers to meet employee education and training needs.

A CASE STUDY IN PROGRESS: DEVELOPING A COLLABORATIVE DISTANCE LEARNING PROGRAM

The organization of this chapter, as well as many of the observations and recommendations, trace this author's ongoing learning experience in coordinating the organization of a consortia of federal partners to implement a nationwide distance learning program for nurse practitioner education. While this project is in the developmental stage, the experiences and decisions made to date may be helpful to others anticipating the development or use of distance learning programs.

The Department of Veterans Affairs (VA), a national health care system employing over 60,000 registered nurses in 170 facilities, has restructured extensively and as a result has an extensive need for increased numbers of primary care providers.

VA nursing leaders were aware that each of the uniformed health services (U.S. Public Health Service [USPHS] and Department of Defense (DoD): Army, Navy, Air Force) also had an increased need for nurse practitioners. In addition, VA leaders were recipients of numerous anecdotal reports that nurse practitioner programs near VA facilities were often filled to capacity with waiting lists of several years. Some VA facilities were not geographically near a graduate school of nursing and some staff were commuting over two hundred miles one way, one or more times a week to obtain nurse practitioner education.

With these facts in mind, the author developed a proposal for a nationwide program of nurse practitioner education, taught over VA's nationwide satellite system. The course would be taught by the Uniformed Services University of the Health Sciences (USUHS) Graduate School of Nursing and students would be VA, DoD or USPHS nurses. Clinical preceptors and on site instructors would come from any of these organizations and clinical practica could be completed in any federal facility or, when necessary, in civilian facilities.

Following rounds of briefings, the proposal was enthusiastically endorsed in concept by VA, and each federal nursing service chief executive. The activities that followed were in many ways typical of any project development, however, they were more complex because they involved coordination of numerous individual and group efforts across several national networks. Work efforts began with the formation of a Steering Committee composed of representatives of each of the project participants. During these meetings it was apparent that each member brought unique expertise needed by others, for example, VA had expertise in television production and media, USUHS faculty were already familiar with certain concepts of distance learning, and all members were familiar with the clinical organization of their national system of field facilities. Potential barriers addressed ranged from identifying contacts at field facilities, identifying VA, DoD and USPHS facilities located in close proximity to each other and identifying equipment available on a national basis.

The Steering Committee determined that the course of instruction to be taught would be a family nurse practitioner certificate program open to clinical nurse specialists. The committee also determined a number of areas in which questions must be answered, the foremost of which was to develop a budget for such a comprehensive project, since cost effectiveness would be one parameter closely scrutinized. Other issues included how to link two or more national broadcasting networks, assuring that the quality of the distance program was equal to the quality and rigor of the residential program; and, how to initiate the collaborative efforts of VA, DoD and USPHS staff for both classroom and clinical experiences.

VA agreed to fund one coordinator/faculty position and to support the costs of a project consultant. Filling the faculty position was a daunting experience. Nurse practitioners of course are in short supply. Finding a certified nurse practitioner with military, teaching and VA experience took effort.

Staff from VA and military hospitals worked with USUHS faculty to develop a pilot project of two phases; the first to test the technology and, the second, teaching of a three credit physical assessment course to determine the feasibility of teaching clinical content via distance learning. Classes for the pilot would be transmitted via videoconferencing that would originate from a Navy hospital studio in suburban Washington, DC. Sites for the pilot would be in West Virginia, Georgia, North Carolina and New Mexico. Phase One of the pilot was conducted successfully. Phase Two is scheduled to begin shortly with students from both the military and VA. If successful, the pilot will generate cost data and other information that will be used to develop a formal interdepartmental sharing agreement. It is anticipated that students could begin a formal program of study approximately five months after the pilot.

The preceding description illustrates several points that can not be emphasized too strongly. Planning is essential to all elements of distance learning delivery. While the author is involved primarily in the technical aspects of the project, faculty are working diligently to adapt the existing curriculum, graphics and handouts. Attention is being given to presentation techniques. Any first effort of this type benefits from consultation and the project is fortunate to have secured the services of an outstanding nurse educator who has extensive experience in distance learning.

Already the project has successfully linked two national telecommunication systems and positive collaborative relations are developing among the VA, DoD and USPHS staff in field facilities. We continue to learn about Local Area Networks (LANs), fiber optics and satellite transmission requirements in comparison to videoconferencing. Professional and trade journals also offer a wealth of education on distance learning and the Internet provides another resource for information, as well as the opportunity to correspond with others involved in distance learning. While it seems that the project will go forward successfully, there is no guarantee. What can be guaranteed is that we will have difficulties, both anticipated and unanticipated—most will be solved at the time, some will require more thought and planning. This project has exciting prospects and potential, and great challenges are anticipated on this new learning horizon.

FUTURE DIRECTIONS

There is sufficient research and anecdotal information to indicate that distance learning is a promising approach to academic and continuing education in nursing. Much of the research though is descriptive, centering around comparisons of traditional learners with their distant counterparts. There are, however, numerous questions which require study. Teaching strategies that work best in a distance learning delivery should be identified, as should those methods that support professional role socialization. Additionally, research is needed to develop theories of learning most applicable to distance learning activities and it is important that student traits that lead to success in distant learning environments be identified. One significant area for study is the effectiveness of distance learning strategies in teaching clinical care concepts as well as methods for assuring the clinical competence of distance learners.

It will also be interesting to note any effect that the growing number of distance learning and virtual education programs may have on accreditation processes or requirements. For instance, will accrediting bodies still require that college and universities maintain a number of volumes and journals in campus libraries if both residential and distance students can download significant numbers of journals and information from computer networks? If indeed we do progress toward virtual colleges, what guidelines will be used to determine the quality and rigor of their academic products?

More stringent methods of authenticating student participation and completion of tests will be needed to support successful expansion of Internet-based activities. In addition, copyright laws and regulations must be clarified with regard to information written for and distributed on the Internet.

There are a number of resources on the Internet to assist teachers of grades K-12 in designing teaching tools, modifying class content in order to use the Internet or distance learning as a teaching tool. While portions of this content can certainly be assistive to nursing instructors at the graduate and undergraduate level, colleges and universities need to collaborate to provide the same opportunity for their constituents. Additionally, innovative models of collaboration in the production and implementation of distance learning programs are needed to maximize this valuable resource.

THE FUTURE OF DISTANCE LEARNING

The preceding description is a snapshot of the future of distance learning viewed from the prospect of today's technologies. These applications, however, will evolve and grow to have little resemblance to what we recognize today. Cutting edge technologies will be combined to result in interactive learning which employs a broad array of approaches. Artificial intelligence, video desktop applications and simulations will be routinely incorporated into distance learning. The distance learning site of the future may or may not be a classroom and the teaching techniques will be less as we know them now and more a reflection of possibilities that will come to be. The only certainty in the future of distance learning is its growing sophistication.

Casmir Skrzypczak, president of NYNEX Science and Technology, describes the use of any new technology as a progression of phases. In the first phase, society uses technology as it has always done but perhaps better. In the second phase, activities become more innovative, taking a familiar course of action several steps beyond familiar parameters. In the third phase, revolutionary actions are taken that have not been known or contemplated previously (*Boston Globe*, 1997). This description of technological evolution is easily applied to distance learning. The designs of existing programs have progressed from simply mimicking the traditional classroom environment to incorporating innovative approaches.

With few exceptions, the current status of design and implementation of distance learning cannot be described as revolutionary. Yet progress is being made. With ongoing research, theories of distance learning are emerging. These theories provide instructional designers and educators with data to stimulate learning such as the use of cognitive tools that encourage students to organize and interpret knowledge (Jonassen, Davidson, Collins, Campbell & Haag, 1995). New theories of collaborative learning will decrease the isolation typical of distance learning and promote socialization (Abrami & Bures, 1996).

Just how nurse educators will employ distance learning technologies to create revolutionary approaches is a question with an infinite number of possible answers. The challenges posed by 21st century health care will create extensive opportunities for entrepreneurial enterprises to impact innovative education.

It will be fascinating to witness the growing sophistication of distance learning as it gains wider use in both childhood and adult education and grows beyond our wildest technical (or should I say Technicolor?) dreams.

REFERENCES

Abrami, P. C., & Bures, E. M. (1996). Computer-supported collaborative learning and distance education. *The American Journal of Distance Education, 10,* (2), 37–42.

Aiken, L., & Salmon, M. (1994). Health Care Workforce Priorities: What Nursing Should Do Now. *Inquiry, 31,* 318–329.

Barry, M., & Runyan, G. B. (1995). A review of distance-learning studies in the U.S. Military. *American Journal of Distance Education,* 9(3), 37–47.

Billings, D. M., & Bachmeir, B. (1994). Teaching and learning at a distance. In L. R. Allen, (Ed.), *Review of research in nursing education, volume VI.* New York: NLN Press.

The Boston Globe (1997). For better and worse, computers change how we learn and live. (February 2, 1997, pp. C2–C3).

Business Week (1995). Virtual B-schools, Oct. 23, 1995.

Cragg, C. E. (1994). Distance learning through computer conferences. *Nurse Educator, 19,* (2), 10–14.

Cragg, C. E. (1991). Professional resocialization of post-RN baccalaureate students by distance education. *Journal of Nursing Education, 30,* 256–260.

Crowley, J. R., Russell, B. L., & Martin, S. M. (1995). Challenges of distance learning for the allied health educator. *Journal of the American Health Information Management Association, 66,* (7), 64–67.

Fulmer, J., Hazzard, M., Jones, S., & Keene, K. (1992). Distance Learning: An

Innovative Approach to Nursing Education. *Journal of Professional Nursing*, 8(5), 289–294.

General Accounting Office. (1995). *Video teleconferencing: A guide to design, development and use.* (Report # GAO/TI-95-1). Washington, DC.

Gurvey, S. (Producer). (1997, February 17). Net effect: Business in the connected world *The Nightly Business Report*. Miami, FL and Washington, DC: Public Broadcasting Service.

Jonassen, D., Davidson, M., Collins, M., Campbell, J., & Haag, B. B. (1995). Constructivism and computer-mediated communication in distance education. *The American Journal of Distance Education*, 9, (2), 7–25.

Keck, J. F. (1992). Comparison of learning outcomes between graduate students in telecourses and those in traditional classrooms. *Journal of Nursing Education*, 31, 229–234.

Lytle, J. S., Lytle, B. V., & Youmans, K. G. (1995). Learning at a distance: People, technology and learning experiments. *Journal of the American Health Information Management Association*, 66, (7), 64–67.

McClelland, E., & Daly, J. (1991). A comparison of selected demographic characteristics and academic performance of on-campus and satellite-center RNs: Implications for the curriculum. *Journal of Nursing Education*, 30, 261–266.

Meister, J. C. (1994). *Corporate Quality Universities.* New York: Irwin Professional Publishing.

Office of Technology Assessment (OTA). (1989). Linking for learning: A new course for education. (OTA-SET-430). Washington, DC.

Penney, N. E., Gibbons, B., & Bushy, A. (1996). Partners in distance learning: Project outreach. *Journal of Nursing Administration*, 26, (7/8), 27–36.

Pew Health Professions Commission (1994, April). *Nurse practitioners: Doubling the graduates by the year 2000.* San Francisco, CA.

Phelps, R. H., Wells, R. A., Ashworth, R. L., & Hahn, H. A. (1991). Effectiveness and costs of distance education using computer-mediated communication. *The American Journal of Distance Education*, 5(3), 7–19.

Satterlund, S. (1993). Fiber goes the distance. *Electronic Learning*, September, 46–47.

Shomaker, D. (1993). A statewide instructional television program via satellite for RN-to-BSN students. *Journal of Professional Nursing*, 9(3), 153–158.

Training. Multimedia Training in the Fortune 1000, 50(9), 53–60.

U.S. Public Law 104-104, *Telecommunications Act of 1996.* February 8, 1996.

U.S. Department of Health and Human Services (DHHS), Health Resources and Services Administration, Division of Nursing. (1994). *The registered nurse population 1992: Findings from the national sample survey of registered nurses, March 1992.* Washington, DC: U.S. Government Printing Office.

US News and World Report (1995). Getting a degree by e-mail, 119(17), 67–68.

Wulf, K. (1996). Training via the Internet: Where are we? *Training and Development*, 50(5), 50–55.

13

Nursing Research—'BACC' To The Future

Paulette R. Cournoyer

Research—

1. It is a state of mind that is discontented with things as they are.
2. It is a pair of eyes that yearn to see through the curtain of obscurity to fact.
3. It is a hand wielding a knife to cut a thing down to its smallest particle—and then to cut open the particle.
4. It is a brain for which there is no peace without knowledge and understanding—and no end to either.
5. It is a soul more concerned with mankind than with self—more anxious for progress than for triumph.
6. It is a man [or woman]—indomitable and uncompromising.
   Gulf Oil Company, 1940, p. 27

These statements on research reflect the sense of adventure, exploration and discovery inherent in the process of research and set a tone readily

---

The views and opinions expressed in this chapter are those of the author and do not necessarily reflect those of the U.S. Department of Veterans Affairs.

applicable to nursing research. The purpose of this chapter is to carefully delineate the importance of baccalaureate nurses to research and to present realistic activities and options to further encourage their involvement with research. This chapter will discuss research preparation for baccalaureate students. Additionally, research utilization and barriers to research in clinical practice settings will be explored. Models that assist research in practice will be presented and suggestions to maximize the contribution of bachelor's prepared nurses to nursing research will be outlined.

BACKGROUND—BACCALAUREATE RESEARCH PREPARATION

The ANA Cabinet on Nursing Research in 1989 indicated that at the baccalaureate level, nurses should be able to "read research critically and to use existing standards to determine the readiness of research for utilization in clinical practice." In addition to understanding ethical principles, especially as they apply to protection of human subjects, the bachelor's prepared nurse: "1) identifies clinical problems in need of research; 2) helps experienced investigators gain access to clinical sites; 3) influences the selection of appropriate methods of data collection; and 4) participates in data collection and implementation of nursing research findings."

In the literature on research preparation of baccalaureate nursing students, multiple articles focus on what should be its purpose, i.e., what outcomes should be expected. There is consensus that baccalaureate nurses should be prepared to be consumers of research (Beyea, Farley, & Williams-Burgess, 1996; Murdaugh, Kramer, & Schmalenberg, 1981). The level of their ability to critique (Overfield & Duffy, 1984; Feldman, 1988; Wheeler, Fasano, & Burr, 1995) still remains to be defined more clearly, though. Additionally, Murdaugh reported that almost one third of the bachelor's programs she surveyed expected beginning research productivity from their students (Murdaugh et al., 1981). These latter two issues continue to be debated by the profession, i.e., what can be realistically expected of baccalaureate students—the balance between reality and the ideal.

A variety of approaches to address the educational objectives set by the profession for research are detailed in the literature. They have been aptly categorized in the following groupings: learning by doing, learning by proposing to do, learning by critiquing (Overfield et al., 1984) and learning by doing in collaboration (Roberts & Crook, 1987). Whether the format should be by individual course(s) in such specific topics as statistics, computers and research (Dvorak, Brophy, Binder, & Carlson, 1993; Murdaugh et al., 1981) or be integrated in the whole curriculum (Beyea et al., 1996) is also a matter of discussion. Issues such as placement/timing in the curriculum (Thiele, 1984; Ludeman, 1979) and teaching methods (Beck, 1986 & 1993; Dean, 1986; Beal, 1989) have been the focus of multiple journal articles.

In sum though, it is evident that there is much effort and commitment to designing excellent nursing research courses. The descriptions of widely varied teaching approaches attest to the aim to engender enthusiasm for research (Beyea et al., 1996), to foster the development of a research attitude (Sakalys, 1985) and to enhance a spirit of inquiry (Fleming, 1980; Larson, 1989) wherein students become excited by research and discover that it can be *fun*. Clearly faculty realize the importance to the profession of turning students on to research at this early stage of their career. Additionally, Werley and Newcomb (1983) noted that the undergraduate experience is a critical time to identify talent and special interests in research and to encourage the pursuit of a research career.

BACCALAUREATE GRADUATE—ROLE IN RESEARCH

From the literature on undergraduate preparation, the faculty authors diligently attempt to delineate realistic expectations for baccalaureate students. This bachelor's education potentially forms the base which instills in each individual nurse the responsibility to, at some level, advance practice through research. Here, in the undergraduate setting, nursing students learn what is expected of them and what they should expect in the practice setting—as it relates to research.

Following graduation though, the baccalaureate nurse's focus is primarily on becoming clinically comfortable by "mastering treatment procedures or acquiring technical competence in using equipment" (Werley et al., p. 206). Technical and skill competencies are the initial focus, the hallmarks of becoming a *real nurse*. Successful skill acquisition, thereby, ensures patient safety and heightens the new nurse's self esteem. Ongoing development of the nurse's abilities encourages advancement to higher level roles and functions (Smith, 1992).

From this point, they begin their progression through the clinical world to incrementally achieve competence, become proficient and also perhaps eventually achieve an expert level of practice. These stages as defined by Benner and colleagues are differentiated as follows: the advanced beginner accomplishes tasks; the competent nurse sets goals and makes plans to achieve them; the proficient clinician perceives situations as wholes based on a deep background understanding of the overall picture; and the expert has an intuitive grasp of each situation and focuses in on the solution without having to belabor a variety of rule out options (Benner, 1984; Benner, Tanner, & Chesla, 1992). It is critical that beginning nurses develop clinical competence before involvement with research is possible.

After attaining a level of clinical proficiency, is it presumptive to assume the baccalaureate nurse has a role in research? While it is unrealistic to portray the bachelor's degree registered nurse as being an independent researcher, the baccalaureate nurse's role in research is important and cannot be overemphasized.

First, the nurse at the bedside or in any clinical setting "is the *only* nurse who can implement significant research findings as an integral part of the care provided" (Welches, 1983, p. 17). While this seems like a simple, obvious statement, it is not. Data about registered nurses employed in clinical settings with position titles of staff nurse and head nurse indicated that baccalaureate nurses represented 33 percent of this population; alternatively, master's prepared nurses comprised only .03 percent and doctorally prepared count for 779 of the total 1,432,827 positions (Moses, 1997). Implementing research into practice serves a significant scientific function; it plays a major role in the development and testing of nursing theories and can foster exploration and adoption of timely practice ideas (Werley et al., 1983).

Secondly, nurses in the clinical setting know the important questions and the patient care problems that need to be studied. In an article titled "The Two Worlds of Nursing," Teresa Chopoorian notes "We, the super-educated professionals, are interested in flashy or *sexy* research projects . . . But what about some of the hard core issues of caring for people [in nursing homes] who have no reaction to us? Who drool all of the time? . . . Who refuse to eat? Who slap and hit . . . nurses? Who scream or yell out constantly?" (1988, p. 450). Answers to these questions would help guide practice and would have a significant impact on day to day nursing care. Without asking these questions, no systematic seeking of answers will likely occur. Practicing nurses are also in the best position to question their practice. By their consistent, objective observations of every day nursing practice, they can easily substantiate the need to reconsider nursing procedures, policies and processes.

Finally, our pool of potential future investigators is baccalaureate nurses. The nursing profession needs to actively attend to this crucial reality. "Research career development is our future. If you say that research provides tomorrow's answers to today's questions, then we're going to have to have investigators tomorrow addressing those questions" (Career Development, 1996, p. 7, direct quote attributed to John Feussner). This stresses, therefore, the need to ensure that bachelor's level practitioners are involved in research.

UTILIZATION OF RESEARCH IN PRACTICE— WHAT SHOULD THE BACCALAUREATE NURSE EXPECT?

The issue of utilization of research in practice has been significantly influenced by the model developed by Rogers describing diffusion of innovations (1983). In Ketefian's investigation of oral temperature practices, she noted that "the practitioner either was totally unaware of the research literature relative to her practice, or, if she was aware of it, was unable to relate to it or utilize it" (1975, p. 91). Similarly, Kirchhoff (1982) who studied the diffusion of knowledge regarding discontinuance of coronary precautions found limited diffusion of nursing research findings into practice. Both of these studies corroborate the gap between research knowledge and nursing practice.

To explore this issue in more depth, a detailed analysis of a more recent survey is in order. In an oft quoted and replicated (Anderson, 1992; Brett, 1989; Coyle & Sokop, 1990) seminal article written by Brett (1987) titled "Use of Nursing Practice Research Findings," five nursing research journals from 1978 to 1983, i.e., *Nursing Research, Advances of Nursing Science, Research in Nursing and Health, Western Journal of Nursing Research*, and *Heart and Lung*, were reviewed and analyzed systematically for their potential applicability to practice. Nine practice innovations were identified from this literature and an additional five findings were added from the research-based protocols developed by the Conduct and Utilization of Research in Nursing (CURN) Project (1982). These 14 innovations related to a range of care issues from positioning of intramuscular injections to passive range of motion activities and intracranial pressure. Brett surveyed 216 hospital-based nurses regarding the extent of their adoption of these innovations. The conclusion indicated that "the majority of nurses were aware of the average innovation, were persuaded about it, and used the average innovation at least sometimes" (1987, p. 344).

This research though, needs to be examined more closely. A MEDLINE search conducted by this chapter's author, selecting one full year (a convenience sample) of each of the previously listed journals during the years specified, showed that 303 articles were published for a total of 2,171 pages including advertisements. Multiplying this by the six years of journals searched, would yield an estimated 1,818 articles. Is it realistic to expect clinicians to read, annotate, compare and critique about 1,818 articles over a six year period to isolate potential innovations? If they indeed were aware of the innovations, what and/or who was the source of the information?

As a further commentary, what is the state of our scientific publications and/or science such that from 1,818 articles from nursing's leading research journals, only nine practice innovations could be isolated? This is made even more poignant by Brett's comment that the "inclusion criteria for this study's research findings were admittedly liberal" (1987, p. 348). To place this dilemma in perspective though, note that even the Agency for Health Care Policy and Research's (AHCPR) *Clinical Practice Guidelines*, which were developed to specifically study significant and well researched clinical issues, state this disclaimer "recommendations . . . primarily based on the published scientific literature. When the scientific literature was incomplete or inconsistent in a particular area, the recommendations reflect the professional judgment of panel members and consultants. In some instances, there was not unanimity of opinion" (Urinary Incontinence, 1992, p. ii). This emphasizes the fact that practice based research has a long way to go and that this is a universal issue for most, if not all, disciplines.

BARRIERS TO RESEARCH—
WELCOME TO THE REAL WORLD!

In considering the paucity of evidence about the utilization of research in practice, investigators have sought to identify the potential barriers to using research. Miller and Messenger (1978) indicated that in response to their survey, employed nurses stated that obtaining research findings was their most frequently encountered difficulty. In another study, investigators found that the two greatest barriers reported were related to the practice setting wherein the nurses felt that they did not have sufficient authority to change patient care procedures and that there was not sufficient time to implement new ideas (Funk, Champagne, Wiese, & Tornquist, 1991). Additionally, this study noted that "lack of cooperation and support from physicians, administration and other staff; inadequate facilities for implementation; and insufficient time to read research" were also rated as top setting barriers (p. 91). These same respondents suggested several ways to facilitate the use of research findings: "increasing administrative support and encouragement, improving the accessibility of research reoprts, . . . improving the research knowledge base of the practicing nurse[,] . . . providing formal mechanisms for colleague support, having more clinically relevant research, increasing time for research review and implementation, and improving the understandability of research reports" (p. 91).

In a similar vein, Ferris clearly articulates a typical reaction about research. "RESEARCH—now there is a paralyzing idea. The thought of even reading research articles conjures up images of forced reading assignments; complicated titles, formats, tables and graphs; boring statistics; and a feeling of 'So what does this mean to me, a clinical nurse?'" (1990, p. 5). Lest you think these thoughts are unique to nursing, Stephen Hawking, a noted physicist, in the introduction to his book, A Brief History of Time, notes the following: "Someone told me that each equation I included in the book would halve the sales" (1988, p. vi).

This partly substantiates that using research can be a challenging task. After determining that practice about a care issue needs to be questioned and investigated, "the problem must be specifically and clearly identified, relevant research-based literature located, and the studies stringently critiqued in terms of both scientific and clinical merit. Additionally, if the research suggests a need to modify practice, all the dynamics of change must be considered, and a plan developed for implementing and evaluating the new or modified approach to care" (Jennings & Rogers, 1988, p. 754). Is this a realistic objective for a baccalaureate nurse?

RESEARCH TO PRACTICE MODELS

There have been a variety of models developed to facilitate the transfer of research knowledge into practice and to facilitate research into practice.

In one such model referred to as CURN (Horsley, Crane, Crabtree, & Wood, 1983), research utilization is described as a systematic series of activities which can be broken down as follows: identify a patient care problem, gather and evaluate research, determine conclusions which can be drawn from the research, i.e., develop a protocol from the research results, design and implement a nursing intervention, and measure and evaluate its effect. After this process, a determination is made regarding whether to adopt the intervention or change it. Then, the preceding process in an ongoing cycle starts again. This model offers a distinct, deliberative process to assist clinicians in translating research into practice and it has engendered broad acceptance as a way to bridge the previously stated gap.

Alternatively, Stetler (1994) delineates a practitioner-oriented model of research utilization which involves six phases. The preparation phase's purpose is to review the research literature on a selected topic. The next phase titled validation includes an assessment of this literature's usability for practice. Next, the model details a comparative evaluation to determine the feasibility of applying the study's result to one's specific setting. Decision making in a cautious, pragmatic way is detailed as the individual practitioner needs to assess whether or not to apply the research to practice; if applied, the approach for utilization can be either informal or formal, e.g., involving organizational processes such as changing policies.

Translation/application involves generalizing the research findings into specific action(s). The final step, evaluation, wherein one assesses if the expected outcome(s) occurred, can be done informally or formally in a rigorous data-based assessment. These two models have been incorporated and/or adapted in a number of clinical settings as a way to increase research's relevance to practice.

To infuse research into practice is the goal of another model which is described by Titler, Kleiber, Stedman, Goode, Rakel, Barry-Walker, Small, & Buckwalter (1994). They delineate a clinical setting which has legitimized research activities by providing "clinical release time for doing research, recognition for participating in research, tuition reimbursement for the completion of research courses, and funding for attendance and/or presentation of research at . . . meetings" (1994, p. 307). In the Titler et al. Iowa model, nursing's research department and division structures are organized to support research in each of the clinical nursing divisions. These activities include reviewing research, disseminating research information, designing and implementing research-based practice and actually conducting funded clinical research. Involvement by nursing students, staff nurses, nurse managers, clinical nurse specialists and nurse scientists are noted. This model includes delineation of a process to determine and implement practice changes based on research throughout the clinical organization. Such an organizational structure with a support system of nurse scientists and nurse consultants provides a valuable resource to bachelor's degree nurses and can indeed make using, and even doing, small scale studies a realistic option.

Many of these described models have been developed and implemented in settings with large research intensive medical centers which have access to nurse researchers, nurse scientists and/or nurse consultants. Scientific nursing expertise though, is not evenly distributed throughout the United States and a significant number of clinical settings do not have such knowledge resources available. Unfortunately, therefore, learning from witnessing the actual performance of research on an every day basis is available to only a small number of baccalaureate nurses. While these models offer promise for the advancement of nursing science, they may have only limited applicability for the majority of health facilities.

RESEARCH ACTIVITIES FOR BACCALAUREATE NURSES

Is it realistic to expect that staff nurses can be involved with research? If there is a commitment to creating an environment where research is seen as integral to nursing practice, there are a variety of activities in which a baccalaureate nurse can be involved. These research activities would require administrative support and some require guidance and assistance from senior staff, but not necessarily nursing staff.

Baccalaureate education can inform nurses that there are a multitude of ways to get involved in research. Their skill, talent, interest and competence can determine the degree of their involvement. As part of an ongoing growth trajectory in the research component of a baccalaureate nurse's career and within the context of the educational objectives specified by the ANA (1989), there are a variety of research activities in which they can be involved. These activities include information seeking, questioning and critiquing, and participating in the research process.

Information Seeking

- Reading the research literature; it is an individual's responsibility to remain current.

- Sharing articles relevant to a clinical area with colleagues; swapping articles.
- Attaching an article specific to a patient's problem to the chart for all of the staff to have easy access to read.
- Arranging for the librarian to regularly photocopy and distribute the table of contents of significant refereed journals.
- Involving nursing students in assisting with literature reviews.
- Getting on the mailing list of research newsletters which are published by a variety of Colleges of Nursing and by hospital nursing research departments.
- Being a member of a 'Brown Bag' Journal Club or starting one.
- Preparing a poster detailing a published research article; posting it to stimulate discussion with colleagues (Sweeney, 1984).
- Attending a nursing research conference; universities, Sigma Theta Tau chapters and large health care facilities regularly sponsor these activities.

Questioning and Critiquing

- Identifying clinical nursing problems, exploring and synthesizing the literature, and discussing with colleagues the applicability and possible utilization of research findings in practice.
- With guidance, determining which symptom(s) occurs most frequently in their clinical care area and searching the literature for reliable and valid instrument(s) to objectively measure that variable consistently to document its response to care interventions.
- Developing a respect for data; when they are required to collect data, determining the reason for the data and ensuring its accuracy.
- Identifying and committing to develop a particular expertise in a clinical interest area; for example, what topic have they found themselves reading about regularly because it peaks their curiosity.
- Actively interacting with faculty at the local university on issues of clinical concern.

Participating

- Joining a research interest group.
- Being knowledgeable of the research being done at their facility.

- Facilitating research done by others.
- Participating on a research project by being a subject, research expediter, data collector, data organizer, data entry person, etc.
- Being a member of a nursing research committee at their facility or offering to assist members of the committee, as needed.
- Exploring their setting and not limiting themselves to nursing service: is there a research laboratory where they can volunteer?
- Cultivating relationships with their facility's research department for information and for potential resources.

Additional activities can be within the purview of the bachelor's prepared nurses when they have achieved Benner's proficient to expert clinical stage (1984). Again, the degree and depth of involvement in these higher level functions are dependent on the talent and special skills of the clinician. These individuals who represent the best, brightest, most independent, resourceful and persevering employees will need the agency's specific commitment to support their success in this endeavor. Many issues will need to be negotiated to make this possible, including of course, workload assignments. (Encouraging these stellar performers to further their education is the preferred option if they desire a research career. For a multitude of reasons though, this may not be a viable alternative for some nurses.) Note that these competent to expert clinical nurses, as categorized by Benner (1984), are most probably only equivalent to advanced beginners in their research role.

Writing

- Starting to carefully delineate in writing their observations and knowledge of care issues, e.g., scientific notebook.
- Summarizing the literature, identifying gaps and questions that remain unanswered.
- Presenting one's scientific paper for discussion at clinical case conferences.
- Publishing in the scientific literature.

While this, in effect, describes some of the steps of the research process, the beginning researcher may be surprised at how receptive senior colleagues will be to giving individual consultation when a written text is available for critique.

Conducting Research—Pilot Work or Small Scale Research Project

The previously noted elements serve as preparation for actually conducting a small scale study. Outstanding baccalaureate-level nurses who have published and achieved a noteworthy level of clinical excellence, i.e., Benner's proficient to expert level (1984), may seek the challenges of conducting a modest research project.

In order to ensure that these proficient clinical nurses remain enthusiastic about research, it is essential that prior to planning a research study, they have a clear understanding of what is entailed in the process. This includes the research proposal paperwork requirements, the levels of review required and the time frame necessary from proposal preparation and approval to final completion of the study, i.e., it can take a few months to several years. These details may differ significantly depending on the complexity of the proposed project, on whether nurses are doing a project which is within the purview of their clinical role, e.g., collecting and analyzing what could be defined as quality improvement data, and whether the individual is seeking funding, either from locally available discretionary funds or from a formal small grants mechanism, internal or external to the agency.

Additionally, *wisdoms* that new nurse researchers need to be aware of include:

- A successful proposal is usually not the work of one individual; a research team, including a statistician, is the norm.
- Pilot testing is essential.
- Mock review(s) of the proposal by objective expert(s) prior to its submission increases its clarity and quality.
- Generally, the more resources requested, e.g., time, supplies and money, the more involved will be the review process.
- For funded research, it takes, on average, three submissions before approval and funding.

What does all of this suggest? A professional nurse prepared at the bachelor's level, now and in the future, is an ongoing learner. Baccalaureate nurses are not to be independent scientists but there is much in the clinical setting to challenge them for the future course of their career. Additionally, such motivated clinicians will be amenable to encourage research in their setting; will seek to maintain an ongoing setting of excellent care and will perhaps more likely be willing to use research in practice. But they must be involved in the process; they must have a role. These listed activities are designed to show practical, realistic ways or activities to increase involvement and to make research, i.e., nursing science, less disconnected from clinician's 7:30–4:00 practice. If clinicians are seen or see themselves as outsiders, we cannot expect research to impact practice to the maximum degree needed and possible.

CONCLUDING SUGGESTIONS

Collaborative Research

To increase the relevance and role of research in practice, collaborative research efforts need to be expanded in order to enhance the baccalaureate nurse's contribution to nursing science. Since the distribution of scientific research expertise is relatively sparse in nursing, joining forces and forming alliances could benefit both academe and practice. While this is not a new idea, it is time to revitalize and forge new or different partnerships.

This process will encourage individuals to "view each other as colleagues with different abilities and expertise" (Stone, 1996, p. 1) and can make research activities happen. As more and more research is done in the practice setting, effective use of baccalaureate nurses as collaborators in research is vital. A notation describing the effective use of students as collaborators was detailed in *The New York Times:* "He is very clever in devising strategies . . . But those strategies wouldn't do him much good if he did not have a large clutch of graduate students who want to work with him and provide essential manpower so that he can get something done" (Severo, 1980, p. A17). The same rationale easily applies to bachelor's prepared nurses. The combination of skills could enable the development of more effective ways to do clinical research and help build a scientific base relevant to practice. Additionally, collaboration would not only share talent but also be an opportunity to maximize resources, especially relevant in these cost cutting times.

Research Literature

If the implications for practice could be distilled and succinctly stated as part of each nursing research article, this would facilitate the clinician's ability to implement research. Perhaps the nursing journal editors included in INANE, International Academy of Nursing Editors, (a very loose, informal organization, B. O'Connor, American Association of Colleges of Nursing, personal communication, March 13, 1997) could adopt a universal format that would instruct authors, i.e., experts in their specific research area, to make specific notations of *current* applicability of their research to practice. Guidelines could specify that practice recommendations be written in language clearly understandable to clinicians. If this could be an expectation similar to abstract requirements, it would greatly assist practitioners in using research.

Additionally, since the practice recommendations would be assessed by seasoned journal reviewer experts, this would ensure a basic minimum level of review. While this would be no substitute for an in-depth critique of the literature, it would minimize the need for each staff nurse, for example, to individually review and critique the research, which is especially pertinent for those with limited experience and expertise. This could also lead to substantive resource savings (Kirchhoff, 1983).

Thunder Project

Nursing organizations could further encourage research by developing and supporting innovative research approaches like that undertaken by AACN's (American Association of Critical-Care Nurses, 1990) Thunder project. This was a multisite research study wherein the research protocol, including education, marketing and data collection materials, was developed, in effect, as a prepackaged, universally transportable research study. Multiple national clinical sites enrolled in this study. This large, nationwide randomized study involved critical care nurses collecting data at their individual hospitals. Its purpose was to develop a research-based standard of practice regarding flush solutions' effect on the patency of arterial pressure lines. It was also designed to generate enthusiasm, i.e., create a *thunder*, for nursing research in clinical settings. Such projects truly encourage research and practice linkages and provide a unique opportunity for individual clinicians to be involved in research.

Research Broker

Joanne Stevenson (1977) noted that the scientific-industrial complex employs brokers whose function is to link the "industrially produced products and marketing activities of the business community [to] form the bridge between research outcomes and changes in practice" (p. 3). Marketing and sales staff bring the product generated from research to the attention of practitioners for their utilization and purchase. If nursing could explore this approach and foster its development by health-related companies, this could assist in mainstreaming our research efforts and decrease the gap between research and health care practitioners. In addition, this could also be a valuable vehicle to increase commercial funding of nursing research.

Best Question Competition

To encourage practitioners to actively think about research questions as they engage in their every day practice, it would be beneficial to have a nursing organization, e.g., Tri-Council[1] or ANA Council for Nursing Researchers, or a nursing publication company sponsor an annual essay competition focused on the best practice question for research. This could encourage inquiry in practice as well as serve as a mechanism to introduce stellar practitioners to a beginning research career. It could be stipulated that each entrant would need the endorsement of a collegiate-level nursing institution; thereby further encouraging an active interface between academe and clinical settings.

Conclusion

The future of nursing research is inextricably dependent on the significant involvement of baccalaureate nurses. Baccalaureate faculty can ensure that their students are fully familiarized with the many options the bachelor's prepared nurse can exercise for their appropriate involvement in nursing research. Additionally, since the advancement of nursing science depends on a strong base of baccalaureate practitioners who value research, nurse scientists have a responsibility and inherent self interest in encouraging and facilitating clinical nurse's vibrant involvement.

---

[1]Includes representatives of the American Nurses Association, American Association of Colleges of Nursing, National League for Nursing, and American Organization of Nurse Executives.

Nursing Research—

1. It is a state of mind—with a spirit of inquiry.
2. It is a pair of eyes—which observe objective data to improve practice.
3. It is a hand—with a gentle touch.
4. It is a brain—open to new insights and interconnections.
5. It is a soul—that cares.
6. It is a woman [, man or team]—that is focused on *The Dream* of better patient care.

REFERENCES

AACN American Association of Critical Care Nurses (1990). *AACN Thunder Project* [Brochure]. Laguna Niguel, CA: Author.

ANA Cabinet of Nursing Research. (1989). *Education for participation in nursing research* [Brochure]. Kansas City, MO: Author.

Anderson, E. T. (1992). Student awareness of research findings. *Nurse Educator, 17*(4), 12–14.

Beal, J. A. (1989). The use of modeling in teaching nursing research on the graduate level. *Western Journal of Nursing Research, 11*, 247–250.

Beck, C. T. (1986). Small group games for teaching nursing research. *Western Journal of Nursing Research, 8*, 233–238.

Beck, C. T. (1993). Integrating research into an R.N. to B.S.N. clinical course. *Western Journal of Nursing Research, 15*, 118–121.

Benner, P. (1984). *From novice to expert.* Menlo Park, CA: Addison-Wesley Publishing Co.

Benner, P., Tanner, C., & Chesla, C. (1992). From beginner to expert: Gaining a differentiated clinical world in critical care nursing. *Advances in Nursing Science, 14*(3), 13–28.

Beyea, S., Farley, J. K., & Williams-Burgess, C. (1996). Teaching baccalaureate nursing students to use research. *Western Journal of Nursing Research, 18*, 213–218.

Brett, J. L. L. (1987). Use of nursing practice research findings. *Nursing Research, 36*, 344–349.

Brett, J. L. L. (1989). Organizational integrative mechanisms and adoption of innovation by nurses. *Nursing Research, 38*, 105–110.

Career development is our future. (1996, October). *U.S. Medicine, 32*(19&20), 7.

Chopoorian, T. (1988). The two worlds of nursing. *Nursing & Health Care*, 9, 450–451.

Conduct and Utilization of Research in Nursing (CURN) Project. (1982). *Using research to improve nursing practice*. (11 vols.) New York: Grune & Stratton, Inc.

Coyle, L. A., & Sokop, A. G. (1990). Innovation adoption behavior among nurses. *Nursing Research, 39*, 176–180.

Dean, P. G. (1986). Participant observation. *Western Journal of Nursing Research, 11*, 378–382.

Dvorak, E. M., Brophy, E. B., Binder, D. M., & Carlson, E. (1993). A survey of BSN curricula: Research content. *Journal of Nursing Education, 32*, 265–269.

Feldman, H. R. (1988). The critique. *Western Journal of Nursing Research, 10*, 515–518.

Ferris, N. I. (1990, Spring). Basic research: Beginning with the abstracr [sic]. *The GNP Newsletter, 27*, 5.

Fleming, J. (1980, January–February). Teaching nursing research content. *Nurse Educator*, 24–26.

Funk, S. G., Champagne, M. T., Wiese, R. A., & Tornquist, E. M. (1991). Barriers to using research in practice: The clinician's perspective. *Applied Nursing Research, 4*, 90–95.

Gulf Oil Company. (1940, June 21). What is Research? *United States News & World Report, 8*(23), 27.

Hawking, S. (1988). *A brief history of time*. New York: Bantam Books.

Horsley, J., Crane, J., Crabtree, M. K., & Wood, D. J. (1983). *Using research to improve nursing practice: A guide*. New York: Grune & Stratton.

Jennings, B. M., & Rogers, S. (1988). Merging nursing research and practice: a case of multiple identities. *Journal of Advanced Nursing, 13*, 752–758.

Ketefian, S. (1975). Application of selected nursing research findings into nursing practice: A pilot study. *Nursing Research, 24*, 89–92.

Kirchhoff, K. (1982). A diffusion survey of coronary precautions. *Nursing Research, 31*, 196–201.

Kirchhoff, K. (1983). Using research in practice: Should staff nurses be expected to use research? *Western Journal of Nursing Research, 5*, 245–247.

Larson, E. (1989). Using the CURN project to teach research utilization in a baccalaureate program. *Western Journal of Nursing Research, 11*, 593–599.

Ludeman, R. (1979). Placement of research content in the undergraduate curriculum. *Western Journal of Nursing Research, 1*, 260–262.

Miller, J. R., & Messenger, S. R. (1978). Obstacles to applying nursing research findings. *American Journal of Nursing, 78*, 632–634.

Moses, E. B. (1997—personal communication). *1996—The registered nurse population: Findings from the national sample survey of registered nurses, March 1996*. (U.S. Government Printing Office). Rockville, MD: U.S. Department of Health & Human Services. Prepublication release.

Murdaugh, C., Kramer, M., & Schmalenberg, C. E. (1981, January–February). The teaching of nursing research: A survey report. *Nurse Educator*, 28–35.

Overfield, T., & Duffy, M. E. (1984). Research on teaching research in the baccalaureate nursing curriculum. *Journal of Advanced Nursing, 9*, 189–196.

Roberts, J., & Crook, J. (1987). Nursing research at the baccalaureate level: A unique teaching/learning model. *Nursing Papers/Perspectives in Nursing, 19*, 43–50.

Rogers, E. (1983). *Diffusion of innovations.* (3rd ed.). New York: The Free Press.

Sakalys, J. A. (1985). Developing a research attitude through questioning. *Western Journal of Nursing Research, 7*, 254–260.

Severo, R. (1980, September 3). A geographer of gene world: Dr. Francis Hugh Ruddle. *The New York Times*, A17.

Smith, B. E. (1992). Linking theory and practice in teaching basic nursing skills. *Journal of Nursing Education, 31*, 16–23.

Stetler, C. B. (1994). Refinement of the Stetler/Marram model for application of research findings to practice. *Nursing Outlook, 42*, 15–25.

Stevenson, J. S. (1977). Nursing research and the industrial community. *Image, 9*, 3.

Stone, K. S. (1986, Autumn Qtr.) Collaborative research: The future. *CNR Voice, 36*, 1.

Sweeney, S. S. (1984). Poster sessions for undergraduate students: A useful tool for learning and communicating nursing research. *Western Journal of Nursing Research, 6*, 135–138.

Thiele, J. (1984). Placement of research: Does it make a difference? *Western Journal of Nursing Research, 6*, 356–358.

Titler, M. G., Kleiber, C., Steelman, V., Goode, C., Rakel, B., Barry-Walker, J., Small, S., & Buckwalter, K. (1994). Infusing research into practice to promote quality care. *Nursing Research, 43*, 307–312.

Urinary Incontinence Guideline Panel (1992). *Urinary incontinence in adults: Clinical practice guidelines.* (AHCPR Pub. No. 92-0038). Rockville, MD: Agency for Health Care Policy and Research, Public Health Service, U.S. Department of Health and Human Services.

Welches, L. J. (1983). The practicing nurse as nurse researcher. *JBCR, 4*, 17–18, 23.

Werley, H. H., & Newcomb, B. J. (1983). The research mentor: A missing element in nursing? In N. Chaska (Ed.), *The nursing profession, a time to speak,* (pp. 202–215). New York: McGraw-Hill Book Co.

Wheeler, K., Fasano, N., & Burr, L. (1995). Strategies for teaching research: A survey of baccalaureate programs. *Journal of Professional Nursing, 11*, 233–238.

Part VII

Enhancing Opportunities Through
Collaborative Initiatives

Nurses *continue to provide* health care services to people oftentimes without an equal place or a well regarded place at the table where decisions are made about health care. Armed with knowledge about the public's need for health care services and what nurses can provide, strategies are emerging that position nurses for influencing the health care agenda in newly emerging partnerships.

Dr. Underwood reminds us that as nursing returns to its roots in the community, challenges and opportunities present themselves. Foremost among them is the shift in emphasis from practicing *in* the community to practicing *with* the community. Coalition building is an integral part of that shift and with it, collaborative leadership emerges. Some examples of successful coalition building are cited which should prove useful in the continued education of nurses for 21st century practice.

A case study from Europe becomes a reminder of the turmoil in health care which is readily recognized by nurses across the world. The outmoded attitudes about nursing and its role in health care are changing, albeit slowly. We are heartened to note the beginning efforts and successes experienced by a committed group of cancer nurses in key leadership positions in Europe as new structures emerge and alliances form. In this new era of cooperation and collaboration it is useful to examine this prototype that gives credence to the potential for greater success when different professional groups work together rather than in isolation.

Mr. Pritchard and Ms. Redmond remind us of the potential influence of nurses as major players in the shaping of health care policy and delivery systems.

14

Building Community Coalitions—A Critical Aspect of Advanced Nursing Practice

Patricia W. Underwood

N*urses of the future* are called upon to contribute to "the health of the community through humane and holistic caring" ("Arista II Envisions Nursing's Future," 1996). Leaders gathered at a conference to plan nursing's future roles in health care echoed the American Nurses Association in affirming the centrality of nursing to the health care delivery system. Melanie Dreher, President of Sigma Theta Tau International, stated that nurses are the first line of care in promoting healthy communities and suggested that nurses will become partners with individuals, communities and colleagues as they fulfill roles in direct care, health promotion, creation of new delivery systems, and social policy development. Nurses' roles in developing partnerships to promote healthy communities is the focus of this chapter.

It is important that nurses in the 21st century accept the challenge to become visible partners in improving health from a community perspec-

Note: The author wishes to acknowledge the two nurses whose projects were cited as examples in this chapter. They are Joni Erlewein, WHNP, RN of District Five Health Department, Michigan and Judith Willink, WHNP, RN who is employed by the Kent County Health Department and Blodgett Hospital in Grand Rapids, Michigan.

tive. Accepting this challenge will reverse the emphasis on practice in acute care settings and bring nursing back to its roots—practice within homes and communities.

The movement of nursing back into the community was highlighted by Nursing's Agenda for Health Care Reform (ANA, 1991). This plan, developed by the American Nurses Association and the National League for Nursing, is supported by more than 70 nursing organizations and calls for a shift in health care to a greater emphasis on the promotion of health and the prevention of illness. The importance of providing health care in the communities where people live is underscored. The vision of a shift of nursing from acute care to community settings was augmented by the reality of the downsizing of many hospitals. In addition, nurses increasingly recognize that community-based practice can afford them exciting opportunities for greater independence and creative entrepreneurial ventures.

Although nursing practice in the 21st century is coming back to its roots in the community, there are important differences and associated challenges and opportunities. A significant difference is that nurses today are challenged to practice not just *in* the community setting but *with* communities. Practicing nursing with the community requires a high degree of collaborative leadership and coalition building and an acknowledgment that the community must play a central role in defining its problems and in proposing solutions appropriate for and acceptable to them. In other words, practicing with the community involves the process of empowerment. Too often health care professionals assess the client's needs and intervene to meet those needs without fully involving the client in the process. When this happens, the client is not the strong partner in health care that is espoused by theorists such as Imogene King (1981) or proposed in models of care such as the Personalized Intervention System (Andersen & Smereck, 1989). Both theoretical perspectives stress the critical, decision-making role of the client in partnership with the nurse.

The effective practice of nursing in the 21st century requires that similar partnerships be extended to the community as requisite to improving the health of community members. This chapter will discuss the implications of the perspective of practicing with the community and the knowledge and skills required for building coalitions as a strategy to effectively address health care problems. Two examples of community coalition building to address specific health needs in underserved populations are provided.

PRACTICING WITH THE COMMUNITY

Practicing with the community as opposed to practicing in communities has two essential components. The first is that the community must have the central role in identifying those issues or problems which it sees as priorities and in selecting the means to address them. A national study that included focus groups in five cities (Atlanta; Boston; Charleston, West Virginia; El Paso; and Muskegon, Michigan) and a random survey of 1000 registered voters, revealed what the public wants in health care (Richards, 1996). Not surprisingly, 54 percent said that it was very important that communities have a say in how health care is delivered. Another 26 percent agreed that this was at least "somewhat important." Too frequently communities have minimal say in identifying health issues and in setting the direction for their solution. The result is that community helping systems are often insensitive to issues of cultural diversity and plagued with inefficiencies including duplication of effort, fragmentation, unproductive competition and lack of planning (Wolff, 1995). The community's ability to *have a say* is no guarantee that problems will be solved, but it increases the likelihood that solutions will be both relevant and coordinated.

The second key ingredient in practicing with the community is an emphasis on assets as opposed to deficits. This means not viewing the community simply as a collection of problems to be solved, and the more the better, but rather seeing the community first as an entity with assets and capacity for finding solutions to its problems. McKnight (1989) emphasizes that outside resources are more likely to make a difference when the capacity of the community is recognized and respected. This perspective of community is consistent with Schlotfeldt's (1978) view of nursing which includes an emphasis on enhancing health assets and health potentials of humans. Schlotfeldt suggests that nurses focus on people's strengths rather than on their problems and pathology in the same way that McKnight underscores the need to recognize community capacity.

The health of communities has received increasing national attention. Foundations, including W. K. Kellogg, Robert Wood Johnson, and Henry J. Kaiser, have committed significant funds to promote healthy communities, to understand health at the community level, and to work to decrease behaviors associated with increased health risk. The discussion of the role of nurses in practice with communities must begin with an understanding of what is meant by community. Taub (1989) defines communities as complex webs of people shaped by relationships, interdependence, mutual interests, and patterns of interaction. Behringer and Richards (1996) further state that the "concept of community encompasses people in a particular place and time, but it also speaks to their history and language and to the shared meaning that develops where history and language intersect." These definitions are useful for nurses because they do not focus on traditional geographic or legal boundaries. It means that nurses can focus their attention more narrowly than an incorporated body. Community, for the purposes of this discussion, will refer to an identified group of people in a given place at a given time who are connected through mutual interests and patterns of interaction. Thus people in a senior citizens' center may be considered a community along with more traditionally defined groups.

Practicing with the community means that nurses will work collaboratively with a group of people in a way that focuses on the assets they bring to solving the problems they identify. It will be important for all professional nurses to critically consider what it means to work collaboratively with groups of people. Advanced practice nurses in the 21st century will need to skillfully use collaborative leadership to build effective coalitions with the community. This focus will afford them the best opportunity to make a difference in people's health and will give them a stronger presence in shaping the systems through which health care is delivered. Communities will be empowered and their capacity for affecting their health will be enhanced.

EMPOWERMENT AND COLLABORATIVE LEADERSHIP

For nurses to practice with the community, they must understand the concepts of empowerment and collaborative leadership. Minkler (1989) defines empowerment as "The process by which individuals and communities gain mastery over their lives." This simple statement belies the complexity of the process to which he refers. Two alternative definitions are slightly more specific. In the first definition, Wallerstein (1992) suggests that empowerment "is a social action process that promotes participation of people, organizations and communities toward the goals of increased individual and community control, political efficacy, improved quality of community life and social justice." In this definition, participation of people, organizations and communities is emphasized, but the nature of the participation is not specified. The goals of this social action are delineated, however. Although political efficacy and social justice are somewhat global goals, they serve as examples of aspects of community life which people may attempt to control.

In the final definition, empowerment is seen as "an intentional, ongoing process centered in the local community, involving mutual respect, critical reflection, caring and group participation through which people lacking an equal share of valued resources gain greater access to and control over those resources" (Cornell Empowerment Group, 1989). As nurses seek to involve themselves with communities, it is helpful to be able to focus more narrowly. The one limitation of this definition is that it appears to focus on deficits, that is, lack of resources. The behaviors of critical reflection, caring and group participation, however, could be viewed as assets. An advantage of the definition is that it emphasizes that the process does not just happen, but is intentional—in other words, planned.

Nurses who agree that empowerment is an intentional/planned process can begin to participate in the process through the exercise of collaborative leadership. Again, this calls for another shift away from the traditional perspective. Traditionally, nurses are accustomed to exercising leadership based on their expertise in the area of health care. Collaborative leadership does not depend on content expertise but does require that the leader focus on the process by which a group comes together as peers to solve a problem. Collaborative leaders may possess particular expertise, but they need to be careful not to impose their ideas on the group. Instead, the collaborative leader assumes a large share of the responsibility for promoting and safeguarding the collective process. Jacobsen (cited in Trasolini, 1996) states that "collaborative leadership requires developing a new notion of power and learning that the more power and control we share, the more we have to use." Many skills are needed for effective collaborative leadership and few individuals possess all of them. For this reason, there is an advantage in shared leadership. When more than one person shares the responsibility for collaborative leadership, the likelihood of the availability of necessary leadership skills is increased.

Historically, much has been written on leadership but only recently has collaborative leadership received attention. Senge (1990) suggests that what distinguishes outstanding leaders is:

"the clarity and persuasiveness of their ideas, the depth of their commitment, and their openness to continually learn more. They do not have

the answer. But they do instill confidence in those around them that, together, 'we can learn whatever we need to learn in order to achieve the results we truly desire.'"

The W. K. Kellogg Foundation, in collaboration with the Health Care Forum, has developed excellent materials to assist individuals in working with communities to promote the development of effective coalitions to increase their health capacity. In the context of a discussion of the requirements of successful collaborative leaders, they suggest that five qualities are essential: flexibility, ability to see the big picture, trustworthiness, patience, and abundant energy and hope (W. K. Kellogg Foundation & Health Care Forum, 1996). Nurses who want to be successful collaborative leaders need to begin through self-reflection to assess their strengths in these areas. They can be encouraged in the fact that the skills needed for collaborative leadership can be cultivated and strengthened. In their book, *The Leadership Challenge*, Kouzes and Posner (1995) provide a thorough discussion of qualities of effective leadership and steps to take to enhance leadership skills.

Chrislip and Larson (1994) identified four principles that are necessary for successful collaborative leadership. They suggest that collaborative leaders inspire commitment and action. While these leaders are action oriented, they do not go into the group to solve the problems identified, but rather to facilitate a process whereby people can solve their own problems. A second principle is associated with the first. The leader must become a peer problem solver. Power is de-emphasized and the leader works to facilitate vision and engender energy and involvement in the solution-seeking process. Broad-based involvement is another principle. Stakeholders are identified and involved people who have differing perspectives are actively sought. The emphasis is on inclusiveness in bringing people together to address an issue of common concern. The last principle focuses on sustaining hope and participation. Collaborative leaders convince people that their opinions are valued, celebrate even small steps toward goals and "help groups do hard work when it would be easier to quit." Although collaborative leadership may require some adjustment, it is an important ingredient in developing effective coalitions as part of practicing with community.

Building Community Coalitions

Definition.   Coalitions have been variously defined in ways that speak to their purpose as well as their composition and duration. Wilson (1973) focuses on the purpose and membership when he suggests that coalitions can be viewed simply as a mechanism for coordinating actions of member organizations. Coalitions offer great potential for coordinating activities, however, their purpose frequently goes well beyond the simple role of coordinator. In addition, restricting the composition of coalitions to organizations does not take into account the hallmark of practicing with community—the inclusion of community members who may represent a point of view rather than an organization. Community coalitions may be defined as "alliances among different sectors, organizations or constituencies for a common purpose" (Francisco, Paine & Fawcett, 1993). This definition clearly expands the membership to include individuals, groups and organizations so long as they have a common purpose.

Brown (1984) suggests that the common purpose of coalitions is to effect a specific change the members are unable to bring about independently. The common purpose whether it is to coordinate, share resources, effect change or achieve a particular political or policy outcome is a major characteristic of a coalition. Shared purpose is not a defining characteristic, however, because other types of groups may have a common purpose.

Likewise, the durability of a coalition is not a defining characteristic. Most early definitions of coalitions considered them temporary in nature (Levine & White, 1961; Aiken & Hage, 1968). Today, coalitions may be considered more durable (Butterfoss, Goodman & Wandersman, 1993), although for the most part they remain time limited alliances (Dluhy, 1990).

It has been suggested that the defining characteristic of coalitions is not in the membership (individuals, groups, organizations) nor in the common purpose but in the ability of members to advocate on behalf of the coalition itself (Hord, 1986; Feigherty & Rogers, 1990). If there is cohesion of the group around single or multiple purposes, the coalition will derive sufficient power to advocate for those purposes in the external world. Advocacy is critical in moving beyond a sharing of resources within the group to the acquisition of resources outside of the group. It is also essential to goal achievement. Advocacy does not need to be on behalf of the coalition. The coalition may act as advocate on behalf of the community. Perhaps the most useful view of community coalitions is one that includes all three aspects: individuals, groups, and organizations coming together to acquire resources (power and material) needed to effect a solution to a common problem within the community.

Advantages of coalitions. Although the process of coalition building can be slow, the outcomes are frequently well worth the effort. Effective

coalitions have the potential for creating a power base sufficient to challenge the status quo and the more traditional sources of power. What
cannot be achieved by an individual or a single group can become a
reality for the coalition. Nurses recognize that coalition building is an
important strategy to achieve political goals at the state and national
level (Campbell-Heider & Hanna, 1993). Coalition building can be
equally effective in achieving change within the local community and
in strengthening the effectiveness of the health care system. In fact,
coalitions can offer a critical avenue for taking programs that arise outside
the community (e.g., Project ASSIST to decrease smoking) and tailoring
them to local conditions (McLeroy, Kegler & Steckler, 1994). Dluhy
(1990) believes that "coalitions can provide one of the most effective
tools available for professionals to use in achieving their objectives"
(p. 17) even in the face of significant opposition from traditional sources
of power. Specifically, coalitions have the potential to foster a health care
system that is accessible, holistic, planned, coordinated, collaborative,
preventive, comprehensive and culturally relevant (Kaye & Wolff, 1995).

Considerations in coalition building.   If nurses are to become vital partners
in building coalitions, they must understand the nature of coalitions and
critical determinants of their success. The literature repeatedly points to
the fact that little systematic research exists to document the efficacy of
community coalitions. However, studies have been conducted to evaluate
specific coalitions (Gottlieb, Brink & Gingiss, 1993; Nezlek & Galano,
1993; Rogers, Howard-Pitney, Feigherty, Altman, Endres & Roeseler,
1993). Review of these studies has led to the suggestion that coalitions go
through four stages of development including formation, implementation,
maintenance, and goal attainment and that different factors may influence
success at each stage (Butterfoss, Goodman & Wandersman, 1993). The
evaluation of funded projects has provided less formal wisdom regarding
the formation and maintenance of coalitions. In this regard, Wolff (1995)
contends that coalitions often work best as catalysts.

Factors leading to coalition success.   Both research and evaluation of funded
projects have contributed to an understanding of factors that can enhance
the success of coalitions. An essential ingredient in this success is maintenance of a strong community base, even if the coalition has sizable
organizational representation. Without strong emphasis, the coalition
will have difficulty in defining the issues and potential solutions from
the community perspective. A planning group or steering committee is

often helpful in the formation of community coalitions that are issue focused. This group can identify all the stakeholders in relation to the issue. *Inclusivity of stakeholder participation* is one principle of coalition success. Powerful community stakeholders are often most visible and frequently recruited. Coalitions composed of the influential can exert significant power, but this power is often directed at symptoms rather than root issues (Wolff & Foster, 1995). It is equally important, therefore, to recruit the least powerful stakeholders. It may take effort to bring these individuals into the coalition and to support their full participation when confronted with people who represent more traditional community power bases. The rewards will be increased ability to get at the roots of the issue and community relevancy of potential goals and strategies. Nurses may be ideally prepared both to recruit the "less powerful" and to facilitate their full participation within the coalition. Coalition members are often selected for their commitment to the issue, enthusiasm, constructive and creative problem-solving, and a capacity for networking. However, the potential for positive political outcome gained by involving stakeholders who may be more resistive to change should be considered.

The inclusivity of coalition membership is closely aligned with the issue of its mission and goals. While inclusivity is necessary to coalition success, it may prolong the process of developing group cohesion and identifying a shared mission. Wolff and Foster (1995) underscore both the difficulty and importance of *developing a shared mission:*

Coalition members must clearly define their shared mission/goals and assure that the identified goals incorporate the self-interests of the various constituencies, plus something larger than those self-interests. Coalition building requires both a realistic understanding that addressing the self-interests of participants is crucial, and a willingness to set aside personal agendas for a common good. Walking the tight rope between these agendas is critical to coalition success (p. 31).

As previously mentioned in the discussion of the concept of empowerment, emphasis on community capacity and strengths is as important as the consideration of deficits and problems. In the process of identifying a shared mission and goals, both perspectives need careful consideration.

Factors related to the *organization* of community coalitions are critical to their success. McLeroy, Kegler and Steckler (1994) found that the literature consistently mentioned the importance of four areas: rules, roles and procedures, leadership characteristics, processes by which decisions are made, and member-staff relationships. Communication processes are inherent in all four areas. Goodman and Steckler (1989) suggest that the more operations become routine, the more likely the coalition will be sustained. The importance of organizational formality is seconded by Gottlieb, Brink and Gingiss (1993). In a survey of 50 state and local coalitions that grew out of the project Smoke Free Class of 2000, they found that members perceived the coalition to be more effective when the coalition was more formally structured. The establishment of rules by which the coalition will operate needs to include not only decision-making, but how conflicts will be resolved. It is particularly important that the latter be given early consideration rather than waiting until the conflicts occur.

The establishment of the Coalition of Michigan Organizations of Nurses (COMON) is a good example of early definition of processes for decision-making and conflict resolution. While COMON is not a community coalition, the process of organization is relevant. The coalition grew out of informal meetings of various nursing organizations in Michigan at a time when legislators were complaining that there were so many organizations, often with varied points of view, that they did not know who spoke for nursing. The formalization of the coalition had as its mission the achievement of a common political agenda for nurses in Michigan. At the onset, COMON organizations agreed that discussion within the group would be free flowing and that political issues would be selected by consensus. No issue would appear on the political agenda if it was potentially detrimental to a particular member. Member organizations further agreed that once an issue had been selected by the group, they were free to criticize within the group potential strategies for goal achievement. What was critical to the coalition's maintenance and success was the agreement to keep silent in public whenever there was a conflict over strategy. It would have been quite difficult to achieve this level of commitment to a process of conflict resolution if it had waited until the conflict occurred.

Collaborative leadership and effective on-going communication are essential to the organization of coalitions. In addition to the aspects of collaborative leadership discussed previously, Brown (1984) suggests that effective coalition leaders are competent negotiators and problem-solvers who are able to garner resources for the coalition. Effective leaders are good communicators and give attention to both the processes and frequency of communication among coalition members as well as the communication that flows outside the group. Communication with the wider community is important, but the timing and framing of communication are critical. Premature disclosure of the coalition's goals may, in some instances, afford opposing groups the opportunity to put the issue in front of the public before the coalition is ready to engage in a full discussion of their plans.

Staff or consultants employed by the coalition need to exhibit many of the same characteristics as the volunteer leadership. It is important for them to have good group and organizational process skills and to be committed to the philosophy of community involvement. Wolff and Foster (1995) caution volunteers against abdicating to staff the responsibility for essential work of the coalition. They contend that to do so diminishes the collaborative, community building functions of the coalition.

In addition to a shared mission, inclusive membership and competent organization, Wolff and Foster (1995) contend that systematic planning, selection of doable actions, optimism, and persistence are crucial to the success of community coalitions. While coalitions usually develop initial plans for achieving their mission and goals, they may neglect to engage in a *systematic evaluation* of progress toward goals and an evaluation of the internal effectiveness of the coalition. Knowledge gained from this type of evaluation is necessary for revision of strategies and modification of processes to enhance the likelihood of goal attainment. Nurses would make excellent coalition members and leaders, because these processes of evaluation and planning are consistently used in clinical practice.

Selecting coalition actions that can be achieved is essential to the viability of the coalition. It is through effective first steps that the coalition can demonstrate its effectiveness in achieving concrete results. Sometimes coalitions choose goals that are very broad and may take significant time to achieve. While this type of planning is not wrong, it must be coupled with short term outcomes so that the coalition can celebrate early victories. Early successes create a climate of optimism and visibility that can serve to sustain member commitment. These early outcomes may be as simple as meeting with important legislators or creating a newsletter. Pressure for immediate results of a more substantive nature may be detrimental to ongoing planning and long-term results. Selection of doable activities is closely tied to creation of an expectation that the coalition can achieve its goals. It is important to sustain this optimism through celebrating small victories. Much energy is needed for a coalition to achieve its goals and celebrations are an important means of renewal.

A final factor in the success of community coalitions is the ability of members to be *persistent in pursuit of their goals*. This is especially crucial when the issues are broad and require more substantive societal or delivery system change. Our society is enamored with the *quick fix* for serious problems. Theories of planned change, however, consistently underscore the need to move slowly and plan carefully, if enduring change is to be achieved.

Although the body of research focused on the factors that predict the success of community coalitions is limited, sufficient wisdom has been gained from funded projects to provide guidance for the establishment of future coalitions. This knowledge can be effectively applied by nurses as they seek to practice with the community.

Examples of Community Coalition Building

As professional nurses increasingly locate their practice within communities, it behooves them to focus attention on the empowerment of clients both at the individual and aggregate levels. Advanced practice nurses will be most effective in creating change within the community and health care delivery system, if they couple a philosophy of empowerment with a commitment to collaborative leadership and a knowledge of coalition building. In a master's in nursing course focused on professional effectiveness, advanced practice students acquire leadership skills and gain knowledge about coalition building, planned change, conflict and negotiation, and effective group communication. They are expected to apply this knowledge through a community coalition project. Each student is required to identify a health need within their local community and form a coalition to address this need or provide appropriate leadership within an established coalition. Specific outcomes related to coalition tasks are not expected. What is expected is that the students critically examine the processes governing the work of the coalition and their application of leadership skills in furthering this work. Two examples of projects with community coalitions are discussed.

Initiating a coalition to increase health care access for minority women. A graduate student employed by a rural health department identified as a concern the limited numbers of Hispanic women who were taking advantage of breast and cervical cancer screening programs (BCCSP). Very low numbers of women were screened despite the existence of a large population of seasonal and resident Hispanic women and despite the fact that the program was funded by the Centers for Disease Control (CDC).

It was apparent to this nurse that the screening program had been planned in the typical fashion—by professionals without the involvement of community members. Acting from a philosophy of empowerment, she visited some of the migrant camps and solicited the perspectives of the women aged 40 to 65, since breast and cervical cancer is highest in this group. As the women discussed the situation, informational, cultural, and logistical problems emerged. First, most of the women interviewed did not recognize the importance of preventive health screening and, therefore, did not see attendance at the clinics as an issue. For them, the issue the nurse identified was not an apparent problem. Secondly, cultural perspectives on privacy meant that certain topics were not freely discussed among the women and that many of the women were ashamed to touch their breasts. Finally, the logistics of getting to the clinic and the times available for mammograms were identified as significant barriers to BCCSP participation.

Since no group within the community was specifically addressing the issue of breast cancer screening for the Hispanic population, the nurse decided to form a coalition to do so. Stakeholders were identified and invited to a preliminary meeting to discuss the issue. Professionals included two nurses from the health department's breast cancer screening program, two radiology technicians from the local hospital that performed the mammograms, two physicians, and the director of the local migrant health clinic. Physicians were important for the power they could bring and because they were frequently in a position to refer patients for screening. The director of the migrant health clinic was an important link to the Hispanic community and critical to the development of health promotional materials that were culturally sensitive. Also critical to the inclusivity of coalition membership were lay representatives of the Hispanic community. Two bilingual women who were past participants in the cancer screening program were asked to join.

The coalition focused on a single issue—that of increasing the participation of Hispanic women in breast cancer screening. Differences in education, culture, and economic level among coalition members, meant that attention had to be paid to rules for the organization that would foster the participation of all members and ensure effective communication. The opinions of the Hispanic women were solicited and respected. Their delineation of the problem and identification of possible solutions were major determinants in the effectiveness of the coalition. Coalition members believed that increasing access to and comfort with screening would increase the attendance at the clinics.

The graduate nursing student was effective in implementing collaborative leadership behaviors and modeled a willingness to critically examine the ways screening clinics had been offered in the past, as a basis for making them more effective. This behavior encouraged other members to examine the ways their agencies were providing services. Persistent use of *we* messages, considering all suggestions, and making decisions as a group facilitated the ability of all coalition members to compromise and to share resources across the coalition (Erlewein, 1995). Planning included setting timelines and identifying small steps toward goals. Small wins were celebrated at each meeting. Another important strategy used by the coalition was to delegate projects to people in the community. This increased the sense of community ownership.

In a remarkably short span of time, the coalition was able to achieve significant outcomes. The Migrant Health Clinic scheduled breast screening clinics on specific dates, the hospital Radiology Department agreed to stay open in the evening on those dates to provide mammograms. Both agencies agreed to adopt a common form for sharing patient information, and physicians found a place to refer women who could not afford mammograms. In addition, pamphlets and other educational materials were developed in Spanish as well as English, Spanish language training materials were obtained; the clinics were advertised in English and Spanish, and the local women were able to make an investment in their culture and community by becoming peer trainers for breast self-examination.

It might be argued that the health department nurse could have achieved a coordination of clinic and mammogram offerings without the effort of building a community coalition. Unilateral action could not have created the degree of community commitment that occurred. Not only was one aspect of the health care delivery system modified to make it more responsive to a particular segment of the community, but important relationships were established and the ability of grassroots members to effect changes was demonstrated.

Joining a coalition.   In the second example, the advanced practice nurse joined a coalition that had been established to decrease high infant mortality rates in the community. The community in question was located within an urban area and exhibited not only infant mortality rates double those of the rest of the county but high poverty levels, high substance abuse, a reliance on public transportation, and a large Native American population. The coalition was formed from people within the area representing businesses, churches, health care providers practicing within the community, neighborhood councils, and other citizens with a concern and passion for the welfare of their community. No one came from the outside to suggest the changes that ought to occur within the community. The diverse grassroots beginning is credited with the continuing interest and energy people have shown for the project.

The coalition defined as its mission that of increasing citizens' access to services that would promote health. Specifically, they wanted to establish a health clinic within the area that would be more culturally, geographically and economically accessible to community residents. Initially, a significant amount of time was spent attempting to gain funding from outside the community. When funding from a major source was denied, the coalition decided to rethink its strategies. This was an important step. If they had simply attempted to solicit other external resources without exhibiting visible achievements within the community, it is doubtful that their level of commitment, energy, and wider community support could have been sustained.

While not entirely abandoning an attempt to acquire outside funding, the coalition decided to see what resources could be mobilized to open at least a prenatal clinic. A small space in a centrally located building was made available by the health department. Supplies were donated by two hospitals that were located outside the community but had a professed interest in community welfare. Volunteer help was obtained from doctors and nurses and the clinic was able to open one and a half days per week. People in the neighborhood were impressed with the personalized service that the little clinic offered and the number of women seeking prenatal care increased. If this concrete step had not been taken, "it would have been difficult to tolerate the time lags inherent in implementation of programs, especially those which depend on the federal government for funding" (Willink, 1995). The community celebrated with the coalition as it saw the ability of their clinic to address "fundamental aspects of bringing new life into their families with less risk to mother and baby, to provide caring people to treat their pregnant teenage daughters, and to be there in instances of physical abuse to pregnant women" (Willink, 1995).

With the help of outside consultation, the coalition eventually obtained a $350,000 grant to open a more permanent clinic able to offer a comprehensive array of services. Several factors appeared to be keys to the success of this coalition. A shared vision, strong involvement of diverse community members, and visible success in reaching short-term goals of delivering vital services to the community were important. The coalition was able to involve other individuals and entities who possessed needed resources not available within the community. Although leadership within the coalition was shared, often passing from one person or group to another according to the need of the moment, the community residents retained ownership of the project. Planning was ongoing and long range and small victories were celebrated with the community at large. The role of the nurse in this coalition was less central than in the previous example, but none-the-less important. She was able to provide services and share her expertise according to the needs of the coalition. She acted on her strong belief that people can identify their needs and plan to solve their problems and that this involvement must occur before any program can be embraced by those it is meant to serve (Willink, 1995).

STRENGTHENING FUTURE PRACTICE

Programs preparing nurses for entry levels of professional practice increasingly provide opportunities throughout the curriculum for community-based practice. In addition to practice opportunities, futuristic curricula will include community-as-partner content so that graduates will be able to assume new roles caring for neighborhoods as a whole (Christopher, Reinhard, McConnell & Mason, 1993). Nurses prepared at advanced levels of practice will assume critical roles in transforming traditional community health nursing by facilitating agency adoption of community-as-partner models of care delivery. Furthermore, to the degree that advanced practice nurses are able to exercise collaborative leadership and embrace a philosophy of empowerment in practicing with community, they will retain a significant role in shaping the future delivery of health care. The outcomes of such practice are aptly reflected in an ancient Chinese poem which begins:

"Go to the people
Learn from them
Love them
Start with what they know
Build on what they have."

The poem concludes with what could be the outcome of the type of leadership that has been espoused in this chapter:

"When their task is accomplished
Their work is done
The people remark,
'We have done it ourselves'"
(Levy, 1996).

REFERENCES

Aiken, M., & Hage, J. (1968). Organizational independence and intra-organizational structure. *American Sociological Review, 63*, 912–930.

American Nurses Association. (1991). *Nursing's Agenda for Health Care Reform.* Washington, DC: Author.

Andersen, M. D., & Smereck, G. (1989). Personalized Nursing LIGHT Model. *Nursing Science Quarterly, 2*, 120–130.

Arista II envisions nursing's preferred future (1996, 3rd quarter). *Reflections,* 26–27.

Behringer, B., & Richards, R. (1996). The nature of communities. In R. Richards (Ed.), *Building partnerships: Educating health professionals for the communities they serve* (pp. 91–104). San Francisco: Jossey-Bass Publishers.

Brown, C. (1984). *The art of coalition building: A guide for community leaders.* New York: The American Jewish Community.

Butterfoss, F., Goodman, R., & Wandersman, A. (1993). Community coalitions for prevention and health promotion. *Health Education Research: Theory & Practice, 8*, 315–330.

Campbell-Heider, N., & Hanna, N. (1993). Nursing's new political era. *Holistic Nursing Practice, 8*, 78–87.

Chrislip, D., & Larson, C. (1994). *Collaborative Leadership: How citizens and civic leaders can make a difference.* San Francisco: Jossey-Bass Publishers.

Christopher, M., Reinhard, S., McConnell, K., & Mason, D. (1993). The community as partner. *Caring Magazine,* 44–49.

Cornell Empowerment Group. (1989). *Networking Bulletin: Empowerment and Family Support, 1*, (1).

Dluhy, M. (1990). *Building coalitions in the human services.* Newbury Park, CA: Sage Publications.

Erlewein, J. (1995). *Community project to increase minority cancer screening participation.* Unpublished manuscript, Grand Valley State University, Grand Rapids, Michigan.

Feigherty, E., & Rogers, T. (1990). *Building and maintaining effective coalitions.* Palo Alto, CA: Health Promotion Resource Center, Stanford University School of Medicine.

Francisco, V., Paine, A., & Fawcett, S. (1993). A methodology for monitoring and evaluating community health coalitions. *Health Education Research: Theory & Practice*, 8, 403–416.

Goodman, R., & Steckler, A. (1989). A model for the institutionalization of health promotion programs. *Family and Community Health*, 11, 63–78.

Gottlieb, N., Brink, S., & Gingiss, P. (1993). Correlations of coalition effectiveness: the Smoke Free Class of 2000 project. *Health Education Research: Theory & Practice*, 8, 375–384.

Hord, S. (1986). A synthesis of research on organizational collaboration. *Educational Leadership*, February, 22–26.

Kaye, G., & Wolff, T. (1995). *From the ground up: A workbook on coalition building and community development.* Amherst, MA: AHEC/Community Partners.

King, I. (1981). *A theory for nursing.* Albany, New York: Delmar Publishers, Inc.

Kouzes, J., & Posner, B. (1995). *The leadership challenge.* San Francisco: Jossey-Bass Publishers.

Levine, S., & White, P. (1961). Exchange as a conceptual framework for the study of interorganizational relationships. *Administrative Science Quarterly*, 5, 583–601.

Levy, B. (1996, December). *The Nation's Health*, p. 2.

McKnight, J. (1989). Do no harm: Policy options that meet human needs. *Social Policy*, 5–15.

McLeroy, K., Kegler, M., & Steckler, A. (1994). Community coalitions for health promotion: Summary and further reflections. *Health Education Research: Theory & Practice*, 9, 1–11.

Minkler, M. (1989). Health education, health promotion and the open society: An historical perspective. *Health Education Quarterly*, 16, 17–30.

Nezlek, J., & Galano, J. (1993). Developing and maintaining state-wide adolescent pregnancy prevention coalitions: A preliminary investigation. *Health Education Research: Theory & Practice*, 8, 433–448.

Richards, R. (Ed.). (1996). *Building partnerships: Educating health professionals for the communities they serve.* San Francisco: Jossey-Bass Publishers.

Rogers, T., Howard-Pitney, B., Feigherty, E., Altman, D., Endres, J., & Roeseler, A. (1993). Characteristics and participant perceptions of tobacco control coalitions in California. *Health Education Research: Theory & Practice*, 8, 345–357.

Schlotfeldt, R. M. (1978). The professional doctorate: Rationale and characteristics. *Nursing Outlook*, 26, 302–311.

Senge, P. (1990). The leaders' new work: Building learning organizations. *Sloan management review*, Fall, 1–16.

Taub, R. (1989, May). *Nuance in meaning and evaluation: Finding community and development.* Paper presented at the Research Conference, The New School, New York.

Trasolini, S. (1996). Leadership: Building capacity to lead a community-based process. In *Sustaining Community-Based Initiatives: Module One, Developing Community Capacity*, pp. 9–28. Battle Creek, MI: W. K. Kellogg Foundation and Health Care Forum.

W. K. Kellogg Foundation and the Health Care Forum. (1996). *Sustaining Community-Based Initiatives: Module One, Developing Community Capacity*. Battle Creek, Michigan.

Wallerstein, N. (1992). Powerless, empowerment and health: Implications for health promotion programs. *American Journal of Health Promotion*, 6, 197–201.

Willink, J. (1995). *Professional effectiveness community project*. Unpublished manuscript, Grand Valley State University, Grand Rapids, Michigan.

Wilson, J. (1973). *Political organizations*. New York: Basic Books.

Wolff, T. (1995). Coalition building: One path to empowered and healthy communities. In G. Kaye, & T. Wolff (Eds.), *From the ground up: A workbook on coalition building and community development*. Amherst, MA: AHEC/Community Partners.

Wolff, T., & Foster, D. (1995). Principles of success in building community coalitions. In G. Kaye, & T. Wolff (Eds.), *From the ground up: A workbook on coalition building and community development*. Amherst, MA: AHEC/Community Partners.

15

Making the Most of Critical Alliances— A Case Study from Europe

A. Phylip Pritchard and Kathy Redmond

As *the new millennium* approaches, health policy and health systems find themselves plunged into a degree of turmoil not experienced in the past fifty years. The reasons for this turmoil are to be found in well known factors common to the developed and developing world—demographic changes, increasing population mobility, the emergence of new and reappearance of old diseases, growing social exclusion, costly new therapeutic techniques and rising public demands and expectations. Unique to the present time, however, is that the pressures the foregoing create are being felt at a time when public and private spending on health is under increasing constraints as governments seek to manage their budgets at a time of international economic recession.

The nursing profession has not been immune to these pressures. Indeed the profession has often found itself at the center of the vortex created by the plethora of health care reforms that virtually every country has initiated in order to try and balance the demands for health care and the funding available to meet these demands—the common objectives of cost control, efficiency and choice that have become the mantra whispered in the corridors of every Ministry of Health throughout the world.

NURSING IN EUROPE

Nurses and midwives are fundamental to health care in Europe. They are the largest group of health professionals on this continent—approximately five million people work in the nursing service of the 50 or so Member States of Europe as defined by the World Health Organization (WHO). The important contribution nurses make to health care is increasingly recognized in the Member States and there is widespread agreement that nursing should be strengthened and expanded in order to provide even better health care for all of Europe's citizens. They promote health, prevent disease and provide care. This important contribution is increasingly recognized in these Member States and there is widespread agreement that nursing should be strengthened and expanded in order to provide even better health care for all Europeans. The cost effectiveness argument that nurses have put forward to justify their value is beginning to be heard, even by the World Bank, which has identified nursing and midwifery personnel as "the most cost effective resource for delivering high quality public health and clinical packages" (The World Bank, 1993).

Nurses were the first group of health professionals in Europe to scrutinize their practice in order to respond to the challenge of Health for All and there is a growing awareness that although nursing "does not grab the headlines like other measures such as the commercialization of medicine or the emergency supply of drugs, [it] could arguably have a greater long term impact on health services" (Salvage, 1993). This awareness is manifest in a number of recent nursing reforms. The starting points and initial conditions for reform differ widely between countries in a continent where even the words *nursing* and *nurse* are used as general terms and applied to all health workers doing nursing related work. It is possible, however, to discern some newly emerging trends. First, there is a deepening commitment to, and proficiency in, evaluating the outcomes of nursing interventions in order to provide a more efficient and effective service. Secondly, there is a growing interest in nursing education, with reform focusing on establishing nurse education within third level institutions, curriculum review with a reorientation to primary health care, new program development, better teaching methods and better training of nurse educators, high quality education materials, continuing education and improving the links between education and service. Thirdly, society's attitudes toward nursing and its role in health care are slowly changing.

The perception of nursing as a low status occupation requiring minimal training and the associated under valuation of humanistic and psychosocial care is beginning to alter although the process is slow and uneven.

Yet these difficulties also offer new opportunities for those with the vision to perceive how the challenges they pose can be overcome with the real possibility of securing substantial future improvements in health. This chapter will describe how one organization, the European Oncology Nursing Society (EONS), represents those nurses involved in cancer care in the geographical region of WHO Europe. By monitoring opportunities closely, EONS has engaged in a number of critical alliances with policy makers, other health care professionals and industries whose products support cancer care, and has become within a period of less than five years, a major player in the politics of cancer care in this region.

Before examining in detail how EONS was able to achieve this remarkable outcome, it will be helpful in the first instance, to describe briefly the organization itself and secondly, in more detail, the wider political, economic, social and professional context in which EONS has had to function. For the most part, the following discussion focuses on those countries that make up the Member States of the European Union (EU)—Austria, Belgium, Denmark, Finland, France, Germany, Greece, Ireland, Italy, Luxembourg, The Netherlands, Portugal, Spain, Sweden and the United Kingdom—since it is in these countries that opportunities to advance the agenda of cancer nursing have been most readily available. There is every indication, however, that with the expected entry of the countries of Central and Eastern Europe into membership of the EU, EONS will achieve similar success for cancer nurses in these countries.

European Oncology Nursing Society

Founded in 1984, EONS is a federation of oncology nursing societies, institutions and agencies involved in cancer nursing. At present EONS has a membership of over 50 organizations which in turn represent approximately 15,000 nurses in 25 European countries. The purpose of the Society is to promote and develop the practice of cancer nursing in all European countries. This purpose is achieved through a number of different activities, many of which will be outlined later in this chapter. The Society has its own secretariat based in Brussels and is in full membership of the Federation of European Cancer Societies (FECS). In addition, EONS has fostered close links with organizations such as the International

Society for Nurses in Cancer Care, International Union Against Cancer, EuroQuan, Standing Committee of Nurses of the EU (PCN) and European School of Oncology (ESO).

EONS is governed by a Board of Directors which meets a number of times per year and the Society meets in General Assembly at least once a year. Each member sends a maximum of two representatives to attend the General Assembly. The working language of the Society is English, although efforts are made to include all European cancer nurses in the work of the Society, regardless of the language they speak. This is one of the greatest challenges facing EONS, indeed any Society which functions in a multi-lingual arena. EONS is responsible for planning the nursing component of the European Cancer Conference (ECCO), a biennial, multidisciplinary conference which regularly attracts over eight thousand participants. In addition, the Society organizes its own biennial Spring Convention. Every effort is made to ensure that all conferences in which the Society is involved has simultaneous translation into at least one other European language.

HEALTH CARE REFORMS

The manner in which health care is delivered in Europe does not differ dramatically from those systems to be found in other parts of the world. Essentially the recent spate of reforms has been directed at four main groups of health care systems:

1. National health services where the health care system is primarily funded through direct taxation (for example Ireland, Italy, Spain and the United Kingdom);

2. Regional health services that constitute a variant of the national health service (for example Sweden) where the country is divided into regions with tax raising powers, sometimes complemented by subsidies from the federal level;

3. Sickness fund systems are highly regulated social insurance systems (for example, Belgium, France, Germany and The Netherlands);

4. Private insurance systems (for example Switzerland) where health care premiums are often risk related and insurance companies distribute money to competing providers that deliver

services. Co-payments usually form a strong element in these systems.

Health care reforms in Europe, as elsewhere, have been driven by two basic objectives: the first is equity; the second, efficiency. In simplest terms, equity means that all members of society have access to the same package of essential health care services regardless of their ability to pay. Efficiency is more difficult to define since it includes elements of the cost effective provision of health care services, discouragement of over and under consumption of health care services, responsiveness to patient's health care preferences, the encouragement and development of new health care treatments and improvement of the health status of citizens.

The impact of these reforms on the nursing profession in Europe has been considerable, as any cursory glance at the editorials of the main nursing journals over the past five years will indicate. The result has been the emergence of a new type of nurse, one who is both political and professional. Cancer, as one of Europe's *big killer* diseases and one that demands high costs if the required standards and quality of care are to be met and delivered, has been a prime target for those seeking ways to cut costs. One has only to understand that four fifths of the publicly funded research and development in countries holding membership in the Organization for Economic Cooperation and Development is spent on two diseases (cancer and AIDS) on which there has been little progress in the last 35 years. It has become increasingly apparent that health care professionals involved in cancer care have had to become extremely focused in arguing the case for securing the necessary funding to maintain and develop cancer services. That nurses in cancer care had begun to organize themselves at the national and European level before the full impact of these reforms began to be felt and had entered into tentative collaboration arrangements with their colleagues from the experimental and clinical oncology community in Europe, who were also being subjected to the same pressures, provided them with a distinct advantage over some of their nursing and medical colleagues when the time came to defend their speciality against these and other threats.

THE EUROPEAN UNION, NURSING AND HEALTH

The EU is a collection of 15 Member States committed to economic, social and political integration (Commission of the European Communities, 1994.) With a population in excess of 400 million, it is the world's largest trading entity. From the signing of the Treaty of Rome in 1957 to the formation of the European Economic Community, now known as the European Union, its aims have been to create a single economic region in which goods, services, people and capital can move freely across national boundaries. But the creation of the EU was also a political act—its founders seeing it as opening the way to an even closer union among the peoples of Europe.

Fulfilling the aims of the EU lies essentially with four institutions—the Council of Ministers, European Parliament, European Commission (EC) and European Court of Justice. Put simply in terms of the government structures of the United States of America, the rough equivalent of the Council would be the President; of Parliament, Congress; of the Commission, the Senate; and of the Court, the Supreme Court. Heads of government of Member States and the Presidents of Parliament and the EU meet at least twice a year as the European Council. Other European bodies include the Economic and Social Committee, Court of Auditors, European Investment Bank and Committee of the Regions.

Nursing is officially represented only in the European Commission through the Advisory Committee on Training in Nursing (ACTN). This committee was set up in 1977 but did not function until 1979. It is responsible for overseeing and making recommendations on all matters relating to training in nursing. The Committee is required to ensure comparably high standards of training across the EU and review the need to amend nurse training in line with developments in nursing and health care science. Similar advisory committees have been established for doctors, dentists and veterinary surgeons. The committee originally met twice a year but this has recently been reduced to one meeting per year. Membership of ACTN is composed of three experts from each Member State, appointed at the beginning of each three-year term. There is one member each for the practicing profession, establishments providing training and the competent authority responsible for regulating the profession in each Member State.

The Standing Committee of Nurses of the EU (PCN) has identified itself as the liaison committee for nurses with the European Commission. Established in 1971, its members consist of representatives from the national nurses' associations in membership of the International Council of Nurses from each Member State of the EU. The purpose of PCN is to bring to the attention of the European Commission the contribution that nurses and nursing can make to meeting health care needs throughout the EU and safeguarding nursing's status and practice. PCN has set itself certain objectives and its priority areas include education, specific health care programs (cancer, AIDS prevention and older people), environmental health, development and implementation of health care technology and the working conditions of nurses.

Nursing in the EU is currently regulated by two directives (a law that binds Member States to an outcome but leaves the method of translating the directive into national law to each Member State), 77/452/EEC and 77/453/EEC. These directives deal with the mutual recognition of diplomas, certificates and other evidence of the formal qualifications of nurses responsible for general care and the coordination of provision laid down by law, regulation or administrative action in respect of the activities of nurses responsible for general care (Pritchard & Wallace, 1994; Quinn & Russell, 1993). As these directives apply to nurses in general care, the needs of specialist nurses, such as those involved in cancer care, are not covered. The role of EONS in highlighting this anomaly is described in detail as follows.

While the EU has taken action in a number of health related areas in the past, such as cancer, its treaties did not give it a specific health competence. Activity in the health field was carried out:

1. By way of articles not specifically concerned with health, such as those providing for the free movement of people or for the single market;

2. Through health related articles, such as that on the environment; and

3. Through "mixed competence," partly based on the treaties and partly by agreements with health ministers.

The pressures created by changing lifestyles, falling birth rates, rising unemployment, movement of people as a result of recent political changes, a growing aging population and ever increasing medical costs brought health a new profile on the EUs during the 80s in a way not previously seen. As a result, the Treaty on European Union (commonly known as the Maastricht Treaty after the city in The Netherlands where the treaty was signed), ratified in October and implemented in November 1993, extended the competence of the EU in health, for the first time, through the inclusion of a chapter on health—Article 129 (see Table 15.1a). This article limits the scope of EU action to public health and prevention

Table 15.1a
Public Health Chapter of the Maastricht Treaty

The Community shall contribute towards ensuring a high level of human health protection by encouraging co-operation between the Member States and, if necessary, lending support to their action.

Community action shall be directed towards the *prevention of diseases*, in particular the major health scourges, including drug dependence, by promoting research into their causes, and transmission, as well as health information and education.

Health protection requirements shall form *a constituent part of the Community's other policies*.

Public Health, Chapter of the Maastricht Treaty

of disease. No mention is made of the harmonization of Member States' laws and regulations in the public health and prevention of disease sectors.

Recent events arising from the threat posed by Bovine Spongiform Encephalopathy (BSE), i.e., a new and so far untreatable form of Creutzfeld Jacobs Disease, have brought public health issues to the fore and major new amendments to Article 129 are now being proposed (see Table 15.1b).

It is important to understand that the new provisions for health in the Maastricht Treaty do not affect the way in which individual Member States finance and deliver health care. It is also important to understand that health protection requirements are to be integrated into other policy areas within the EU's competence. Consistent with the spirit of the Treaty, Article 129 reiterates the principle of subsidiarity—decisions should be taken at the lowest level consistent with effective action within a political system. (The principle of subsidiarity finds a parallel in the Tenth Amendment to the United States of America's Constitution and Article 30 of the German Constitution both of which reserve to the states of *Laender* powers not specifically allocated to the federal government.)

The EU has the responsibility, in liaison with the Member States, of coordinating policies and programs. The EU might initiate such coordination but, in this context, the EU and Member States are also encouraged to coordinate their work with developing countries and international organizations, such as the WHO, United Nations agencies and nongovernmental organizations, such as the Red Cross and Red Crescent. There is no intention that the EU would become involved in national health

Table 15.1b
Proposed Revision of Article 129

(The words in bold type highlight the proposed amendments to the current Article 129)

1. **As part of its powers** the Community **shall ensure a** high level of human health protection. **It shall, in addition,** encourage cooperation between the Member States in this field by lending support, if necessary, to their action.

   Community action shall be directed towards **any measure liable to prevent human illness or to obviate sources of danger to public health. The action shall cover the fight against** the major health scourges, including drug dependence, by promoting research into their causes and their transmission, as well as health information and education.

   Health protection requirements **must be integrated into the definition and implementation of the Community's other policies.**

2. Member States shall, in liaison with the Commission, coordinate among themselves their policies and programmes in the areas referred to in paragraph 1. The Commission may, in close contact with the Member States, take any useful initiative to promote such coordination. **The Council shall, on the basis of a report from the Commission, undertake a comprehensive annual evaluation of the results of such coordination.**

3. The Community and the Member States shall foster cooperation with third countries and the competent international organisations in the sphere of public health.

4. In order to contribute to the achievement of the objectives referred to in this Article, the Council:

   — **acting in accordance with the procedure referred to in Article 189b, shall adopt measures regarding the approximation of the Member States' laws, regulations and administrative actions designed to protect human health, especially in the veterinary and phytosanitary fields;**

   — acting in accordance with the procedure referred to in Article 189b, after consulting the Economic and Social Committee and the Committee of the Regions, shall adopt any incentive measures capable of lending support to efforts made by Member States in the context of coordinating their policies.

   — acting by qualified majority on a proposal from the Commission, shall adopt recommendations.

systems and certainly not directly involved in the delivery of services, treatment or care.

While the preceding may be official policy, however, there is every reason to suppose that the introduction of the Single Market might have consequences on health issues beyond the control of any one country. Greater mobility of people who work and live in or retire to countries other than their own could make differences in the health care standards more obvious and bring demands for even more convergence in both health services and social policies, even though there might be resistance to such views at the moment. In addition, political changes in Central and Eastern Europe also mean that public health and prevention of disease problems in one country are affecting other European states to a greater extent than before. It is becoming even more urgent, therefore, for the EU to consider the effects of public heath and disease prevention activities in all its institutions on other European countries, particularly when it is likely that many of the countries of Central and Eastern Europe will be members of the EU by the year 2000.

Given the preceding information, it is not difficult to understand that there is a growing body of opinion within the EU that there needs to be a single focus within the EU with responsibility for coordinating health issues. Although a small Public Health Unit has been established in the Directorate General (DG) V of the European Commission responsible for employment, industrial relations and social affairs, there is no one department within the entire EU set up that deals specifically with health issues. (Table 15.2 illustrates those directorates general that are concerned with health.)

If Article 129 is to become a reality then one of the first matters to be addressed should be the radical restructuring of the administrative infrastructure and the allocation of sufficient resources to ensure that agreed programs and projects are implemented. One argument is for the setting up of a separate Directorate General for health issues but in a recent interview, the Commissioner responsible for DG V appeared to indicate that this was not yet the time to move forward on this matter (Belcher, 1996). There are indications, however, that the European Commission is taking a more broad-based and integrated approach to programs based on the health needs of each Member State. Two reports on the integration of health protection requirements in Community policies have already been published (Commission of the European Communities 1995a, 1996b) as has a report on the state of health in the European Community (Commission of the European Communities, 1995b).

Table 15.2
Directorates and Other EU Funded Agencies of Relevance to Health Care

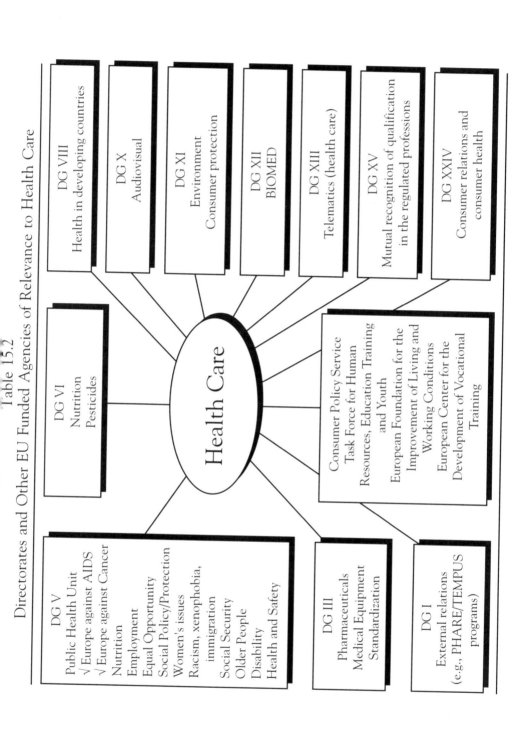

Health Care

DG VIII
Health in developing countries

DG X
Audiovisual

DG XI
Environment
Consumer protection

DG XII
BIOMED

DG XIII
Telematics (health care)

DG XV
Mutual recognition of qualification
in the regulated professions

DG XXIV
Consumer relations and
consumer health

DG VI
Nutrition
Pesticides

Consumer Policy Service
Task Force for Human
Resources, Education Training
and Youth
European Foundation for the
Improvement of Living and
Working Conditions
European Center for the
Development of Vocational
Training

DG V
Public Health Unit
√ Europe against AIDS
√ Europe against Cancer
Nutrition
Employment
Equal Opportunity
Social Policy/Protection
Women's issues
Racism, xenophobia,
immigration
Social Security
Older People
Disability
Health and Safety

DG III
Pharmaceuticals
Medical Equipment
Standardization

DG I
External relations
(e.g., PHARE/TEMPUS
programs)

"Europe Against Cancer" Program

Cancer is a major world health problem. In 1990 there were seven million new cancer cases worldwide and before the year 2000 over 60 million people will die of cancer and over 80 million will die of cancer in the first decade of the next century. While cancer is known as a major cause of death in developed countries, Stjernsward and Teoh (1993) have reported that it is predicted that in 2015 two thirds of all cancers, an estimated 10 million of 15 million new cases, will occur in the developing countries. At the same time although more than half of the world's cancer patients presently live in developing countries, less that 5 percent of the resources committed to cancer control are available to them. While infectious disease and perinatal and maternal mortality have usually received more attention, it is a little known fact that once an individual has survived the first five years of life, cancer also becomes one of the major causes of death in developing countries.

Moving to the EU, cancer is responsible for one quarter of all deaths within this geographical area and has always been a central concern of national health authorities. Along with accidents, it ranks as the main cause of early death (prior to the age of 75). In recent decades there has been a significant increase in mortality due to cancer and the average age of the population has increased. The most recent data from 1990 show an annual rate of 1,300,000 new cases of cancer and 840,000 deaths due to it in the EU (Esteves et al, 1993). The incidence of cancer is increasing rapidly among those over 50 years of age; the median age at which cancer is diagnosed is approximately 65 years of age in the EU. It is anticipated that mortality due to cancer will increase over the next 15 years in the absence of strategies to combat cancer, which include effective measures for prevention and treatment.

The European Council took note in May and December of 1985 of the concern shown by the competent national authorities and their citizens in the face of this disease and decided to establish a "Europe Against Cancer" Program (EAC). An initial action plan was successfully implemented in 1987–89. In light of the encouraging results obtained, the Council of Ministers and European Parliament approved the implementation of a second action plan for 1990–1994. These action plans have been the subject of annual reports by the Commission. In addition, an evaluation report on the first six years of operation of the program was approved by the Commission on March 15, 1993 and forwarded to the Council of Ministers and European Parliament for examination. In its resolution of December 13, 1993, the Council recognized the importance of continuing the "Europe Against Cancer" Program and asked for a third action plan to be drawn up. The third action plan, while ensuring continuity with the preceding plans, was to take into account other activities undertaken by the EU in the field of public health, particularly those to be implemented in the context of the new Article 129.

On March 29, 1996, the European Parliament and Council of Ministers approved the third action plan. The objective of this plan is to contribute toward ensuring a high level of health protection and will consist of actions aimed at preventing premature deaths due to cancer; reducing mortality and morbidity due to cancer; promoting the quality of life by improving the general health situation; and promoting the general well being of the population, particularly by reducing the economic and social consequences of cancer (Commission of the European Communities, 1996a).

Whatever is done to address the cancer problem, be it prevention, screening, diagnosis, treatment or care, all the agencies involved understand that the nurse is the common denominator wherever there are patients with cancer. Many cancers are preventable and cancer nurses are taking a leadership role in patient and public education and public health initiatives to address cancer prevention. When this is not possible, emphasis is placed on early detection. Cancer nurses are responsible for providing quality cancer patient care, treatment, monitoring and preventing side effects of therapy and involvement in clinical trials research. Improvements in the supportive care of cancer patients have taken place mainly through nursing research addressing pain control, quality of life, symptom management and control of nausea and vomiting. Supportive care provided by cancer nurses is a common goal, even in developing countries, although the major focus may be quite different due to lack of resources. Cancer nurses are there with the patient providing care and counseling across the life span, at every stage of the health-illness continuum and in a variety of settings. The potential contribution of the nurse in the fight against cancer across the globe could be seminal. But if this potential is to be realized it is essential that the voice of cancer nurses is heard in the corridors of power where cancer policy is determined at the highest levels.

Before the strategies EONS determined and implemented to bring this message to these corridors of power are described in detail, one further development, referred to earlier, occurred at the level of the professional groups involved in cancer care that would lead to an important critical alliance.

Federation of European Cancer Societies

Founded in 1981, FECS is registered as a non-profit making international organization with scientific purpose with the Belgian Ministry of Justice. Currently, the full member societies of FECS are the European Association for Cancer Research, EONS, European Society for Medical Oncology, European Society of Surgical Oncology, European Society for Therapeutic Radiology and Oncology and the European branch of the International Society of Paediatric Oncology. The European Society for Psychosocial Oncology is an affiliated member. The primary aim of FECS is to promote and coordinate collaboration between these societies in the different fields of experimental and clinical oncology and cancer nursing. In further-ance of this aim FECS encourages the participation of its member societies at intergovernmental level in collaborative ventures and every two years organizes ECCO, the European Cancer Conference.

Through its federated structure FECS now represents the greater num-ber of basic research scientists, medical oncologists, surgical oncologists, radiation oncologists and nurses working in the geographical region of Europe as defined by WHO. FECS also works closely with the European Organization for Research and Treatment of Cancer and European School of Oncology and has informal links with WHO, the Organization of European Cancer Institutes, Association of European Cancer Leagues and International Union Against Cancer. FECS offers its member societies a number of services aimed at raising their profile with those governmental (IGOs) and nongovernmental organizations (NGOs) with a responsibility for health at the European level. Among these services are:

1. The dissemination of relevant information produced by the institutions of the EU and other organizations highlighting the implications for and impact on their work;

2. Coordinating contacts between the full member societies and the institutions of the EU, IGOs, NGOs and commercial con-cerns,

3. Raising the media's awareness of the European experimental and clinical oncology and cancer nursing community; and

4. Developing contacts, particularly with the European Commis-sion and Parliament.

FECS's multi and interdisciplinary structure is unique. In the United States of America the experimental and clinical oncology and cancer nursing community is represented through a number of large and powerful organizations that include the American Association for Cancer Research, American Society of Clinical Oncology, American Society for Therapeutic Radiology and Oncology and Oncology Nursing Society. These organizations are roughly the same as their European counterparts apart from the fact that they function primarily at the national level, have a monodisciplinary focus and have been in existence for more years. Despite the fact that these organizations are powerful and well organized in their own right, it could be argued that their attempts to foster closer cooperation and collaboration with each other have not been as obviously successful as those of their European counterparts. Recognition of the benefits of such collaboration are recognized and understood, a fact recently acknowledged by Glick (1996), but rarely acted upon.

EONS became a full member of FECS in 1993 and this has conferred on the Society a number of benefits, including the services previously mentioned. As stated, the status of nursing varies considerably across Europe and the fact that a nursing society was accepted as an equal member of a multi and interdisciplinary federation sent an important message to European health care professionals and has done much to raise the status of cancer nursing in a large number of European countries. Moreover, EONS's membership in FECS has provided the clinical and experimental oncology community with an opportunity of gaining a greater understanding of the wide ranging contributions nurses can make to cancer care. Such understanding has resulted in improved collaboration between European scientists, doctors and nurses and an acknowledgment that for some issues success is more likely when these different professional groups work in tandem rather than in isolation. This new era of cooperation and collaboration was demonstrated when EONS signed a collaborative agreement with ESO, an organization which to date had focused on medical education, to work together on various educational initiatives that have applicability to a medical and nursing audience.

Further details about FECS and its activities can be found on its web site (http://www.fecs.be).

MOVING THE EUROPEAN CANCER NURSING AGENDA FORWARD: A CASE STUDY

It is clear from the above that many challenges face European cancer nurses in moving their agenda forward, not least the significant cultural and language diversity in Europe and wide spectrum of opinion as to how nursing and nurses are perceived. One of the most important functions of the institutions of the EU is to break down the many barriers to economic, social and political integration which exist both within and between Member States. In order to move the European cancer nursing agenda forward it was critical that EONS formed alliances with these institutions. One of the greatest difficulties in forming such alliances is identifying which EU DG is important in terms of both cancer and nursing. In the late 1980s the EC facilitated EONS in this respect by focusing on the problem of cancer through the establishment of EAC. Improved training of health care professionals was one of the key elements of the first action plan (1987–89) implemented under this program. In the document announcing the action plan the European Commission stated:

> *Of all health care professionals, it is the nurses who are the most frequently in contact with patients. Accordingly, they play an important part in the fight against cancer, especially in the treatment field* (Commission of the European Communities, 1986).

As a result the ACTN established an *ad hoc* working party to study the present situation with reference to the teaching of cancer care at the basic and postbasic nurse level. The establishment of this working group provided EONS with the first opportunity to collaborate with the EU and the outcome of this collaboration was a series of recommendations on the training of nurses in the matter of cancer at a basic, postbasic and advanced level (Commission of the European Communities, 1989). EONS acted on these recommendations by bringing together a group of cancer nurse educators, representing each Member State, who were given the brief of developing a core curriculum for a postbasic course in cancer nursing. The extensive differences in both cancer nursing and nurse education within Europe made this a difficult task. These differences also meant that the curriculum had to be flexible enough to allow local interpretation, yet comprehensive enough to include all of the important dimensions of cancer nursing practice.

The workshop, which was funded by the Marie Curie Memorial Foundation, a British charity, resulted in the production and subsequent publication of a core curriculum for a post-basic course in cancer nursing (EONS, 1991). The next step was to gain a pan-European consensus on the content of the core curriculum. This step was vital in ensuring that the curriculum was both accepted and utilized in each Member State. In

1989 the EAC program decided to accept a proposal from EONS to convene and fund a consensus conference with a view to gaining agreement on the content and implementation of the published curriculum and EONS was asked to organize this conference on behalf of the program. The consensus conference was a historic first for European cancer nurses since it provided the first opportunity to agree on ways of achieving some degree of harmony of training in a particular clinical specialty in the EU. This conference brought together cancer nurse experts, cancer nurse educators, members of PCN, ACTN and other interested persons from European governmental agencies. Following three days of debate and discussion, a consensus was achieved and the curriculum was unanimously endorsed for flexible implementation according to each country's basic, post-basic and continuing cancer nursing education needs. This agreement signaled an important victory for EONS since it provided tangible support for the argument in favor of recognizing cancer nursing as a distinct and important nursing specialty. Prior to this, the move toward developing nursing specialties along the lines of diseases was resisted vigorously by various European and national nursing organizations in the membership of the International Council of Nurses.

The core curriculum has stood the test of time. Since its endorsement by the EU the majority of cancer nursing courses supported by the EAC have been based on the core curriculum (Jodrell, 1996). It has clearly demonstrated its acceptability and usefulness to European cancer nurses. This positive feedback enabled EONS to enter another critical alliance; this time with a member of the industries whose products support cancer care. In recent years there has been increasing awareness of the pivotal role cancer nurses play in ameliorating distressing symptoms which result from cancer and its treatments. Nurses need to be adequately prepared to undertake this role. With this in mind and with a substantial educational grant from Smith Kline Beecham Pharmaceuticals, EONS was able to organize a series of roundtable discussions which were convened with the purpose of developing educational materials for use in national training courses in different aspects of cancer care. The project, known as Cancer Care: Priorities for Nurses, has resulted in the production of educational materials on subjects as diverse as altered body image, emesis, pain, psychological disorders and infection. These subjects develop areas already identified in the core curriculum. For each subject a curriculum and educational supplement has been produced. These materials have been used extensively throughout Europe to develop short courses at a national and local level.

At present, EONS is involved with a number of projects which are funded by the EU. Not all of these projects are funded by the EAC program. EONS has sought funding from Commission DGs other than the DG which is directly responsible for health (DG V) and recently, in cooperation with a number of partners, the Society was successful in obtaining funding from DG XIII for a pan-European project assessing the utilization of computer information systems in harmonizing cancer nursing practice.

One EONS project of note which has been funded by EAC is the pan European implementation of Dr. Gertrud Grahn's "Learning to Live with Cancer" Program. This program is based on the American Cancer Society's "I Can Cope" Program originally developed by Judi Johnson and Pat Norby (Johnson & Klein, 1994). Grahn saw the potential of implementing the "I Can Cope" Program with a population of Swedish cancer patients and their relatives. Following a learning needs assessment and testing of a more extensive patient education program with a Swedish audience, "Learning to Live with Cancer" was developed (Grahn & Johnson, 1990; Grahn, 1993). It was felt that a program, developed originally in the United States and modified in the light of the needs of Swedish patients and their relatives, would be applicable in all European countries. As a result EONS, in collaboration with the University of Lund, sought and was successful in receiving funding from the EAC Program to run a series of training the trainers programs. The first training the trainers workshop was held in March 1995 with representation from Belgium, Estonia, Ireland, Italy and the United Kingdom.

During this workshop the enormous diversity in the provision of information and patient education throughout Europe became apparent. In some European countries, for example, it is culturally unacceptable for patients to be provided with information about their disease and treatment (Glaus & Grahn, 1995). Despite this barrier, nurses who attended the workshop gave a commitment to implement the program in their own country. Two further training the trainers workshops were held in 1996 and two more are planned for 1997. Bristol-Myers Squibb has supplemented the grant from EAC to ensure that nurses from outside the EU can attend the workshops and, to date, participants have come from over 20 European countries. All participants have attempted to implement the program in their own countries with varying degrees of success; progress can be slow. Nevertheless, "Learning to Live with Cancer" is now well established in Ireland, Italy and Norway and plans for its implementation are well advanced in other countries. This clearly demonstrates that, despite huge differences in culture, programs developed in one European country can be implemented sensitively and successfully in many others.

The success of the preceding initiatives has given EONS the confidence and impetus to move forward with its political agenda. In recent years EONS has established a sound reputation within the EU and its contribution to the improvement of cancer services in the EU is now readily acknowledged. However, a constant source of discontent for European cancer nurses has been that nurses are not represented on the various EU committees, including those of EAC. Each Member State is allowed to nominate a representative and an alternate for each EU committee. EONS was aware that it would need some leverage to motivate national governments to nominate a nurse so a decision was made to approach a Member of the European Parliament and request that a question on lack of nurse representation be put to the Commission. In answering this question, Padraig Flynn, the Commissioner for DG V, was placed in a position where he had no option but to emphasize his support for nurses and the importance of their representation on EU committee. His hands were tied, however, as he could not force a national government to nominate a nurse.

EONS then used this reply to raise the awareness of each Member State's government to this anomalous and unjust situation. The responses from each Member State were mixed; most indicated their willingness, in principle, to listen to the nurses' viewpoint yet were unwilling to nominate, at that stage, a nurse to any of the committees. Nevertheless, an important political point had been made and a number of changes have taken place recently in respect to the various committees. Most significantly, the President of EONS is now invited as an observer to the meeting of the newly established Advisory Committee on Cancer Prevention. One of the key reasons EONS has been able to influence the EC is the quality of the information on the EU and other organizations which the Society receives regularly as a service from FECS.

It is clear from the preceding example that EONS has started to influence the EC's thinking in matters relating to cancer. However, EONS also believed it had an important contribution to make to the EC's thinking on other matters relating to health and nursing in general. Despite the fact that PCN has established itself as the official liaison committee with the EC on all matters relating to nursing, a number of different specialist nursing groups, including EONS, have begun to liaison with the EC. There was a risk, however, that the EC would receive conflicting messages and a wide range of viewpoints from all of the different nursing groups. It is, of course, *sine qua non* that if nurses really want to influence the EC's thinking on health matters, than they need to speak with one voice and that this voice needs to be representative of all nurses in Europe (Redmond, 1995). PCN has facilitated this process by establishing a European Nursing Forum, the first meeting of which was held in Madrid in November 1996. The meeting was attended by representatives from PCN, other non-EU national nursing associations and a number of specialist nursing groups, including EONS. The purpose of this forum is to provide an opportunity for discussion and debate on issues confronting all European nurses and achieve consensus on the way forward. One of the most important issues confronting specialist nursing groups is the fact that many nursing specialties are not recognized at either a European or national level. This has implications for the freedom of movement of specialist nurses within the EU, an anomaly which EONS has brought to the attention of the European Nursing Forum. EONS, in collaboration with other specialist nursing groups, now intends to bring this matter to the attention of the EU.

The fact that the majority of European nurses only speak one European language competently has been the most significant barrier to collaboration and cooperation among European nurses. For many years EONS has given consideration as to how to overcome this problem. The provision of translation at conferences or for written materials is prohibitively expensive. EONS's burgeoning reputation as the most eminent nursing specialty group in Europe has raised its profile with the pharmaceutical industry and thus, provided the Society with a new and extensive source of funding. A number of exciting critical alliances have been made with members of the pharmaceutical industry, the most noteworthy have resulted in two projects which will have a profound impact on cancer nursing in Europe.

The first project, *Action on Fatigue*, is based on the Oncology Nursing Society of the United States of America's FIRE (Fatigue Initiative Through Research and Education) project. This project, supported by an educational grant from Janssen Cilag consists of educational and research dimensions. In September 1996, 200 nurses from 32 countries worldwide attended a professional education course on cancer-related fatigue. This was a landmark event since, for the first time, a European cancer nursing conference was simultaneously translated into five European languages. This meant that nurses who previously could not attend European conferences because they did not speak English were given the opportunity to attend an international meeting. This opportunity provided them with a new vision of cancer nursing practice. All the participants have agreed to run an educational program on fatigue in their country of origin, ensuring that the problem of cancer-related fatigue will be highlighted to many more nurses involved in cancer care.

The second, and probably most significant, project that EONS has become involved with is the launch of a journal entitled *Oncology Nurses Today* (ONT). This journal, supported by a grant from Bristol-Myers Squibb, is published in nine European languages and distributed to 25,000 nurses throughout Europe. Although not a peer-reviewed journal, it will provide European nurses with a forum for debate and exchange of information which until now was unavailable, indeed, to many, unimaginable. ONT will provide European nurses with their first glimpse of the nature of cancer nursing in different countries and of the many developments in health care which are impacting on cancer nursing at both a national and international level. The potential impact of this journal in terms of empowering European cancer nurses is enormous and in the future this power may mean that the cancer nursing agenda will move forward at a much more rapid pace; indeed it may become unstoppable.

Conclusion

At a time when demand for health care now outstrips the available financial resources, it is inevitable that the impact this will have on the way health care professionals are able to carry out their responsibilities will be dramatic. In a world where difficult choices in health care are likely to be based on cost analyses without due consideration of the gains in effectiveness, or political considerations without due reference to the scientific analyses that should inform policy, the traditional roles of professionals in the health care field will come under increasing pressure. New ways need to be found to ensure participation in decision making processes at the highest level if cancer patients and their families are to continue to receive care that is both efficient and equitable. The cancer nursing community in Europe has been and continues to be acutely sensitive to the winds that are changing the face of health care in that continent. This awareness has led them to understand the importance and benefits of forging critical alliances with other major players—other professional groups, patients, industry and politicians—with the result that they have been able to demonstrate unequivocally their seminal contribution to cancer care. It is a lesson from which nursing as a whole could learn.

REFERENCES

Belcher, P. A. (1996). Padraig Flynn, European Commissioner responsible for employment and Social Affairs (including matters related to public health). Interview. *Eurohealth*, 2, 2–3.

Commission of the European Communities (1986). *Europe Against Cancer Program: Proposal for a plan of action 1987–1989.* COM(86)717 FINAL. 16.12.1986. Brussels: European Commission.

Commission of the European Communities (1989). Commission recommendation of November 8, 1989 concerning the training of health personnel in the matter of cancer. *Official Journal of the European Communities*, L346/4, Vol. 32, 27.11.1989.

Commission of the European Communities (1994). *European Union.* Luxembourg: Office for Official Publications of the European Communities.

Commission of the European Communities (1995a). *Report from the Commission to the Council, the European Parliament and the Economic and Social Committee on the integration of health protection requirements in Community policies.* COM(95) 196 final. 29.05.1995. Brussels: European Commission.

Commission of the European Communities (1995b). *Report from the Commission to the Council, the European Parliament, the Economic and Social Committee and the Committee of the Regions on the state of health in the European Community.* COM(95) 357 final. 19.07.1995. Brussels: European Commission.

Commission of the European Communities (1996a). Decision No. 646/96/EC of the European Parliament and Council of March 29, 1996 adopting an action plan to combat cancer within the framework for action in the field of public health (1996 to 2000). *Official Journal of the European Communities*, L 16.4.96.

Commission of the European Communities (1996b). *Second report from the Commission to the Council, the European Parliament, the Economic and Social Committee and the Committee of the Regions on the integration of health protection requirements in Community policies (1995).* COM(96) 407 final 04.09.1996. Brussels: European Commission.

European Oncology Nursing Society (1991). *A Core Curriculum for a Post-Basic Course in Cancer Nursing.* Revised Edition. Luxembourg: European Commission's Europe Against Cancer Program.

Esteves, J., Kricker, J., Ferlay, J., & Parkin, D. M. (1993). *Facts and Figures of Cancer in the European Community.* Lyon: International Agency for Research on Cancer.

Glick, J. H. (1996). American Society of Clinical Oncology: A society in transition. *Journal of Clinical Oncology*, 14, 8, 2387–2398.

Glaus, A., Grahn, G. (1995). Information, education and counseling: Essentials of supportive cancer care. In Klatersky, J., Schimpff, S. C. & Senn, H. (eds.) *Handbook of Supportive Care in Oncology.* Basel: Marcel Dekker.

Grahn, G., & Johnson, J. (1990). Learning to cope and living with cancer: Learning needs assessment in cancer patient education. *Scandanavian Journal of Caring Sciences, 4,* 173–181.

Grahn, G. (1993). Learning to cope—An intervention in cancer care. *Supportive Care in Cancer, 1,* 266–271.

Jodrell, N. (1996). *An assessment of activities in the area of training in oncology for nurses: Interim report to the Europe Against Cancer Program.* Luxembourg: Commission of the European Communities.

Johnson, J., & Klein, L. (1994). *I Can Cope: Staying Healthy With Cancer.* Minneapolis: Chronimed.

Pritchard, A. P., & Wallace, M. J. (1994). Moving around Europe–An overview of European Union nursing legislation. *Accident and Emergency Nursing, 2,* 211–215.

Quinn, S., & Russell, S. (1993). *Nursing in Europe.* London: Scutari.

Redmond, K. (1995). Do nurses influence the European Union's thinking in matters relating to health? A commentary. *European Journal of Cancer Care, 4,* 104–105.

Salvage, J. (1993). Raising the nursing profile: The case of the invisible nurse. *World Health Statistics Quarterly, 46(3).*

Stjernsward, J., & Teoh, N. (1993). Current status of the Global Cancer Control Program of the World Health Organization. *Journal of Pain and Symptom Management, 8(6),* 340–347.

The World Bank (1993). *Investing in health: The World Bank Development Report.* New York: The World Bank.

Part VIII

Roots and Resonance of Responsive Care

Observations about change as described by Dr. Valentine are all too familiar to us. When one examines the evolution of the American health care sector over 200 years and the magnitude of the rapid escalation of today's changing scenario, there is hope and new meaning of what is possible.

The author believes that this is a good time for nurses to master personal characteristics such as risk taking, problem solving and dedication as the perspective of the corporate world is gained, while still holding on to those values which are our legacy—patient advocacy, intimacy in caring during life's crises and dedicated public service. This is a great challenge for nurses in a dynamic environment such as ours. Dr. Valentine offers guidance in this important undertaking as nurses take professional and personal responsibility to improve health care in the 21st century.

16

Nursing's New World— A Guide for Taking Professional and Personal Responsibility to Make Health Care Better in the Next Century

Nancy M. Valentine

SURVIVING VERSUS THRIVING: HOW TO MAKE SENSE OUT OF ALL THE CHAOS

Most people resist change and certainly nurses are no exception. Questioning and exhibiting skepticism about change is considered and generally accepted to be part of human nature. Yet it has been the experience of many seasoned participants and observers of the change process, no matter where the changes may occur, that this is not a linear process and without a certain degree of chaos, fundamental change is simply not possible since the forces of resistance will eventually wear down and outweigh the energy and risks involved in experimenting with new approaches. A status quo environment at best allows for small, incremental change, often orchestrated by dynamic, committed leaders, unafraid to color outside the lines, who enjoy doodling in the margins and pushing whatever envelopes happen to be around to push. These individuals unfortunately are usually in the minority; no doubt attributable to the

The concepts for this paper were developed and first presented at the Dr. Maryann Fralic Endowed Lectureship at the University of Pittsburgh School of Nursing, October, 1996.

fact that unless one is positively encouraged and rewarded for taking risks, the behavior is either extinguished in organized bureaucracies and the individual is controlled by the system and eventually becomes compliant, or alternatively, the individual ultimately leaves the organization in frustration to pursue new challenges and takes on a new system, or perhaps ventures on to become an entrepreneur. In a health care organization that is fundamentally committed to no major changes in how to do business, the few changes that do occur are often personality driven and the long-term impact relatively isolated. Unfortunately, even for changes that have made important differences in critical areas such as quality of care, staff and patient satisfaction, or marketing for example, without the support of an organization that actively fosters change and rewards innovation, there is the risk that these contributions will never become part of the fabric of the operation and all too often evaporate as soon as the visionary and risk-taking leader exits.

For the health care industry, this has been a typical scenario, even in settings that were considered relatively dynamic. Until recently, much of the complacency and limited influence of competition in how the health care system has been managed in the United States was the result of a system of private and public financing that ensured continuous survival by supplying additional capital based on an escalating cost-based reimbursement policy. This period of sustained growth launched new technology, supported treatment programs, funded enormous research endeavors and employed the staff necessary for successful implementation. Consequently, today's efforts to curtail growth in the progressive escalation in the percentage of the gross national product dedicated to health care particularly over the past thirty years, has catapulted consumers and providers alike into a new era of health care reforms. The need has never been greater for nursing to actively participate and take a leadership role in reshaping health care both today and for the future. The changes in financing, expectations among consumers and the practice patterns of all providers are fueling a new definition of health care in the United States. As health policy debates have become a priority among national issues, nurses now find themselves in the middle of swirling agendas. Heated debates within the discipline focus on the attempts to balance the needs of the consumer with the professional politics of how the profession will be changed, perhaps for both better and possibly worse, or at the very least radically different, as a result of a national trend in system reengineering.

If one were to ever question the power of public debate, a stunning case example would be to study the impact of the *failed* health care reform legislation on the American health care system. Although the proposed legislation was not enacted in 1994, the rhetoric and debates took hold in the consciousness of the population. For the first time since the enact-ment of Medicare and Medicaid in the mid 1960s, there was the gradual but nonetheless populace-charged, grassroots momentum that created the political will necessary to change the existing system. Managed care has been one of society's ultimate contributions to the end of the 20th century and has shifted the thinking and the ways in which we are approaching health care problems and solutions; thus signaling a new era of multifac-eted reforms in the entire approach to the financing and delivery of care. Through a complex matrix of borrowing from corporate business principles that includes finance, focus on accountability for outcomes, health care value and the desire to meet the needs of the customer, (ranging from both predicting and achieving the desired cure to decreasing the waiting time in a clinic), the introduction of a free-market competitive model into the health care equation has resulted in an entirely new and future determining role for how health care will be changed in our society between now and the dawning of the next century. Through the impact of high profile public debates, it is ironic, in retrospect, that rhetoric and the public sharing of data related to cost, access, and policy alternatives rather than legislative mandates began to get the voter's attention and ultimately influenced one of the country's largest industries to change. By introducing the idea that health care had the capability to operate like any other business, and that more federal legislative mandates were unnecessary to further burden the industry to be accountable to the public, change indeed began to take flight at near lightning speed. The desire to save money by concentrating on reducing waste, duplication and employing cost-benefit analysis methods, to name simply a few strategies, captured the imagination of enough opinion makers to collectively force all participants engaged in the system to operate as a business enterprise based on observable and measurable quality outcomes that demonstrated to multiple audiences—policy makers, payers, providers and clients alike that health care savings and value is indeed attainable. Within only a few years time, radical, new assumptions have found their way into nearly every care giving arena that previously had operated in comparatively blissful isolation. Prior to this, the United States health care sector had evolved over the past nearly 200 years, shaped by a combination of professional education and socialization processes that had successfully transformed American medicine into a sovereign profession and signaled the making of a vast industry (Starr, 1982).

To support the expansion of the health care enterprise, as well as to take on the missions of professional health education and scientific inquiry, this industry, unlike any other, was kept apart from the influences of the free market system through a not for profit system of revenue generation and accounting. The medical-industrial complex grew virtually unchecked and essentially unaccountable according to the same market forces and standards utilized in the for-profit business sector where revenue, expenses and profits are carefully balanced and controlled. During this period, the for-profit sector in health care, in which share holders can participate in the risks, rewards and growth of the company, was small as compared to the not-for profit sectors and was traditionally viewed as not relevant and potentially destructive to the complex decisions and need for resources to be directed back into the multiple missions of the system. Making money from people who are ill did not hold a great deal of social appeal. Much of the activity to remain not profit-driven reflected values firmly anchored in a shared social contract based on the belief that it is essential to do whatever is best for the patient, irrespective of cost. Times have changed dramatically in less than a decade; hence the chaos of how to best deal with these changes has confronted everyone involved in the health care industry from chief executive officer to housekeeper; public policy analyst to consumer. Change of this magnitude is the making of multiple paradigm shifts; raising every conceivable issue and calling into question all previously held assumptions beginning for some with cost of care, and cost-benefit analysis of one treatment over another, and for others, quality of care, access to services and continuity of care. Depending on one's professional perspective the challenges involved in interpreting and implementing these often sharply competing choices and changes in both an organizationally and socially responsible manner spark unending debates, ranging from the moral choices involved from the viewpoint of the health care ethicist, to the challenges involved in how to provide quality care for less cost from the vantage point of health care administrators and corporate trustees.

It is no wonder that nurses often experience an overwhelming sense of disempowerment, confusion and openly react to what can only be concluded to be a chaotic and unresponsive environment in which their opinions, concerns and proposed solutions simply get lost in the swirl of issues, rhetoric and activities. These are indeed physically, emotionally and spiritually demanding times and call for great curiosity, courage, tenacity, skill and a fundamental understanding of the forces of change. There is also a pressing need to identify strategies that can be used to frame and create a context for the many issues with which the industry and thereby, their employees are struggling. It is vitally important that nurses be included in a manner that invites the participation of not only the seasoned professional, but most especially the neophyte nurse. Rather than to be caught unaware and overwhelmed with the frenetic activities associated with change, it is critical that nurses anticipate the scope of the changes ahead and engage in active, meaningful and productive participation as opposed to exclusion; to experience the spark of excitement and adventure in being a meaningful participant in this age of health care renaissance as contrasted with reacting out of anger and despair. Especially for the beginning practitioner of nursing what better time to respect, mentor and nurture the importance of mastering those personal characteristics sometimes underestimated, such as risk-taking, problem-solving and dedication? Nursing's greatest legacy is one of patient advocacy, intimacy in caring during life's crises, and dedicated public service (Gordon, 1997).

What a tragedy it would be if these values were fundamentally altered or eventually lost in the midst of attempting to accommodate, understand, adopt and be socialized into a new corporate world. Perhaps the greatest dilemma facing each individual nurse and the nursing profession as a whole today is how to carefully and thoughtfully transition into the perspective of the corporate world, without sacrificing the values, standards, social relevance and positive aspects of a proud professional identity that has evolved through the educational and practice-based experience, characterizing today's nurse as an extremely valuable resource and asset to the American health care delivery system and to the public.

The dynamic and daily challenge before us is how to gain, even if a slow and incremental process, the sense of mastery and control at a time when there is great uncertainty and fear about the future and where these many changes will lead us. There is no curriculum that has provided us with the answers we must search out. Knowledge, mentorship and a belief in the power of self will give us the foundation for meeting the problems at hand. At the beginning of one's career, as well as periodically throughout one's work life, it is essential to nurture the adoption of an unrelenting belief that you do, and will continue to make a difference in the lives of people from whatever vantage point you may find yourself, no matter how difficult the circumstance may seem at any given time. This respect and belief in self is a critical variable that cannot be underestimated. It is the force that fuels the momentum to move forward and not lose the values clarification essential to preserve the image and ethics of what nurses offer the public. At a time of such dramatic change and reformulation of a system in transition, each individual, most especially those involved in the early stages of learning the art and science of nursing, must take care to inventory two very fundamental areas and ask the questions: Do I have a thorough knowledge of the global phenomena of change which is essential for becoming a relevant participant in the drama that is unfolding in the world in which we live? and secondly, Do I have a commitment to the importance and value of expanding, using to the fullest and preserving the intellectual, psychological and physical capital essential to making a thorough, meaningful and sustained investment in a profession that is anticipated to be rewarding over the course of one's career?

For many, these are not easy questions to answer in the tumultuous workplaces in which many nurses find themselves. New assumptions require individuals, organizations and the profession whether in a clinical, educational or research setting to adopt new behaviors in order to survive and thrive in a changing world. Five years ago we were operating under different assumptions such as the belief that the nursing program curriculum whether ADN, BSN or beyond provided us with the foundations we would need to successfully cope with the employment setting over the course of a professional lifetime. Since nursing was steadily growing in stature as a profession and jobs were plentiful, the potential for job mobility, promotion and satisfaction were virtually limitless. In the health care employee driven marketplace of yesterday retraining and cross-training were largely by choice, not by employer driven mandates. Nursing as a discipline and nurses as individuals must learn to be innovative in today's highly volatile environment. Yet, what an adventure and personal opportunity to meet the challenge and grow beyond one's expectations. Attitude is key as we face how to develop a perspective that allows that adventure to unfold in ways that lead us to new discoveries, stretch us to leave safe havens for unexplored shores, force us to continuously question the status quo and energize us to take the necessary action to quest for new and innovative solutions to old questions. An application of this attitude shift, for example, is the notion of professional survival, although a real question and issue to be concerned about on one hand, narrowly focusing on this question in the abstract leaves one with a sense of energy drain and fear of the possible outcomes. Whereas the idea of a profession advancing in new and previously undreamed of directions portrays an entirely different and certainly more hope giving impression. Few would debate the fact that the latter is worth striving for even at a time when traditional nursing roles and organizational structures appear to be under siege and future opportunities for nurses in some situations less optimistic. In fact, if not for the fundamental questions being raised today, major paradigm shifts for nurses might not even be an option to consider. Comfortable and content to continue with the familiar, no real and lasting progress would be made. Therefore, rather than shun the chaos, we must gain an affinity for and comfort in embracing it as a tool to be used right at the beginning of one's career. This attitude of adventure, *can do*, and developing the related ability and willingness to confront adversarial experiences as new learning opportunities has a much greater chance of affording the new nurse a long and successful career as contrasted to a professional image of succumbing to and eventually facing extinction as a consequence of negative predictions, of which there often seems to be an endless supply.

The strategic goal is to be in a position of knowledge-based self confidence, greater self determination in a changing world, and maximizing the value of our efforts and skills to benefit clients, families, communities and the health of the nation. The strategic question is how to move from where we are in today's environment, often buffeted by the changes, to where we want to be in the future. Transitioning to reconsider old beliefs based on incorporating learning from new experiments in how we can make our contributions count is a significant dilemma at times and also an opportunity for the individual whether in clinical practice, education or leadership positions (Rosenthal, 1997).

Unfortunately, there are no straight forward formulas or patently simplistic solutions. Several strategies are offered for nurses, both students and seasoned practitioners, to consider in order to better sort out and understand the contradictory and confusing landscape of health care reform implementation. The first is to have a context for interpreting the broad scope of these reforms and secondly, to gain a perspective for understanding the multiple political and economic forces that drive the decisions and policies that we observe in our work worlds and lastly, to underscore the critical importance of discovering, developing and actively nurturing an internal sense of professional and personal balance based on an appreciation for the growth potential that this chaos brings into our lives. Acknowledgment of the personal patience and courage necessary to confront rather than retreat from the challenges at hand and beyond brings us unparalleled learning opportunities for which we need to reach out and grasp.

TODAY'S CHALLENGES AND TOMORROW'S OPPORTUNITIES FOR NURSES IN THE NEW HEALTH CARE MARKETPLACE

The Basic Economics Underlying Health Care Policy Shifts and Reforms

Individuals choose nursing as a career for many reasons, not the least of which is the opportunity to make a contribution to the humanitarian objectives of society. This sense of altruism is a noble one and is chiefly the reason why patients and their families trust nurses above other health care providers. Although job security and compensation is of importance, it is rarely the number one factor in making this particular choice of career. Since nurses focus primarily on patient care, most do not look at their career choice or the workplace as a business, yet it is and we need to become more comfortable with this fact. At first glance, a discussion of economics and finance seems foreign and unrelated and is usually unpalatable to many nurses who given a choice would rather focus on quality and practice issues, which is their comfort zone. Money somehow seems to taint the picture and blurs the focus on caring and social welfare. Ironically, shunning knowledge in these areas does not serve the nurse nor the profession well. A working knowledge of the financial transactions and economic realities provides valuable information for making choices both for nurses and their patients in an increasingly complex world. Knowledge in these areas can also serve to decrease anxiety about the changes we cope with every day. Understanding how nurses contribute to the health care marketplace is one avenue for appreciating the broader perspective necessary for gaining experience and accuracy in analyzing the present revolution in health care. The basic principles of microeconomics and macroeconomics, as applied to understanding basic concepts such as competition and supply and demand, provide a new lens in order to view self interests in the marketplace, as well as to view the broader horizons of tomorrow's predicted changes. Application of this body of knowledge, coupled with gazing into the foreseeable future to view the vast array of technological changes spurred by knowledge explosions in complementary fields are anticipated to occur within the professional lifetime of today's new graduates.

These knowledge explosions will further contribute to a context for explaining today's health care struggles and will offer a greater appreciation for the evolving role of the nurse. This perspective is not expected to change the concerns expressed regarding practice, staffing, and quality of care issues that nurses on the front lines are confronting on a daily basis. It will hopefully provide, especially to a nurse new to the field, an expanded vantage point and appreciation for the multiple and sharply competing challenges and concerns, many of which are rooted in economics, that are driving the paradigm shifts we are living through during these revolutionary times.

THE TRADITIONAL VIEW OF SUPPLY SIDE NURSING: THE MICROECONOMICS PERSPECTIVE

Where Nurses are Typically Factored Into the Health Care Finance Equation

Hospital redesign, restructuring, and reengineering often leave nurses wondering, where are we going in this tumultuous period of change? Why are nurses suddenly no longer in such high demand? Why are nursing services being replaced with service line managers? What will the job market look like in the next five years? How can a nurse possibly feel empowered in such a volatile state of organizational upheaval and job market uncertainty? What are the opportunities and threats that exist which allow for predicting the future? To construct answers and develop hypotheses for the future, economics can be a useful tool for analyzing these current events.

Economics is the science that deals with the production, distribution and consumption of commodities or services (Webster's, 1994). As in any other field, moving from the general to a specific aspect of the science depends on what perspective is chosen. From the interests of the individual nurse or nursing as a profession, a place to start is the microeconomics perspective. The microeconomics view looks at the basic definition of economics from the specific vantage point of an individual consumer, person, firm or business (Heilbroner & Thurow, 1984). In contrast to what Heilbroner and Thurow refer to as the *worm's eye* view of microeconomics is the *bird's eye* view of macroeconomics, which is essentially the bigger picture of looking at problems from above and following or forecasting the trajectory of events and trends as the economic system moves into the future, which can be explored as a second level of analysis (Heilbroner & Thurow, 1984).

Exploring each component from the vantage point of the individual nurse and the profession at large offers a balanced view of the conflicts today and how trends in health care may very well offset what appear at first glance to be downward trends. In both of these viewpoints, an important related concept is the market forces that influence supply and demand, essentially the relationship between quantities and prices. For example, we have all experienced in everyday life the effect of a particular price on our willingness to either buy or sell a service or commodity and the influence of this relationship on the quantity demanded or quantity supplied (Heilbroner & Thurow, 1984).

If we think about today's managed care marketplace, we can readily appreciate and no doubt identify many examples of supply and demand in action, such as consumers making more choices in the marketplace simply because more exist, or an employer, through the opportunity to make a purchasing decision among a wider array of health insurance options, choosing a lower cost provider i.e., a nurse practitioner versus a physician for a procedure or treatment that has the same quality outcomes. In this case the cost for the service provided by a nurse practitioner may be much less than the same service provided by a more expensive physician provider and as consumers and employers alike have to make more out of pocket decisions, it can be anticipated that over time the demand for nurse practitioners providing primary care for a population of subscribers will increase, whereas the demand for physicians doing these same activities will decrease (Winslow, 1997).

Another familiar example is the many redesign projects that substitute non-licensed personnel for registered nurses. Although nurses have been very vocal in their opposition to this trend, if outcomes can be demonstrated to be as good or better than the previous organization of the nursing team, or if the patient satisfaction is determined to be the same or better, there is the marketplace pressure to change the supply and demand for a different mix of nursing staff. "The competitive marketplace is not only where the clash of interest between buyer and seller is worked out by the opposition of supply and demand, but also where buyers contend against buyers and sellers against sellers" (Heilbroner & Thurow, 1984).

Applying these basic economic concepts to the nursing workforce today and on into the future is relatively simple. Beginning with the basic definition of economics and isolating the three key variables of *consumption, production* and *distribution*, and combining these with the dimension of *supply* and *demand*, an explanation and trend analysis begins to develop which views the nurse as an economic contributor to the whole of the production of health care as contrasted to only looking at the world from one's professional and discipline-specific bias. Critically analyzing the nurses' contribution to the marketplace asks us to consider the health care reforms that most impact on the nurse's practice and work and provides information on alternatives and opportunities where new growth is possible.

Starting with the microeconomics viewpoint, a picture from the *worm's eye* point of view begins to take shape as viewed by how the economics of health care impacts on the nurse. In this model, for example, *consumers* are defined as patients and their families, *suppliers*, the current model of health care delivery composed of hospitals, clinics, doctors, nurses, etc. and *distribution* as largely determined by a variety of insurance arrangements or entitlement such as Medicare and Medicaid. General trends in each of these areas can be described as follows. *Demand*, in the most recent past used to mean simply the desire on the part of both consumers and providers united to use the maximum amount of services that were most often prescribed by one's physician. Therefore, to be admitted to the hospital and the length of time spent there was largely determined by the treating physician and more care, tests, and consultations were generally determined to be better than less. The definition of demand today is changing and these new definitions of demand are significantly different than the demands upon which we have operated in the past. From the consumer's point of view, demand is the gradual but consistently emerging trend to have a more independent role in determining options, be they services, providers or costs associated with purchases in an expanding marketplace. Not only do consumers want quality of care, they are demanding information that is indicative of how quality will be measured in advance of a treatment or procedure. In most cases, gone are the days when the consumer trustingly left the decisions about care in the hands of the physician or other health care provider, for that matter. This is the information age and with access to information systems becoming readily available in the home, workplace, library and senior citizen centers it can be anticipated that the demand for information and quality will only increase and become the norm as consumers both gain independence and establish increased expectations based on self-acquired knowledge. Many are already *surfing the net* to study their illness in order to make health care decisions *with* their providers and not simply be content to follow *doctor's orders*. Consumers also are demanding that the health care system provide increased access to services, organized for their convenience and covered by insurance that is affordable and portable. Patients and their families are no longer satisfied with traveling long distances, waiting for an appointment at the convenience of the provider or dealing with complex insurance issues and forms. One might describe this relatively recent and heightened sense of demand for fast, convenient service and a quality product at a good price as the McDonald's approach to consumer demands. This approach connotes a changing health care marketplace where quality, timeliness, a consistent, and reasonably priced, known product (with few or preferably no surprises), begin to influence the system to change by adopting free market values in order to meet new and quickly emerging demands. Demand on the part of the customers we serve is signaling the need to rapidly accommodate these needs, wants and desires because choices can now be exercised in the marketplace related to access, cost, quality and the perception of satisfaction. Emerging consumer demands and the realization that they cannot be dismissed, nor are they going to disappear, has put every facet of the production end of health care on notice.

Meeting these demands is a tall order for a system that until recently was still a largely cottage-based industry that took pride in establishing positive relationships between treaters and patients and getting the desired response to treatments, and much less concerned with efficiencies and hotel services, for example. Today, the bar has been raised via marketplace demand which requires a new emphasis that embodies both quality, and a tighter control on the cost implications of care. Hence, the term patient-centered care has come to mean reengineering specifically to meet the demands of patients. Most systems are trying to catch up with this notion and are not readily designed for putting the patient first.

To achieve this goal requires a sociological shift away from behaviors that are determined by the hierarchical and bureaucratic customs of putting the doctor first, or expecting the patient to comply with nursing routines, to one that has to consider instituting training programs that orient the physicians and nurses, as well as all other members of the team and/or organization, to listen to what the patient and family wants and to use this feedback to redesign the system of delivery. With this rather novel idea of customizing care, eliminating unnecessary routines and schedules, and redesigning to focus on what will satisfy the patient and not the staff as the priority, an entirely new paradigm has been created.

To meet those demands, all of the suppliers of services from nurse to receptionist; physician to phlebotomist must be re-trained to adopt an approach of conscious and consistent effort to provide customer satisfaction at every juncture in the care process as an expected and measurable outcome and product in itself. In essence, whether redesign is focused on patient satisfaction, finance, or developing a seamless system of care delivery, one can argue that despite many who point accusatory fingers at accountants and highly paid executives for overhauling and disrupting the health care system, the strongest impetus for health care reform has come largely from grassroots efforts among citizen consumers, certainly not from providers who more often lobby for few if any changes. Therefore, it is the consumers who are in truth shaping a new system based on their needs and demands and thereby are turning the tables on a system that grew up largely at the discretion of physicians, administrators and yes, even nurses. Since modern day health care began in the early 1800s the trends in treatment models have been those of systematically moving care out of the home and into institutions. Over time, complex systems were created to treat infectious diseases, house technology, and conduct professional education and research in central locations starting with community-based hospitals that eventually grew into large, medical center complexes (Starr, 1982).

Today, the trend is just the opposite and the competing demands are requiring the systems to reverse many of their priorities and traditions thereby destabilizing a system that had become comfortable and affluent in some sectors with uncurtailed growth and expansion into a marketplace cushioned by the willingness on the part of the public to pay more and more for services on an annual basis. In sharp contrast, other sectors, principally those in urban and rural settings, were frightfully underprivileged and grossly underserved. With an escalating gross national product dedicated to health care, coupled with ominous predictions about the consequences of a burgeoning budget deficit, the average citizen, through a combination of public debates and polling of the populace, made their claim known primarily to public officials. The message that was carried on a national scale was that voters had finally had enough, principally of the lack of access and the inflationary price tag being assigned to both services and in turn, the insurance coverage necessary not to be at risk.

How to satisfy demand, or *demand management* as it is often called, has cast the spotlight on the economics involved in the production of health care. Efforts to re-tool the production side of the equation are directly related to attempts to meet the demands of consumers as interpreted by health care leaders, and consequently this is where nurses have primarily felt the greatest upheaval and stress. Production is the arena where the potential for labor cost savings has been targeted as one of the best opportunities to cut costs while building efficiencies into an otherwise uncontrolled and costly system. Hence, redesign, restructuring and reengineering efforts have often focused primarily on cost savings as a first step with a keen eye on the nursing expense side of the ledger. In this analysis, nurses are seen as an expensive input into the production of the product, not as revenue generating or cost-saving. However, as the analysis becomes more sophisticated and innovative solutions are designed to meet consumer demand in less costly ways, alternatives such as nurse managed telephone triage programs have flourished. Nurses are readily employed in such arrangements since in this application, their services are far less expensive that a patient's trip to an emergency room (Anders, 1997).

Aggressive efforts to streamline the production of services has flourished in an attempt to meet several objectives: determine the actual cost of care, control these costs once determined such as employing less costly labor substitutes and eliminating unnecessary waste and duplication. The basic concept underlying managed care is to create a system of accountable care where the buyer understands the service delivered based on the actual costs involved in determining a market value price paid for the product. The momentum to produce quality care at a cheaper price has been paradoxical as both a risk and an opportunity of managed care. Most will agree that there has been waste and duplication in many health care systems for years but the rapid turn around to tightly control these costs has been viewed by many as unnecessarily aggressive and potentially dangerous. Emotionally debated issues range from professional substitution with multiskilled workers to denial of care passionately considered necessary by providers via managed care gatekeepers. Remedies in the name of cost conscious management without equal emphasis on quality has left many providers and consumers very dissatisfied and angry. Yet the realities of competition predict that organizations will learn to successfully compete among themselves in order to be positioned to win lucrative contracts, demonstrate to managed care companies that their organization has developed a comprehensive program of cost containment, and be able to boost profit potential in order to stay in business. Early lessons in the transition to a managed care model underscore just how critically important it is in striking a balance between quality and cost, otherwise the health of the business (based of course, on the health outcomes of the population served) is in jeopardy. In accountable health systems that work, quality issues must be addressed and corrected, otherwise the business will eventually fail.

Demand, from the perspective of those who *distribute* the dollars to finance care, such as large insurance companies or employers who have elected to self-insure or managed care organizations, all operating on performance-based fiscal incentives have as a goal stretching premium dollars over the largest number of interventions (episodes of care) for the greatest number of people (subscribers) at the lowest possible price. Attempting to reduce risk (by enrolling more healthy people in the group than those with pre-existing conditions), decreasing exposure to catastrophic care (through a combination of prevention and early intervention), and work to increase profits, (especially for shareholders, where applicable in for-profit enterprises which have begun to proliferate at a phenomenal rate in a fluid and entrepreneurial marketplace) has made those who distribute the finances more entrepreneurial and sophisticated in their negotiations with providers and others involved in the production end of the business. For the consumer, belt-tightening responses to their demands, primarily through the changes that have been made in the production of care as a result of new behaviors on the part of the financiers have functioned to decrease premiums in an increasingly competitive insurance market, (which is the good news). It is equally important to recognize that the cost savings are a result of a combination of factors such as contracting with the lowest priced provider, managing the costs of care through careful case management, contractually limiting certain benefits such as those for substance abuse and mental health treatment, and reducing adverse selection of those included in the insurance pool, among others.

The feasibility of any one of these interventions merits evaluation in order to determine the impact on quality and cost over time. Depending on how well these measures stand up to evaluation, the cost savings can either be justified based on achieving the desired health outcomes or may ultimately be considered penny wise and pound foolish if, for example, denial of care leads to a more costly (i.e., hospitalization) and poor outcome (continued illness and complications) for the patient. Frenetic marketplace activity indicates that the race is on for exploring all alternatives for achieving the desired balance between health and expenditures. As the private sector has experimented with these models of care, the

public sector has increasingly taken a keen interest in applying these
same cost management approaches to a population of patients and families
who often have a history of chronic illness due to a complex set of factors
that are both health related and consequences of economic hardships,
such as job loss and/or loss of insurance, among a host of other social
welfare circumstances. As the tax base is predicted to continue eroding
for both federal and state level welfare and health care programs, managed
care becomes a politically attractive alternative. Therefore, nurses and
all other health providers will be seeing the proliferation of managed
care and soon to follow, capitation models of financing care, in both
private and public sectors within the next five years.

On the supply side of the care equation, individual consumers in
managed care arrangements have received on average less expenditures
for care per capita, but these changes have also resulted in providing
an opportunity for more individuals in the marketplace to be enrolled
(primarily because insurance premiums were lowered as a result of competition) and to have at least a minimal amount of care. Suppliers of services
such as nurses indeed have seen both the best of times and the worst of
times, depending on the ability of any given organization to respond to
the changes. Success or failure depends on many factors but there are
cases where the difficulties encountered are far greater for some organizations than for others. For example, entrepreneurial organizations without
teaching and research missions are able to flexibly respond to the market's
demand and have flourished precisely because they are developed and
organized to be solely service providers. Whereas in startling contrast,
prestigious, university-based teaching hospitals with a research enterprise
have had a much more difficult task of preserving their multiple missions in
an era of ferocious competition with their less academically distinguished
neighbors. Although there may be respect and admiration for the labors
entailed in education and research activities, typically when payers of
services sit at the table to negotiate contracts with the suppliers of services,
their interests are strictly focused on the cost and expected outcomes of
treatment. Remembering that the goal is to get the most value for the
dollars paid on behalf of their subscribers the focus is on the details of
what is provided and for what price. In negotiating these contracts with
a facility or provider group that is solely in business as a health service
provider, the costs for these services are easier to determine than when
the costs associated only with the care delivery are being determined in
a complex organization and budget such as a teaching hospital. In the
latter case, the costs only to deliver the services contracted for requires

that these costs be carved out of what it may actually cost to run a health care facility when the expenses of clinical care, teaching and research are added together. Formerly, in a system of cost-based reimbursement when insurance companies would agree to pay whatever the provider charged for the services, this was not an issue since insurance rates were simply adjusted upward to absorb the increases. Under this arrangement, often all of the costs of direct health services, and much of the indirect expenses such as overhead related to teaching and research activities were simply added to the daily bed rate to simplify accounting and generate enough income to cover expenses.

Under managed care, there is no longer this agreement. As managed care moves into communities with teaching and/or research facilities facing off in stiff competition with other, less complex organizations, one of the early signs of heated competition is the heavy *discounting* of the daily bed rate particularly in teaching hospitals, which results in the more expensive institution risking generating less income than it actually requires to run the institution in order to compete for managed care contracts. On behalf of their subscribers, executive managers, stock holders, and managed care negotiators are not adding on dollars to these contracts for the cost of teaching residents, nurses and other allied health professionals, nor are they footing the bill for research laboratories, the institution's library, or other academically-oriented interests. Financing for these interests must come solely from other sources such as the government, foundations, and private fund raising efforts, all of which have experienced similar cutbacks. University-based institutions in particular have had to face the realities associated with either substantially cutting their costs or simply going out of business. Mergers and acquisitions that assist in cutting overhead and duplication of services, all of which impact on the number and type of providers, have been interventions used to *cut the fat*. In summary, the result is both less dollars in the system and a substantial redistribution of funds, resulting in more active competition on the supply side of the economic equation.

From the nursing perspective, as a major supplier of services, it has been a confusing, tense and painful transition. There has been extensive disruption in the equilibrium of current manpower supply with a variety of trends emerging such as competition with physicians, unlicensed assistants, and other providers. New skills are demanded and new stratifications have emerged between the generalist and advanced practice nurse, job titles have been eliminated and the flattening of organizations have been frequently accompanied by concurrent flattening of salaries. The results have included role confusion, in some cases, layoffs, a sense of diffuse anger unable to be focused on any one factor, and motivation to strike back at the changes fueled by a combination of fear and cynicism. Questionable professional opportunities for growth and personal anxieties relative to job security and survival, as well as a strong sense of obligation to patient advocacy in a competitive world have added to the turmoil. Most who are involved in these changes will attest to the fact that the transition is at times overwhelmingly stressful, difficult, and costly with purpose and outcomes often uncertain. Although there is data to counterbalance many of the negative anecdotal experiences reported in the workplace by nurses, results of surveys vary according to the researcher's interest and methodology (Canavan, 1996). The question still unanswered is what will the future bring?

TOMORROW'S HEALTH CARE MARKETPLACE: A MACROECONOMICS VISION OF THE FUTURE

Preparing to Meet the 21st Century

Surprisingly, it is the musing about the many changes predicted to occur in the 21st century that provides the macroeconomics or *bird's eye* view which shifts the analysis into a very different, more hopeful and potentially exciting future for nurses to expand upon their abilities to serve their patients and communities. Gaining an understanding of the community, national and world-wide shift in health care demand and supply allows for a shift away from focused self interest to a more objective appreciation for today's flaws in the system and the pressing need for innovation and creativity on a larger scale than we may have ever dreamed possible. Especially promising are the breakthroughs in technology and biology. Thinking beyond the conflicts of today helps to renew the spirit of commitment to programs for people that do make a profound difference. Shifting the discussion, using the macroeconomic lens to re-examine the demand from the three perspectives of the definition of economics, we can now see a clearer message about what the future may hold and how nurses can prepare for these changes.

Demand, from the *consumer's* perspective, is for consumption of *caring*, not necessarily more institutionally-based care or emphasis on cure. The ability to be objective enough to perceive the difference and to shift resources accordingly to achieve a different balance between the classic medical definition of care, which is to do more testing or interventions, to a holistic approach which truly centers on patients and their desire for increased self determination will be essential. Consumers want to be healthy, not to be labeled patients. People prefer not to be in any kind of institutional setting if other alternatives can be devised. Therefore, approaches that capitalize on independence, quality of life, access to information and allow individuals the greatest degree of freedom to be in control of choices even in circumstances where choices are limited, have a better chance of meeting the consumers' needs as they define these for themselves, not as decided by providers.

Demand, from the *production* perspective, requires not only continuing to reengineer our current delivery systems, but to actively create entirely fresh approaches based on a new set of assumptions. Primary care services that focus on prevention, wellness, independence and personal choice for distinct and specialized populations such as women, adolescents, single parents and the elderly will be in greater demand. Consequently, producers will be compelled to continue the process of retooling existing systems to deliver different health care products and services, systematically moving nearly every service into the community. Providing new technology, new pathways to access providers and information sources as well as linking resources globally, will be the basis for accelerating the momentum to design the innovations of the future.

Demand, from the *distribution* perspective, will force new alliances that will be more global and spur more creative financing options. An illustration of this evolutionary thinking is where creative mental health commissioners have begun to engage in early experimentation in commingling separate funds that if left in their specified accounts to be managed, would suffer varying degrees of mounting fiscal constraints, and would result in more limited rather than expanded opportunities. Alternatively, available money is pooled so that new options for creative financing emerge. For example, funds for housing are added to the budget for mentally ill, retardation and other categorically funded populations. The money is then used to purchase goods and services for a population in much the same way a budget is devised for a household. As a result there is more opportunity to design creative options, such as taking the full array of case management services for keeping a population healthy directly to a housing project where clients are in need of services, rather than expecting these same individuals to seek services at a variety of community clinics inconveniently located many miles away from their

residence. In new alliances such as these, bureaucratic controls are replaced with financial incentives to develop a seamless, integrated system
of care. In considering the scenarios of various financial, provider, and
political options available as well as those that could be created, there
is an interesting and dynamic shift in thinking to less fear of letting go
of the past and increased receptivity to an open, *politically will-driven*
discussion of options and choices developed jointly among consumers,
providers and payers. A spirit of joining forces rather than splintering
into factions will set the stage for the team efforts necessary to create
nursing's new world.

The macroeconomics view allows for the envisioning of the future
with great excitement and anticipation. This *bird's eye* view lets in the
needed fresh air to move beyond the frustrations associated with a system
in transition. We will have our work cut out for us but will have more
flexibility to encourage nurses to take on the responsibility to make change
happen. The work and the roles for nurses may be similar in some cases,
and may be very different in others, but no doubt will be expanded greatly
based on the forecasts of many health care experts. In a recent publication
entitled *Preparing to Meet the Health Care Challenges in the 21st Century*
(*U.S. Medicine, 1996*) a wide variety of noted health experts were asked
to describe the future. The result is an impressive scope of anticipated
scientific breakthroughs that will fundamentally redefine how health issues will be managed and the kind of systems that will be necessary to
support these new advances. The systems of tomorrow may look very
different than those we have today. Each forecast has specific challenges
to be met and it is interesting to ponder how individually and collectively
they might influence the nursing profession in the arenas of education,
practice and research. Certain prognostications echo the problems we
have already identified, only on a larger scale, and others introduce nearly
unimaginable alternatives to the *primitive* practices we utilize today.

Highlights of such forecasts for the next millennium start with demographic shifts. Population growth will be dominant leading to mega-cities
with millions of inhabitants. These environments will have increased
cultural diversity and poverty is anticipated to persist. Disease vectors
such as rats and mosquitoes will flourish in these compacted environments
and the diseases they carry will be widespread. Travel will increase, putting
these large populations at risk for worldwide spread of exotic diseases
that previously had been contained in remote regions of the world.
Biological warfare is predicted to spread across political borders. Therefore,
the roles that nurses will play in community settings will evolve into

roles that will have to expertly manage increasing levels of violence, cultural diversity and poverty. The ability to assist communities to network and share resources and to support the need for community-wide stress management as well as proper sanitation will be in demand. Cross-training in these settings will include the need for increasing knowledge in cultural variations, languages, epidemiology and the sociological and psychological stressors associated with population density.

More and more chronic diseases will be found to have an infectious etiology. Antimicrobial resistance will be chronic. Breakthroughs in genetics will be profound. Currently, genetics account for an estimated 3,000–4,000 heredity-based illnesses. Advances in vaccinology will make prevention possible through immunization. While we are presently occupied with trying to reengineer traditional health care systems, scientists are busy reengineering the human body. As a result, blood products will eventually be manufactured, xenotransplants will be commonplace, and organ replacements will be based on miniaturized functions rather than actual replacement of parts such as heart, liver, and lungs. One of the most fascinating developments is the possible emergence of a new field referred to as nanotechnology which is based on advances in physics which entail the manipulation of matter at the atomic level for reconstruction and then reordering of the atoms through a device referred to as an assembler to have the reformatted matter produce specified functions. Applications of this technology, although in the very early stages of experimentation, may lead to extraordinary changes such as non-invasive diagnostics where ultra-miniaturized blood analysis technology could perform hundreds of analyses on a single pinprick of blood, pharmaceutical production meeting near flawless standards, and applications such as nanocomputers applied to a *smart* mouthwash able to distinguish and destroy pathogenic bacteria and leave the healthy flora in tact just to name a few simple applications. Assuming this capability were to be developed and became more sophisticated over time, the potential for drug actions to specifically target diseased organs or tumors would have profound implications for non-invasive treatment of illnesses. Roles for nurses will focus on the application of these new technologies and the management of the many psychosocial and ethical considerations that will be associated with treating genetic illnesses and the prolonging of life. Working closely to interpret to individuals and families the scope of the technology and bringing much of these advances directly into the homes of patients will be a major challenge. As consumers have more control over life and death choices and options, nurses will function in a counseling role to assist individuals and families to process the information and make the best possible choices. Nurses will need to understand the emerging field of genetics and knowledge and skills in the area of informatics will be a valuable asset.

Other factors will change the world in new ways, such as global warming predicting new patterns of disease, automated telemedicine redefining how and where we supply services and increased application of cyberspace; introducing new sources of information to people in any region of the world. These are but a few of the changes on the horizon that will help to reframe today's concerns into opportunities for improvement. Based on these predictions, nursing's future will no doubt be different but potentially more challenging than ever before. To prepare for this future today will require a resocialization process in order to unleash the creative potential of each nurse. The most meaningful application of the concept of empowerment is not simply striving to gain or retain a degree of empowerment within our present day workplaces, but to apply the meaning of the term to actively using self to create the future. Nurses cannot simply wait for the future to arrive, and then try to figure out how best to respond. If there is a lesson for nurses in the managed care shift we are experiencing today, it is that once change takes hold, it happens very quickly and is experienced as a virtual *overnight* phenomenon. Planning for the future with the larger picture in mind and the ability to rapidly respond to the needs of people, both locally and globally is where we need to be headed.

DEVELOPING STRATEGIES FOR GAINING PERSONAL MASTERY OF HEALTH CARE'S FUTURE WORLD

Nurturing and Respecting the Power of Self to Create Solutions for the Future

Being controlled by change never feels good. Optimally we all strive to be in control of our lives. The personal transitions that nurses are being called upon to make can run the spectrum of emotions and for the individual are as threatening as well as challenging as those encountered in any other major industrial change. Bridging the gap between yesterday, today and tomorrow begins with letting go of the natural tendency to cling to the past. The sense of loss and mourning is to be expected and must be dealt with as in saying good-bye to any person, place or experience we hold dear. Although easier said than done, the assumption that we can create a future if we have a vision of what we want firmly fixed in our mind's eye eventually forces us to let go of the past in order to have the necessary energy to envision what is coming next. This does not have to translate into a loss of identity and the discarding of all the many fine traditions of the profession.

As we once gave up the status and prestige associated with the symbolism attached to the nursing cap, we must think about how to build upon rather than fight to retain those traditions that no longer fit the present circumstances. A second step associated with this change is the ability to live fully in the present. Rather than looking backwards or focusing too far into the future, the road from here to there is surprisingly available to us every day. If we are willing to acknowledge the realities that we encounter as opportunities rather than threats, new opportunities come into focus. Each day, as we move little by little, the future will arrive in ways that are amazingly similar to the future we had envisioned all along. Living fully in the present allows us to absorb, act on and evaluate all the information that is available to us, if we take the time to turn our attention to what really matters. Every action and circumstance needs to be reframed into an opportunity for growth and development, especially those involving conflict. This requires re-training ourselves to be less attuned to over achievement and perfection and more thoughtful about how the lessons of today can be applied to future problem-solving. The outcomes of this daily exercise will be to conduct a thorough inventory of personal and professional strengths, considered to be essential stepping stones to determining what you do best, and then fostering the personal freedom necessary to pursue the dreams that will best utilize your unique talents.

This, in time, may be one of the most freeing lessons to be learned as a result of the revolution in health care today. Since business as usual is no longer an option, we are pressed to move on. As a byproduct of all of the paradigm shifting and the new assumptions for which changes are being devised, nurses actually have more freedom than ever before to create solutions to the problems that we are being forced to face today.

Paying attention to growth on a personal level and not limiting or narrowing the focus to work life issues is an essential part of the transition. A few things do remain constant and one is the fact that there will always be a need to have well balanced people in the workplace. This degree of personal growth and reflection requires time and attention to the daily stresses that once again, act as energy draining obstacles, rather than facilitating a healthy approach to dealing effectively with people and problems. Therefore, planning to give this effort priority and taking action in order to attain balance will require time to read, think, and dialogue with all available sources in order to expand your knowledge and horizons and ability to take risks, both small and large. Balancing a life requires dreaming, rest, relaxation, and periodic physical and mental health checks. The outcome to be achieved with these many avenues for exploration is the development of a keen ability to focus. Focus is a fundamental ingredient for success since without this ability, jobs are half-done and important solutions and contributions are not brought to fruition. It is a talent and skill that can be developed in each person with the proper attention paid. In addition, developing a core belief in the process and meaning of change functions to provide a catalyst as well as a bridge to the future and gives a clearer and more positive approach to interpreting the events of the day. No one describes this cultivated affinity for change better than Deepak Chopra in his thesis *The Seven Spiritual Laws of Success* (Chopra, 1994). Describing the sixth law, "The Law of Detachment," he counsels:

The search for security is an illusion. In ancient wisdom traditions, the solution to this whole dilemma lies in the wisdom of insecurity, or the wisdom of uncertainty. This means that the search for security and certainty is actually an attachment to the known. And what's the known? The known is our past. The known is nothing other than the prison of past conditioning. There's no evolution in that—absolutely none at all. And when there is no evolution, there is stagnation, entropy, disorder, and decay.

Uncertainty, on the other hand, is the fertile ground of pure creativity and freedom. Uncertainty means stepping into the unknown in every moment of our existence. The unknown is the field of all possibilities, ever fresh, ever new, always open to the creation of new manifestations. Without uncertainty and the unknown, life is just the stale repetition of outworn memories. You become the victim of the past, and your tormentor today is your self left over from yesterday.

Relinquish your attachment to the known, step into the unknown, and you will step into the field of all possibilities. In your willingness to step into the unknown, you will have the wisdom of uncertainty factored in.

This means that in every moment of your life, you will have excitement, adventure, mystery. You will experience the fun of life—the magic, the celebration, the exhilaration, and the exultation of your own spirit. Every day you can look for the excitement of what may occur in the field of all possibilities. When you experience uncertainty, you are on the right path—so don't give it up. You don't need to have a complete and rigid idea of what you'll be doing next week or next year, because if you have a very clear idea of what's going to happen and you get rigidly attached to it, then you shut out a whole range of possibilities.

One characteristic of the field of all possibilities is infinite correlation. The field can orchestrate an infinity of space-time events to bring about the outcome that is intended. But when you are attached, your intention gets locked into a rigid mindset and you lose your fluidity, the creativity, and the spontaneity inherent in the field. When you get attached, you freeze your desire from that infinite fluidity and flexibility into a rigid framework which interferes with the whole process of creation.

From the book *The Seven Spiritual Laws of Success* © 1994 Deepak Chopra. Reprinted by permission of Amber-Allen Publishing, Inc., P.O. Box 6657, San Rafael, CA 94903. All rights reserved.

This is a good example of the kind of personal paradigm shift that must occur before we can hope to make progress with the paradigm shifts and new expectations we are encountering in the workplace. With the combination of personal beliefs and good health maintenance strategies in mind, one can frame a whole host of professional strategies that are sure to balance the economics entailed in achieving personal and professional success. The development of positive, growth-producing professional strategies begins with an attitude of embracing the commitment to lifelong learning. For example, one must be open to thinking beyond one's discipline. To work toward attaining comfort and enjoyment with interdisciplinary thinking and collaboration is the key to healthy team spirit and cooperation. Learning the skills of collaboration requires effort in addition to practice on a daily basis. Computer proficiency opens up new avenues of knowledge and communication that are unparalleled in the history of the world. This technology is creating the opportunity for innovation development and sharing at an unparalleled rate. It is both fun and frustrating at times, but a tool to be mastered so that new horizons can be explored on an information highway that can visit corners of the world one might never otherwise reach. Never losing a sense of curiosity supports a commitment to lifelong research, which reinforces and strengthens the commitment made to lifelong learning and the use of available technology. Reading and contributing to the professional literature supports active networking with experts across the discipline and beyond and joining professional associations allows for additional engagement with those of like interests that can move a specialty or special interest group ahead. As an added benefit, building alliances outside of work allows for the development of new friendships and opens new doors. Finally, adopting a colleague to mentor and allowing for the reciprocity of being mentored yourself is a special personal journey that can unlock new understandings and insights into the creative process, as well as support the development of your special role in creating the health care system of the future. Utilizing all of these strategies will serve to leverage creativity and satisfaction to new heights. Enhanced career satisfaction through a combination of strategies that support continued self-development, engagement in multiple arenas of activity and a conscious effort to acquire the skills to foster positive growth and effective communication will be vitally important in sustaining our efforts in new circumstances.

Nursing's new world offers opportunity, uncertainty, growth and challenge. Preparing ourselves for this new world by re-framing the economic equation so that nurses move beyond only the supply side of the equation is possible. We play significant roles in the analysis and meeting of the demands of the many populations we serve. Nurses can and no doubt will expand their influence to contribute to the production, distribution and consumption of health care goods and services by applying knowledge broadly to solve even the largest problems facing the industry. Re-framing new horizons will require that nurses view themselves as architects, not victims of the changing system. Continuing to be patient advocates is our greatest strength and we must recognize the power this commands in effectively negotiating for those we serve. We must continue to return to our roots and stay close to our practice base which advocates holistic, patient-centered care. Being fully informed of the changing world will assist in our determination to be heard as an important voice in the change process. Above all, despite the complexity, pace and enormity of the changes today and on the horizon, we must not lose hope for ourselves or for our patients. Nursing's new world has a lot to offer and nurses have a lot to offer in return. It is our challenge to journey on, find new pathways and work to create the changes we have longed for. The new world awaits our imprint. The time to begin is now.

REFERENCES

Anders, G. (1997). How Nurses Take Calls and Control the Care of Patients From Afar: They Ask About Symptoms Much as a Doctor Does, Hold Down HMO Bills. *The Wall Street Journal.* February 4, 1997.

Canavan, K. (1996). Nursing Addresses Troubling Trends in Managed Care. *The American Nurse.* October, 1996, p. 19.

Chopra, D. (1994). *The Seven Spiritual Laws of Success: A Practical Guide to the Fulfillment of Your Dreams.* San Rafael, CA: Amber-Allen Publishing, The New World Library.

Gordon, S. (1997). What Nurses Stand For. *The Atlantic Monthly.* 279(2), pp. 80–88.

Heilbroner, R. L., & Thurow, L. C. (1984). *Understanding Macroeconomics* (pp. 3, 70–71). Englewood Cliffs, NJ. Prentice-Hall.

"Preparing to Meet the Health Care Challenges in the 21st Century," *US Medicine, 32*(15)(16). August, 1996.

Rosenthal, E. (1997). Senior Doctors and Nurses See Threats to Jobs: Big Paychecks Become Cost Cutter's Targets. *The New York Times.* Jan. 26, 1997, 1, 24.

Starr, P. (1982). *The Social Transformation of American Medicine.* New York: Basic Books, Inc.

Webster's II: New Riverside University Dictionary. (1994). *The Riverside Publishing Company,* Houghton-Mifflin.

Winslow, R. (1997). Nurses to Take Doctor's Duties. *The Wall Street Journal.* February 7, 1997.

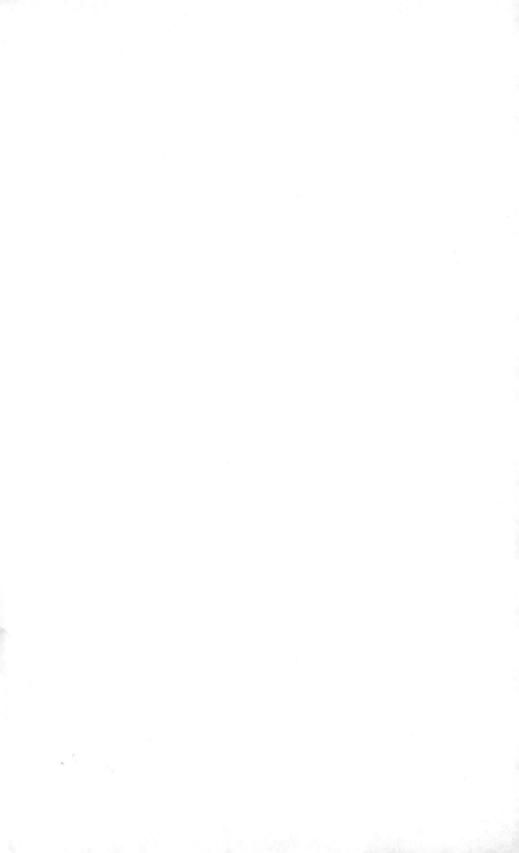

Part IX

Engaging New Strategies for Change

*T*he demographic changes that are evident and which will accelerate markedly early in the 21st century require attention to power relationships and influence as public policy is shaped. We are reminded that the workforce now and into the 21st century will change considerably. Johnston and Packard predict that only 15 percent of the net new entrants to the labor force will be native white males, compared to 47 percent presently. Eighty-five percent of the new entrants will come from the ranks of women, ethnic and racial minorities and immigrants, groups which are not viewed as influential in shaping the economy or public policy.

Dr. Fleming offers the battlefield as a metaphor for the worksite and victory as achieving successful outcomes. In this instance, it is winning the battle for recognition and influence of those who have not been viewed as powerful. Winning battles is about winning strategies. Some of the weapons of the new warriors and the traits exemplified by them are described and are instructive to us.

Johnston, W. and Packer, A. (1987). *Workforce 2000, Work and Workers for the 21st Century*. Indianapolis: Hudson Institute.

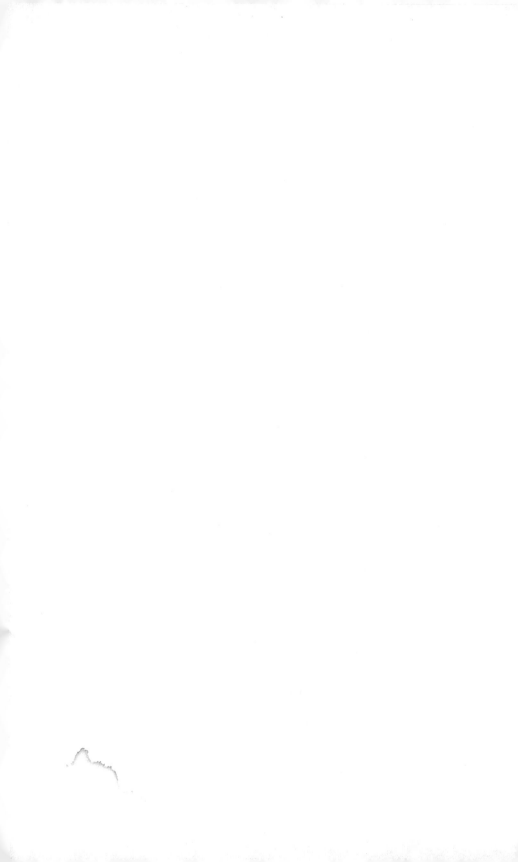

17

New Warriors

Juanita W. Fleming

D_{umas} (1978) *noted that* neither women nor ethnic minorities of color are among the powerful in America. They have, she said, through the years of gallant and courageous struggles been moving little by little toward a middle level position. This middle level position of power is below the elite. They are for example members of Congress, pressure groups and members of the upper class. Those in the middle level are able to gain the ear of those who hold positions of power and who can exercise direct power on their behalf if they chose to do so.

If the statistics are correct, the largest workforce this country will have in the 21st century will likely be women and minorities. Their struggles for positions may not be as difficult as they have been in the past. The *ethnic upsurge* in America has some healthy consequence, including long overdue recognition of the achievements of women, Black Americans, Indians, Hispanics and Asians among others (Schlesinger, 1991). Probable factors contributing to this are 1) what appears to be a decline of white male talent to fill the multiple roles that are emerging; 2) a decline in the average wage of 25–44 year old white males and the increase in the workforce participation of women (Peters, 1987); 3) the technology revolution; 4) the rapidity of information generated and altered that results in the multiple roles; 5) the globalization of the economy; and 6) the recognition that all the talent of this nation is needed if it is to remain competitive. Thus, it appears these groups will have a greater role in performing the work that is needed to assure that this nation continues as a viable entity. Controlling costs and increasing productivity may be one of the major strategic challenges facing the nation in this and the next decade.

The purpose of this article is to introduce the idea of a different type of warrior that will be needed to address the types of conflict that are likely to be more evident in the 21st century. Conflicts in the health care industry make this notion particularly relevant to nurses, many of whom are women, and to other health care professionals.

The transition from brute force to brain force economies necessarily invents what can only be called brain-force wars. "In the past when diplomats fell silent, guns very often began to boom. Tomorrow, according to the United States Global Strategy Council, if diplomatic talks fail, governments may be able to apply non-lethal measures before engaging in traditional, bloody war" (Toffler, A. & Toffler, H., 1993).

Toffler (1993) describes *knowledge warriors* as intellectuals in and out of uniform dedicated to the idea that knowledge can win or prevent wars. I believe knowledge will cover a broad array of areas including the global interest in communication and information technologies. The computer will be to the information age (21st century) what the automobile was to the industrial age. Toffler's description of these warriors is in keeping with his conceptualization of the information age and the shift of power. His treatise, *Power Shift* is a remarkable one, in that he helps the reader understand that conflict is an inescapable fact and that force and wealth are lesser powers than is knowledge. They are finite and can be used up. By contrast knowledge is not finite and does not get used up. It is the most democratic source of power; it can help avert challenges that might require the use of violence or wealth and can be used to persuade others to perform in desired ways out of perceived self interest. Consequently, knowledge yields the highest quality of power. Given, in my estimation, one knows how, when, where and why it is being used.

Toffler (1990) noted three assumptions about power:

> Inequities at one level can be balanced out at another level. For this reason, it is possible for a power balance to exist between two or more entities, even when inequalities exist among their various subsystems.

This assumption seems to provide a perspective on equilibrium and parity.

The existence of some degree of inequality is not, therefore inherently immoral, what is immoral is a system that freezes the maldistribution of those resources that give power. It is doubly immoral when that maldistribution is based on race, gender, or other inborn traits.

This assumption may help in weighing traits that affect the distribution of power.

Knowledge is more maldistributed than arms and wealth. Hence a redistribution of knowledge (and especially knowledge about knowledge) is even more important, and can lead to a redistribution of the main power resources.*

This assumption seems to strengthen the importance of knowledge if used properly.

War has been defined by Webster's dictionary in the context of the agricultural and the industrial age. It is said to be a state of open, armed, often prolonged conflict carried on between nations, states, or parties; the period of such conflict; a condition of active contention or antagonism. Warriors are defined as those engaged or experienced in battle. Women because of their psychophysical characteristics may be best suited to conduct certain aspects of war or engage in battle in the information age because the combat arena is likely to be both more psychological as well as physiological and have a minimum of physical weapons. Wars in the information age will be unlike the industrial age wars where warfare dealt mostly with geographic resources and physical resources such as capital (money) and iron-based physical weapons. Agricultural age wars used human resources in the context of large armies and increasing dominance of the seas.

Peters (1987) notes that to meet the demands of the fast-changing competitive scene we must simply learn to love change as much as we have hated it in the past. Loving change is a prerequisite for survival, let alone success. The fast changing macro and micro economic environment necessitates organizations becoming fast changing, high value adding creators of niche markets.

The psychophysiological characteristics of women which make them

---

* From *Power Shift* by Alvin Toffler. Copyright © 1990 by Alvin Toffler and Heidi Toffler. Used by permission of Bantam Books, a division of Bantam Doubleday Dell Publishing Group, Inc.

the most suitable and capable of engaging in war in the information age are the following:

1. The physiological and psychological make-up of women. The possession of a large quantity of some hormones (e.g., estrogen and progesterone) may give them stamina as they seem to be able to withstand physiological stress over a long period of time. Women have more progesterone than men. The principal target organs of progesterone are the uterus, the breast and the brain. The feedback effects of progesterone are complex and are exerted at both the hypothalamic and the pituitary levels. The development of the female hypothalamus may depend simply on the absence of androgens in early life (Ganong, 1991). They live longer for the most part and are generally healthier than most men.

2. The maternal skills used in child rearing such as patience, nurturing, caring, thoughtfulness, healing, ability to deal with chaotic situations; dealing with new and changing circumstances and behavior which necessitates being flexible, deliberate, alert, anticipatory, and tolerant, as well as skills in negotiation and mediation.

3. Caring that protects, enhances and preserves human dignity.

4. The ability to attend to detail as well as more than one activity at a time, and

5. Recognition that little things may make a difference in the outcome.

Hormones do not appear to be necessary for the occurrence of maternal behavior, but prolactin which is secreted in large amounts during pregnancy and lactation facilitates it (Ganong, 1991).

These *new warriors* are highly likely to be women who emerge from various disciplines, fit Toffler's definition of *knowledge warriors* and possess the preceding characteristics. Many professional nurses epitomize well *new warriors* based on their educational preparation and the other preceding characteristics. This is not to suggest that there will not still be roles for male warriors. The overlap of the agricultural, industrial and information ages as described by Toffler (1990, 1993) assures this. It too is logical to assume that the need for balance in combat will be essential. Resolving conflicts will be complicated and solutions may necessitate a combination of skills, some of which may be reflected in each of the ages. Women are likely to possess more of those skills that would fit the information age than are men. The attributes of both men and women like other phenomena will likely reflect a normal distribution, as illustrated by a Gaussian curve (Abdellah & Levine, 1979).

EXAMPLES OF *NEW WARRIORS*

There are a number of women who could be identified as new warriors. The examples provided in this article are limited, however, they make the point that there are women who are exhibiting the traits needed for warriors in the information age. On the January 22, 1990 cover of *Business Week,* in large letters, was a headline that read "Trade Warrior." The inside story was about Carla Hills, an attorney who served as a U.S. trade negotiator. She must, according to the author battle Japan and Europe and keep U.S. Protectionism at bay. She is described as a "stiff-backed, no-nonsense person with a relentless bargaining style (which) is a sharp break from the mold." She "has proved herself to be a quick-study." Her style of negotiating is termed "extremely tough and calculating." She is thought to be "intense, brainy and argumentative." She has juggled careers as a lawyer, corporate director and government official. "Hills certainly does her homework . . . Some complain she loses the big picture in her attention to rules and minutiae." Mother of three children, she is said to have never missed a school play.

On May 2, 1990 *USA Today* reported that in Houston the University President (Barnett), the mayor (Whitmire), the police chief (Watson), the chamber chief (Crowley), the school's chief (Raymond) and the hospital chief (Moore) were women. The article noted that Houston, often thought of as a *good ol' boy* city had these women leaders. Some women command top posts in important federal agencies presently. Four of those with high visibility who have been successful in their roles are Health and Human Services Secretary Donna Shalala, Madeline Albright, the first female Secretary of State, Janet Reno, Attorney General and Shirley Chater (who has a background in nursing), Commissioner of Social Security Administration. Nurses make up the largest group of workers in the health care industry (the third largest industry in the United States) and are another example of *new warriors.* They combat health problems in their roles as practitioners, educators, researchers, administrators, consultants and policy makers; and they are becoming more effective in participating in coalitions, in bargaining and negotiating, and in entrepreneurship.

Women are increasingly assuming posts that clearly require those skills necessary to resolve the types of conflicts that are occurring in the age in which we are living. They are functioning in public and private organizations and an array of various societies, associations and organizations such as the military, government, education, health, business and industry, foundations, and professional and social agencies.

FUTURE

Women are sometimes placed in particular positions of authority, but due to multiple factors, the most salient one being lack of support, they are sometimes unsuccessful and are eliminated by one means or another. To eliminate women from positions of power, however, is an increasingly hollow victory. Exerting power and fighting in the traditional manner no longer work.

The measure of the character of a people is how they respond to what appears to be a defeat. Networks have been formed which are designed to support women (e.g., National Network of Women Leaders in Higher Education, and The American Council on Higher Education Identification of Women in Higher Education). Programs designed to help women obtain the skills they need to be successful in leadership positions are being offered, and a number of men are serving as mentors to women and making efforts to facilitate their success. The talents of women continue to gain prominence in a variety of ways.

More women are becoming successful entrepreneurs. While most businesses are likely to fail within three years of start-up, women-owned businesses have a much better survival rate, according to the National Association of Women Business Owners. Women entrepreneurs are as credit worthy as the typical U.S. firm. Ninety-two percent of women business owners pay their bills within 30 days of the date due (*Black Enterprise*, 1996). Wells Fargo is one of a number of supporters of women entrepreneurs. It has put one billion dollars into a loan fund and teamed up with the National Association of Women Business Owners to hunt for credit worthy female entrepreneurs (*Black Enterprise*, 1996).

The traits of new warriors are not exclusive to women, but it is likely that more women will have skills that will help them function effectively as *new warriors* in terms of their knowledge based on the number of women, as compared to men, completing graduate degrees. According to data from the Council of Graduate Schools more than half of the master's degrees awarded in 1993–94 were earned by women. In the fields of health sciences and education women accounted for 70 and 76 percent of the master's degrees granted, respectively. Men accounted for approximately three-fifths of the 39,800 doctorates awarded in 1994. Although they were the majority of doctoral degree recipients, women earned more than 50 percent of the doctoral degrees in education, health sciences and public administration and one half of the doctorates in the humanities and the social sciences.

Toffler notes that places will be found for people who are good conciliators and mediators, able to move back and forth among conflicting organizations, listening to each side and interpreting the other. Future oriented individuals will be favored over those who live primarily in the past. The art of listening to others is critical. DeMare (1968) delineated well how to listen to the future. The high profile, arrogant, *know it all* attitude can no longer be tolerated in a society that must compete globally. The importance that communication plays in influencing others cannot be ignored or neglected. *New warriors* must try to master the secret of reaching people and display that crucial ability that Plato called "the art of ruling the minds of men" (DeMare, 1968). The human mind is the most complex and most marvelous tool ever created, far more powerful than any computer or other machine devised by man, and it influences everything we do. It is always active, with or without our awareness of it and it cuts both ways; either to facilitate accomplishment of our goals or to block it (Zilbergeld, 1987). In almost every single area of life that we can think of, the mind is what makes the difference between winning and losing any battle.

REFERENCES

Abdellah, F., & Levine, E. (1979). *Better patient care through nursing research.* New York: Macmillan.

Black Enterprise. (February, 1996). 26(7), 29.

DeMare, G. (1968). *Communicating at the Top.* New York: John Wiley & Sons.

Dumas, R. (1978). Black Women and Power. *Nursing Digest*, pp. 77–81.

Ganong, W. F. (1991). *Review of Medical Physiology*, 15th edition. Norwalk, Connecticut: Appleton & Lange.

Peters, T. (1987). *Thriving on Chaos.* New York: Alfred A. Knopf.

Schlesinger, Jr., A. M. (1991). *The Disuniting of America.* Knoxville, Tennessee: The Larger Agenda Series, Whittle Books.

Syverson, P. D., & Welch, S. R. Early data release from 1995 CGS/GRE Survey of Graduate Enrollment. Washington, DC: Council of Graduate Schools.

Toffler, A. (1990). *Power Shift*. New York: Bantam Books.
Toffler, A., & Toffler, H. (1993). *War and Anti-War*. New York: Little, Brown and Company.
U.S.A. Today. (May 2, 1990).
Zilbergeld, B. (1987). *Mind Power*. New York: Ivy Books.

End Note

Constance Holleran

This is indeed a varied and interesting book. The thought provoking ideas expressed throughout, as well as the discussion of already evident and rapidly moving trends in health care are viewed from a variety of perspectives. Clearly, it will help us to prepare for the next few decades.

As fate would have it, the first chapter manuscript reached me just three days after the front page news stories of the cloning of *Dolly* the sheep. That story has fired the imagination, to say the least! The implications for health care could be scary or stupendous! There could be animal transplants to humans or cloning of humans! The initial fear of the potential of such a phenomenon was followed by fascination with the possibilities. Ethical issues we were told must be anticipated far enough in advance to provide guidance to policy makers. The time for that is now and nursing needs to be involved in those discussions.

The reason for commenting on the *Dolly* case is that it is only one of the many unforeseen events that will occur as we move into the next century. Health care and nursing must be flexible and alert enough to make adjustments in a timely way in order to meet the real needs of people of all backgrounds. This publication presents a timely variety of views of the near future. There are many points discussed to ponder and reflect on relative to how nursing practice and nursing education must evolve to meet those changing needs.

Kathleen McCormick has given us a historical flashback and flash forward. She reminds us that Isabel Robb in 1909 was urging the use of an international nursing language, and today the International Council of Nursing is getting close to accomplishing this with its work on the International Classification of Nursing Practice (ICNP). American nurses have contributed greatly to that effort.

In reading Elizabeth Dickason's chapter one has to wonder why our society, as we have observed in many states, has cut back on the number of nurses in the school systems. It is no wonder our child and adolescent health and violence statistics are so poor when compared with the Nordic countries, for example. Dickason's emphasis on the need for school nurses to have a good education, including assessment skills preparation that encompasses experience with children of many different racial and cultural backgrounds is helpful. Now we need data that can be used to influence policy makers to get more qualified school nurses into the schools.

Gloria McNeal and her co-authors describe a concrete, operational mobile health service that is realistically meeting the service needs of a large group of generally underserved people. They describe a theory to practice approach that works well and is a model others should consider adopting. Corporate funding has also been a factor in this project's success.

The sensitivity of the providers of care in this mobile unit comes through repeatedly. For example, the need to select a culturally appropriate interpreter is particularly important, as communication is especially vital when one is ill. References to the *dominant society* add clarity to this chapter as well. The mobile units described are providing very good nursing education experiences that will better prepare future nurses to give culturally sensitive care.

Freida Outlaw presents "A Call for Scholarly Inquiry on Human Diversity" that will inspire a wide range of responses among nurse researchers. She points out the fluctuating status of our perceptions of *cultural diversity* and the responses of young and older nurses to provide appropriate care.

The need for awareness and understanding of the usual practices of various groups is vital. For example, the people of Western Samoa generally do not make eye contact during discussions or regular conversation. To do so is considered very rude or impolite. Yet when a young nurse from Western Samoa studies abroad she may find herself being told that she must be hiding something or that she is not telling the truth because she averts her eyes. Cross-cultural challenges are always present when one enters another country's health care system.

Dr. Outlaw calls for action and suggests some of the steps to be taken. She addresses the importance of calling on experienced nurses to help neophytes in this crucial area and for solid research to be undertaken as soon as possible.

Dolores Patrinos reminds us of the financial pressures of nursing (and other) students today. I am reminded of my past work with the American Nurses Association and the success of the (Senator) "Javits Amendments" that provided financial and other types of assistance to disadvantaged students and enabled them to enter and succeed in nursing schools.

Federal funding cuts have deprived many of today's students of such opportunities. Yet, Andrea Mengel and Susan Sherman, in their discussion of community colleges remind us of the current federal tax policy discussions concerned with making community college education available to all. Should that become a reality will nursing be ready to meet those new challenges? Should it change curricula? How should those first two years be developed to provide the best basis for nursing education?

Dr. Beatrice Adderley-Kelly has presented a good overall perspective on the cultural aspect of nursing care and of the need to strengthen that component of the nursing curriculum. Her description of some well developed teaching modules is very helpful as is her discussion of her own research approach. Nurses are being openly challenged to improve their skills in caring effectively for people from very diverse backgrounds. This is essential for each of us. We must provide competence in this aspect of care as well as in all others.

Dr. Drayton-Hargrove's discussion of cultural diversity prompted reflection on my own firsthand observations of nurses providing care in all parts of the world. Most of that care was being provided to the underserved. The common threads of our practice were there in each case. Nurses must continue to develop more appropriate cultural awareness about health and the impact of illness on people of all cultures.

The course structural design included in Shirlee Drayton-Hargrove's chapter presents timely information which will be of great value to teachers who are refocusing their own courses to better reflect multicultural aspects of care. It is interesting to see the findings that reveal the reasons why students would or would not choose to work in underserved areas. While not surprising, perhaps the question is, how can the situation and the students' perception be changed to help get health care into those communities? Dr. Drayton-Hargrove has invested her chapter with the enthusiasm needed to motivate well prepared nurses to meet the challenges ahead.

I found the chapter by Dr. Jane Brennan to be quite thought provoking. Teachers of nursing (or any other subject) can surely benefit by studying from the check list at the end of the chapter. Yet one has to wonder what is wrong with teachers who discourage individual students from seeking help. As one who had to repeat courses at the very start of my nursing career I well remember the pain caused by such situations. Further, as a student who encountered difficulty learning languages I could sympathize with the examples given of the bilingual nursing students.

Racism is unfortunately still very prevalent. Students facing it need support and open discussion of the situations as they occur. Teachers, therefore, must be self aware and able to enter fully into such discussions. I was reminded of a young student with whom I shared clinical experience, and the distasteful experience she had with a disturbed, racist patient. It was important to be there with and for the student, and to discuss it once she left that room. Awareness on the part of the nurse faculty members must be increased and Jane Brennan provides a good push in that direction.

The Givens' and DeVoss' chapter reminds us of changing demographics and that family caregivers are becoming even more essential. Nursing's guidance and assistance must be appropriate in such circumstances. Culturally specific and acceptable care in the home will become an expectation we must be able to meet routinely.

Interesting isn't it that six months before the establishment of the Nightingale School at St. Thomas' Hospital in London, a school of nursing was started in Lausanne, Switzerland and its focus was community and home care and not hospital nursing! That school is still graduating nurses, but unfortunately it lost its independence many years ago when it was moved into a hospital setting. That is the La Source School of Nursing.

Moving to the area of chronic illness, Dr. Donna Tartasky offers quite a change of pace as she focuses on an increasingly prevalent and important clinical condition for which the nursing role can be crucial. Stated to be one example of the many chronic illnesses for which nurses are increasingly assuming more responsibility, she provides specifics helpful to any nurse starting a plan of care for someone with a chronic condition such as asthma. In light of changing demographics, the need for nurses to provide appropriate patient education as well as adequate clinical management of care are points to be broadly applied.

Information revolution, and information overload are both terms currently in use, sometimes with abandon. Yet the ways in which our lives have been improved by such technology is evident daily. Dr. Charlotte Beason, in her chapter, describes the information technology already in active use for distance learning. It makes one realize the need for teachers of nursing at all levels to drastically alter their approaches *now*. Cost pressures, need for better prepared practitioners, and changes in the health system demand such changes.

The Washington Post, on March 27, 1997 ran a feature story on the rapidly expanding opportunities for obtaining a respected degree from a wide variety of universities, some requiring only periodic face to face sessions, and based mainly on courses being taught via internet. The implications of such changes for faculty and their universities are tremendous. Issues such as relationships, validity, costs, physical plant requirements and student performance are a few of the factors needing prompt study. Nursing has a lot to gain if it plans for such programs carefully, evaluates their progress and documents their results.

Charlotte Beason presents useful data which may be implemented as plans for changes in the future of nursing education are made. Distance learning will become an important part of every nurse's career. Let us hope it will not lead to distance nurses, meaning emotionally distant. That will be an important part of the challenge—to retain the caring component by caring a bit for the students' personal needs for assistance and support. It is important to determine how that can best be accomplished.

Those of us who remember the really early days of nursing research in this country are amazed and thrilled at the progress that has been made. Nursing practice has clearly benefited from the clinical research results we have long sought. How to speed up and expand that process is, however, a continuing problem.

Dr. Paulette Cournoyer spells out the importance of the involvement of the young BSN nurse in research activities in the clinical areas. She also stresses the need to find ways to assist young nurses to utilize the results of research as it becomes available and makes suggestions useful to others, especially to teachers of basic students and clinical mentors to the young graduates. Her points should serve to remind each of us of our responsibilities to this important aspect of career development.

Dr. Patricia Underwood's discussion of community coalitions brings out many of the points emphasized in the World Health Organization's documents on effective primary health care. Village leaders, if consulted early enough, can greatly assist health care providers to be more effective by conveying to the population the support of that leader and the importance of cooperation on health matters.

I was privileged to observe such assistance in a small rural village in Pakistan. A community nursing faculty member from the Aga Khan University made her very first stop in the village at the home of the village elder. He was so positive and warm in his greeting that it was obvious that they had a good working relationship. In that short visit the elder brought the nurse up to date on health matters of the village. Next, village women brought the nurse to the home of a baby about whom all were worried. They seemed to work as a team and to recognize the role of each of its members. That was an effective community nurse.

Coalitions of many types have been put to good use by organized nursing and by nurses in practice. The increasing requirements for such efforts are well substantiated in Pat Underwood's chapter.

The Phylip Pritchard and Kathy Redmond chapter offers another change of pace by providing a quick look into the structure of nursing in the European Union, as well as the nursing clinical specialty development on that continent. Having participated in several of the European wide nursing meetings I can attest to the increasing political sophistication of its efforts to have the nursing contribution to health services recognized in other than a paternalistic way. The examples stated have significance for nursing in the United States as well, as our legislative and political efforts require constant awareness and effort. Globalization of health services is coming and it is coming from a variety of sources.

The statistics given for the uneven allocation of resources for cancer research and care globally are much too familiar and can be compared with data from some sections within any major U.S. city.

I was especially pleased to see the point made that nursing must be of one voice to have real influence. That is a lesson European nursing has learned from seeing the confusion created here in recent years by competing, often conflicting voices speaking out. There is no doubt we will have strength in numbers. Everyone knows that but us.

At a time when we all bemoan the rapid pace of change Nancy Valentine encourages us to see the "excitement and adventure." Having herself been involved in an organization undergoing drastic change, it is encouraging to see the positive attitude she conveys in her chapter. It causes one to think that her "call for curiosity, courage, tenacity, skill and understanding of the forces of change," can indeed be met.

Nursing must of course change, but it can control some of the changes to be enacted if it knows itself and what it values as its most critical contributions to the health of the people. Nursing cannot simply be buffeted by the winds of change, complaining and undercutting what others propose.

We can do what Dr. Mahler, former Director General of the World Health Organization, has called on us to do in his speech on "Nurses Lead the Way." Likewise, Dr. Nancy Valentine has exhorted us to take similar steps by urging nurses to "gain the sense of mastery and control" that are part and parcel of the process of change.

The need to be able to fully participate in discussions of cost, finance and value of care components in an economic sense is good advice in these days of *bottom line* policy makers. As Dr. Valentine says, change will continue. I believe she is telling us that if we wish to continue to exist as a profession we too will continue to change.

Dr. Juanita Fleming refers to Toffler's *knowledge warriors* and surely we in nursing need those who will lead us forward.

Ideas abound throughout these many chapters and there is much to explore and implement. In closing, let me say I have the greatest confidence that nurses and nursing will continue to adapt to meet changing needs. Whether they will do that in a timely and enthusiastic way is up to all of you.

Lately I have caught myself saying that my years in nursing were better than today's seem to be. Really that is not true. Tomorrow offers some great beginnings. *Dolly* is one starting point toward future changes. How exciting to see what else will come along! I look forward to the creative care that will be available in the years to come.

Index

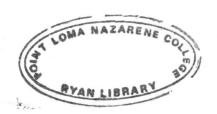